Ashes to Dust

A Memoir

Melody Rising Star

Ashes to Dust

Copyright © 2023 Melody Rising Star

All rights reserved.

No part of this book may be reproduced, distributed, or transmitted in any form or by any means, including photocopying, recording, or other electronic or mechanical methods, without the prior written permission of the author, except in the case of brief quotations embodied in critical reviews and certain other noncommercial uses permitted by copyright law. For permission requests, write to the author, addressed "Attention: Permissions," at the email address books@melodyrisingstar.com or use the contact form on my website www.melodyrisingstar.com

Legal Disclaimer: This memoir is based on my personal experiences and is intended for mature audiences only. The opinions and statements expressed in this book are solely my own and do not represent any legal or medical advice. The information presented in this memoir is based on my personal experience and is provided for educational and informational purposes only. The author is not a healthcare professional and the information presented in this book is not intended as medical advice. Readers should consult their healthcare provider or legal counsel for advice and guidance on any healthcare or legal matters. This book contains descriptions of experiences with hospital abuse, including physical abuse by a nurse. I have changed all names in the book to protect privacy. While I have taken every effort to ensure the accuracy of the information presented in this book, I make no representations or warranties of any kind, express or implied, about the completeness, accuracy, reliability, suitability, or availability with respect to the information, products, services, or related graphics contained in this book. Any reliance you place on such information is therefore strictly at your own risk. In addition, I cannot and do not guarantee or warrant that the actions I took to seek justice against those who wronged me will have the same results in any particular case. Any actions you take after reading this book are solely your responsibility and at your own risk. The author and publisher are not liable for any damages or negative consequences from any treatment, action,

Ashes to Dust

application, or preparation, to any person reading or following the information in this book. The reader should regularly consult a physician in matters relating to his/her health and particularly with respect to any symptoms that may require diagnosis or medical attention.

Book Cover by Midjourney AI

Illustrations by Midjourney AI, and Melody Star

ISBN-13: 978-1-7389706-1-2 (paperback)

ISBN: 978-1-7389706-0-5 (ebook)

PART ONE
THE CIRCLES

Ashes to Dust

1

Author's Note

Through these events and trauma, my birth name became ashes to dust. I change the names (including my old one) in my re-telling of my story to protect the privacy of the people involved. Here's a disclaimer, it's not for kids even if it reads as fiction, it's for mature readers. It's my 2021 story arch, and it was so awfully eventful that it took me a long time to write out. Excuse any simplicity, I forgot things, yay trauma! (Sarcasm).

I'm not sure what to call my imaginative experience during my dehydrated state, since it wasn't something I ever experienced before, and it wasn't hallucinations where you could see or hear things. There were no voices in my head, or in my room, only my own voice projecting different sounding characters. It was rare for a true hallucination from the days of being dehydrated from food poisoning and lack of sleep it caused. It was more like a one-woman-show. Where I was both the ventriloquist and the dummy. The voices came out of me. Like if a voice actor were voicing different character parts.

Since I could not physically see what characters were suppose to look like, I used Midjourney AI to create photos of the written version my brain at the time had informed me characters were meant to appear as. Some of the "characters" like High Priestess for example, change in appearance throughout the story. In the beginning she appeared similar to me, but not. Her hair was black, and her skin was paler than mine. But as the story goes on and my "intuition" grows, she changes to what she "truly" looks like.

This also happens with the "Lucifer angel" where in the beginning he is old, with grey hair. But then after he changes too many times for me to describe properly. When I was writing the story it did not occur to me to include what they "looked" like most times since I was not actually seeing them. I'm almost certain he became younger as soon as he became "attached" to "Ash", and then changed in appearance again, but never old and withered like he first was.

I'm glad AI came out before I published so I could show what my imagination was trying to create in its many days of story telling. Since AI recently came out in 2023, I don't remember what a lot of things like Gods and Goddesses were suppose to look like, so I did not attempt to re-create them.

Here's my nightmare of a journey to the new me, with a new name. Call the old me Ash Dust.

2

My head nods to an internal question I have. It-scares-the-pants-off-of-me! I freeze, and then I ask something else to confirm it wasn't just my imagination. When I nod again, I slowly close my computer and back away as I say my thanks and leave my room. It was a lot for me to handle.

The new head motions of nodding or shaking my head no, were from my spirit guides. I find out they are all-loving, Spirit Guides. They can't tell which thoughts you actually feel are true. But it doesn't matter to them because they apparently love you and want to help you anyway.

I feel bad knowing that and try to say which thoughts I actually mean and don't, but it becomes too hard. There are too many thoughts and they said I shouldn't try because it's normal and I can't control thoughts or Ego. I wasn't too sure what Ego was, just that it had something to do with the darker thoughts.

I wanted a easier way to communicate with them than shaking my head yes or no, so I asked if they wanted me to spell out a answer.

Yes.

But it had to be a clean, quiet place with a lit white candle. I went into my bathroom, where I previously did my spiritual bath, (awkwardly naked, surrounded by three white candles for fifteen minutes of soaking in Epsom salt after showering beforehand). I lit a

Ashes to Dust

candle and took out my cat notepad.

The letters that they say yes to end up making no sense. I keep trying, but I quit after they say the three letter ones are important.

I feel this strange pressure of energy in my eyes, left or right, depending on which spirit guide is closest (I'm assuming). Since I don't know how many guides there are, I guess left is a different guide from the right, since the feeling is less intense, almost milder compared to when I feel the energy in my right eye. I blink a lot now because of the spirit guides. The best way to describe the energy in my eyes from them is like if you had allergies and your eyes wanted to water but never did. It didn't hurt. It was just strange.

I follow their meditation video suggestion. They make my head nod when it was the right one. The video is to learn who your spirit guides are. I discover I had three. Their names are Brandon, Miranda, and Penny. I couldn't see them. I can never see things when I meditate or visualize. It was just a knowing. And it took more than one "knowing" guess sometimes.

It eased my worries to know that Spirit Guides were all loving and would do you no harm, only help guide you, even if you thought hateful things at them unintentionally or intentionally.

My beautiful cat Lovie gave me inspiration to ask about cats.
Can she see Spirit Guides?
No.
Can she see bad things?
Yes.
Does she want babies?
Yes.
That made me reconsider the fixing my mom wanted me to do to her. Does she want them now?
No.
Soon?
Yes.

Ashes to Dust

Next year?
No.
This year?
Yes.
After we move?
Odd pause, and then a yes.
Will she be happy if I keep just one of her babies?
Yes.
That's it I'm letting her have kittens and keeping one when we move.
I saw my sister's baby and asked if babies could see Spirit Guides.
No.
It made me feel better as I wave to her cute face and she smiles at me. It makes me think it's genuinely for me and not towards the all loving Spirit Guides like I thought it was.

I was in the kitchen as I remember the spooky Hecate tarot card I got for what Goddess is trying to reach out to you. It was the second time I saw her come up. The first being a random YouTube video of a ritual to summon her with a dagger in the ground. I asked before if she was nice but something didn't feel right, so I ask something else.

Can she hurt me?
Yes.
If I don't want to worship her as my Goddess and reject her, will she hurt me?
Yes.
Can she kill me?
Yes.
That terrified me. Can you protect me from her?
No.

I remembered my mom saying I used to talk about my past life when I was a kid and knew where things were without ever being there before. I found it weird that the High Priestess Tarot card kept coming up in my tarot video searches. So I ask, did she try to contact me in a

Ashes to Dust

past life?
 Yes.
 Did I reject her?
 Yes.
 Did she kill me?
 Yes.
 I ask if the Gods can harm cats out of spite for saying no?
 Yes.
 Can she hurt Spirit Guides?
 Yes.
 Can she kill Spirit Guides?
 Yes.
 Doesn't something stop her?
 No.
 Why?
 No answer. It's not a yes or no.
　It reminded me of all the issues people in blog posts have said about having troubles with Gods and Goddess that won't take no for an answer. Especially Odin, who someone said left their house filled with bugs and kept sending ravens to them all the time.
　It made me wonder why they could do whatever they wanted, but humans had to have bad karma and consequences for their bad behaviour. I thought of a new question.
　Is there a way to create a new rule for the Gods and Goddesses so they would get karma for harming any living being like humans, animals, and Spirit Guides?
　Yes.
　Is there something I can ask that is higher than the Gods and Goddesses?
　Yes.
　I remember all the inspirational videos I watched, like Abraham Hicks who mention the source, and the meditations that mention

Ashes to Dust

Higher Power. The Spirit Guides wanted me to believe there was a Higher Power, so I chose that wording.

Do I ask the Higher Power?

Yes.

I thought of all the candle magic I've been looking at, and ask if there was a spell involved.

Yes.

Was it simple?

Yes.

Based on the videos, I guessed some ingredients. White candles? Yes. One? No. Two? Yes.

I thought of the salt circles used in witchcraft shows. Circle of salt? Yes.

There was nothing else I could think of other than spell words.

Yes to spell words.

New problem, how would they tell me the spell words. I ask if I could search it up.

Yes.

I wanted to make sure the ingredients were right, so I went over them again. My spirit guides shook my head no at all but the circle.

I try to guess new ingredients like flowers (what I saw used in a spiritual cleansing bath).

Yes.

I ask if one's like roses from the grocery store were okay.

Yes.

Did I need a quiet place?

Yes.

I ask if a field will work. (It's the only empty place I can think of.)

Yes.

I thought of the darker aspects of witchcraft shows. Do I need a animal?

Yes.

Ashes to Dust

A darker aspect. I ask if it needs to be dead.
There is a strange pause with no response.
I quickly say I'm not willing to harm an animal.
There is another strange pause, and then my head shakes in understanding (what I assume is understanding).
I think of the poor squirrel that was left run over by the road, and ask if roadkill worked.
A pause, but then a yes.
I ask if that's what my electric bike is for.
A quick nod.
Ugh. That is disgusting. I don't want roadkill on my bike. And I certainly don't want to touch one. But I might consider using a cloth.
I think of the blood in used in the darker witchcraft shows. Blood?
No response.
A little blood?
Silence.
I wasn't sure if they were waiting for me to guess right, so I ask if a finger pick (like diabetics use) would work?
No.
I am surprised they responded to that so fast. I ask if it was a lot of blood.
That would probably be my blood! There's no way I could do what they do in the shows and slice their palms open. Right after I finish my thought, my head shakes no in response to my question.
I'm wondering if it was a no because I didn't want to hurt myself. I think I remember something in that spooky summoning ritual of Hekate with a dagger. I ask out loud if a dagger is needed.
A quick yes.
I didn't have one, so I asked if a kitchen knife was okay.
Another yes, but less quick.
It's confirmed to be the same as the video I saw. I ask the last question. Do I plunge the knife into the ground with my blood?

Ashes to Dust

Yes!
I don't understand why my spirit guides would want this.
Are we summoning Hekate?
Another nod.

Whoever this is, it isn't my loving spirit guides. No wonder the ingredients changed from simple to dark. I say the first thing that comes to mind as I grip the counter, "I banish you from me." I keep saying it with as much strength as I can until I feel lighter.

They're gone, and I don't know how I know.

I quickly ask my guides what happened.

I break it down to a simple yes or no, and find out my guides were taken over by a God named Odin.

I remember a blogger saying names have power, so I give him the nickname Bird Boy when mentioning him. I ask if more would come, and I didn't like the answer.

Yes. All the Gods and Goddesses who disagreed and didn't want to be held accountable will come to attack.

From all the myths and different beliefs out there, I don't know which is fact and isn't. I just know there are way too many for me to handle. I didn't like the surprise intruder in my head, so I give a secret code for my spirit guides to use when they are compromised. I tell them to nod three times (since sometimes they nod twice if it's really important or to confirm better).

They shake no.

I ask if it's too long, and they nod yes.

I think of something they have never done before. I tell them to nod and then shake my head no. They demonstrated with the nod turning into a half head shake no, so it seemed like they were making a backward "L" when they did it to the left.

Right after demonstrating I feel an odd sensation. Almost like the pressure in my eye had changed. I could feel the difference a bit. There was this odd silence. The feeling from the silence was like when you walk into a funeral when everyone is looking at the closed casket in a room.

My head nodded and then quickly went into a half head shake.

Oh shit! I felt my face fall. Not again! It was fainter and had moved into my right temple instead.

I remember the dream I had of Odin disguised as an actor who plays Odin from a TV show. He wouldn't leave me alone and kept sending his birds (crows) to spy on me. I tried to call Hekate for help to banish him in the dream, thinking she was a step above him and would do that for justice when he was doing wrong. But she didn't show up, and I ended up setting Odin on fire, and his birds were all bloodied on the windowsill. In the dream I stopped him myself with my own power.

Later when I told my spirit guides about the dream they said Hekate never showed up when I summoned her in my dream. Which was a good thing because her and Odin work together. So Odin was trying to get me to summon Hekate in the dream too.

It's how I know the first attacker was Odin, and this second one is Hekate. I don't know the rest. I remember Hekate used with torches and dogs, so I nicknamed her Torch Lady.

My body is shaking like I'm having a seizure. I have to hold onto the counter sometimes as I'm banishing. It's terrifying. After I successfully banish Torch Lady from me, I know I need help. I ask my untainted spirit guides if I should ask my mom.

No.

I knew that but I'm so desperate for help. Then I look at my sister Kat. I feel like she would be my only choice. Maybe she could understand and help me. I ask them if it would be okay to tell her because I need help.

Yes.

I call Kat into the kitchen and tell her about waking up to the spirit guides and how they make my head nod for yes or no. I know it's weird, and she surprises me by saying she believes me. She even smiles and laughs when my spirit guides nod my head or shake it at a question she asks or something I say. It's such a huge relief that she believes me and wants to help me.

I tell her that the Gods and Goddesses are mad because I'm trying to make it so that they get karma for doing wrong deeds like harming humans, animals, or spirit guides. Because I want them to be held accountable for their actions. They're mad about it and attacking me.

I'm so thankful she's so open to all of this without judging me. I feel less alone and maybe I can make it through it. I'm glad I asked her because I had no one else and I know my mom wouldn't have been the right choice to go to. I need to do this without being seen, and Kat is willing to help me figure it out.

I'm attacked by a God again, and my body shakes, making a weird vibrating of my body like I'm having a standing seizure. My head bobbed uncontrollably. I managed to banish the attacker and went upstairs with Kat. She let me use her room so she could help me.

I had another God jump in that I had to banish them while Kat was making a post for me on Reddit. She was asking for a witch who didn't have the Torch Lady or Bird Boy as their worshiping choice to ask their spirit guides for help (they have free will) and if they can speak directly with them to ask for the spell to complete it.

I read Kat some of the ingredients and had to give her the paper because I was attacked by a God again, and had to banish it. If I tried to talk to Kat I would lose a bit of energy and felt the God overpowering me. Bad for me, but I still had to get a few words in so Kat could finish putting it on social media and post it to a YouTuber as well.

I told all the Gods and Goddesses listening multiple times that there was no point in attacking me since it was posted on the internet now. And someone, somewhere, would finish what I started and do it properly, where Gods and Goddesses would get karma and consequences for their actions.

Ashes to Dust

They don't let up and keep attacking. Kat has to go downstairs to take care of her baby because Barb (our mom) is mad and doesn't want to watch her.

I sit up for a while banishing, but then I have to lie down on Kat's bed. I'm worried I'll fall asleep and a bad God will take over, so I have to keep switching positions. This one is taking a lot longer to banish than the rest. I'm not sure if it's because I've done a few already or I'm running out of energy to banish them. I'm so tired and have been banishing for over thirty minutes.

I grab my iPod and message Kat that I need some white candles and for her to look up how to help me. She is worried because our mom is upset, but I beg her and she comes soon after.

She found one that told her to make a salt circle and use two white candles and light them in it. I was still banishing and felt like I was moving through an energy-sucking goo every step forward, but I went to my room to look for the stuff she needed. I found two small white candles, a lighter, candle extinguisher, and grabbed my container of sea salt. I gave them to Kat, and let her set up while I went back on her bed banishing.

Kat stood in a circle of sea salt, holding two white candles (I just bought from Dollar store) while saying, "I banish you from Ash," over and over like a mantra. She changed it to just, "I banish you," sometimes.

I've been saying, "I banish you," for hours now, but I was glad she was helping me. I knew I couldn't ask mom for this kind of help.

I finally get through to my spirit guides, and Kat asked if her banishing was working.

They said yes.

I didn't get to talk to them much, since they got tainted really fast again. I was worried that Kat was going to get burned as I heard the candles dripping onto the tiled floor. At least Kat was safe in her circle so the Gods couldn't hurt her or jump into her.

Ashes to Dust

The candles burnt out one at a time with Kat shouting, "Ouch," as it naturally extinguished itself and fell to the floor. Kat said it was natural, and they were meant to do that.

I got through to my spirit guides again, and Kat asked if she should keep doing it, and they said yes. So Kat grabbed the last two little white candles left and lit them. She started banishing at the same time I had to start banishing. By the time they burnt out, Kat had to lookup, "How to banish," videos while she stayed in the circle.

Mom tried to come in and we told her she had to leave (she almost wrecked the circle from the door being so close). Mom didn't like that, and she got really pissy. She made a remark, then left. Kat had to go get the baby so mom wouldn't complain.

I sent Kat the two videos I looked up while she was getting the baby ready for bed. I was trying to watch the baby on the bed so she wouldn't cry (like last time, which was distracting). I asked her if one of them could help since I couldn't watch anything or pay attention.

Kat sat beside me and watched the videos. She managed to find one and started reading what to do. She cleaned up the old circle and candles, and then set it up for me with new salt, and carved in the symbols you needed for the candles. I strengthened the circle salt with more salt.

I managed to find two more white candles, and she carved the banishing symbols in them.

While in the middle of the new circle of salt, I did as Kat instructed. I lit the two candles and repeated the words Kat said to me.

The Gods and Goddesses were still attacking me, and I didn't feel much of a difference between no circle and a circle.

Kat wrote down the words so she could repeat them to me. I repeated them back, facing north (what I assumed). I choke up at times reading it, as the Gods are fighting me and wanting me to stop so they can take over.

I try a different tactic, telling them they, the intruder, are the weak ones, growing weaker and weaker and me stronger and stronger. I do this for a while, envisioning it true. It angers them because I feel my stomach rumble and I suddenly have to go poop really badly.

I could feel it with every word, and I warned Kat as soon as I could to look away. I grab a grocery bag just outside the circle and bring it in next to me. I feel it wanting to turn into diarrhea, and I squat down, careful not to leave the circle, and then I shit on the bag.

I'm still banishing, inhaling the smell. It came out instantaneously, and I waited in case they wanted me to diarrhea. The poop was large, thick, and a little too dark looking. Not quite black, but grainy. They changed the feeling of diarrhea to pee, and I asked my sister for her big blue plastic cup. I pee in it and wait for more, but they are silent.

I get a small break window, then they pounce again.

I then repeat the words my sister says, but I turn east. After I say the words, I stop, turn to the next direction clockwise, and say the words. Kat is excited about the flames going higher when I speak. She says she read about it and it's a good thing. It means it's working.

I do this again and again while fighting the Gods that choke off my words and throat pipe. They really don't want me to say the words needed to banish them. I keep getting brain fog even though my sister has repeated the same words for hours now. I can never remember them. It's the Gods and Goddesses.

I'm exhausted, and it's not looking good for me. I'm scared of what will happen if they take over. There are too many and they're stronger combined than just one human me. I feel their anger directed at Kat now for helping me. I warn Kat in between the same monotone words.

If I don't win, whoever walks out of the circle won't be me, and to stop me if I come towards her.

Kat said no, she wouldn't, and that there was nothing to use.

I worried she'd be too weak to stop me and I looked around her room. I saw the heating lamp for her lizard and said, "Grab the lamp and bash me over the head with it."

Ashes to Dust

It's been a long time and I'm on the ground, struggling to stay awake as I watch Kat fall asleep. She is being put to sleep by the Gods and Goddesses. Even Kat's baby was being put to sleep. I keep waking Kat, but it's hard because my voice gets choked off and I can't think. She keeps falling asleep in the middle of the spell words, and I need her to stay awake.

I ask the higher power to come and bestow karma on the Gods and Goddesses. And that it is given to them with consequences, and they feel the weight of it for what they have, and are doing to my family right now.

It feels like it's working and I keep going as Kat cheers me on saying, "You got this Ash. You can do it. I believe in you."

I can tell she's worried for us if I fail. I don't know if her cheering is helping or making me worry more about letting her and her baby down. I am trying so hard to find the right words to direct at the Gods. Words are power.

I finally get through to my Spirit Guides, untainted, and ask if it worked.

They shake my head no.

I don't know how, but the Gods are blocking me from reaching anything else to help us. I can feel Kat's devastation. We both are right now. One of the two candles goes out and we both panic.

Kat asks my spirit guides if we can still do it with only one, and they shake their head yes. Then they shake their head no.

Oh no. I ask if they're compromised and they give the head signal.

Kat asks again if it'll work with just one.

I don't know, so I tell her it will have to do for now.

We both look at the last candle worrying when it'll go out.

I'm banishing the intruders, all but my loving spirit guides. They are shaking my head a lot more intensely with nos. It's their anger. When I say they're banished or Kat says they're banished, they start shaking my head no.

Kat says they are coming faster now before I speak it.

I know, and I hate it. I don't know what to do except go round and round in circles, saying the same thing over and over. I have to sit down again. My legs are tired from standing for hours. I see the light through Kat's curtain, so I know we've been at this all night. Which means I haven't slept for a day. The only one getting sleep is Kat's baby.

I sit in the circle repeating the words, realizing I have to pee again. I grab the blue cup and fill it up. I then ask Kat for another drink of water.

I was so thirsty from talking nonstop for hours, but I couldn't waste our only water bottle. I drank the little remaining and now I dread how long it's going to take without a drop of water to drink.

I keep banishing. Kat keeps falling asleep. I switch from standing to sitting multiple times. Then I accidentally hit the candle, and the liquid from the melted candle extinguishes it. No! I don't know how I could be so stupid. The Gods made me hit it on purpose knowing it would go out. I did what they wanted and now I don't know what to do.

Kat was hard to wake up before the last candle went out. I don't think we will make it now. We're humans who tire, and they aren't.

I finally get through to my Spirit Guides, and desperately ask them if there is a God who will help get rid of the other Gods and Goddesses, and help put the new law in place.

They nod yes.

I hope there aren't requirements like they said before about a God needing worship before doing such a big favour.

I ask my Spirit Guides if Isis, the one who healed me before, would be one of them.

A yes, then a no.

I get confused, and Kat's hopes are dashed too. They're compromised again. I start banishing again. Kat helps with the words, and I change

Ashes to Dust

the ending a bit for more power.

I tell Kat to look up how to contact Isis, just in case it was a true yes. But we realize she would have to stop helping me with the words. The shakes and head jerking seizure like movements are so intense, I'm worried they will take over and erase me and my family from existence before we can stop them.

I ask her to give me my iPod so she can still say the words to me and I can repeat as I look it up. She does, and it's hard to multitask with the body movements and remembering to repeat the words Kat says.

I find a site that says to look at a photo of Isis and call on her. It seemed simple. Apparently, a tarot card of her was preferred, so I look up tarot card images of Isis/Aset. I find one of her with a darker skin tone, and her golden wings spread out.

I keep banishing with the image in the middle. When I finally get through to my temporarily untainted spirit guides, I ask them if Isis is safe for real. I need clarity.

Quick nod yes. I think it was an excited nod.

Then I ask if this tarot picture I found was good enough.

Another yes.

I double check to make sure that I don't need to worship her first.

A no.

I'm so happy to have a confirmed answer. They get tainted right after, and I knew it was now or never. I was desperate.

I stop banishing and look at the picture of Goddess Aset, and call on her to help protect me and my family. I say it a few times. Kat also chimes in. She needs it to be over too.

It was quick, and suddenly I felt everything be lifted. All the anger from the Gods and Goddesses, and all the shaking and hurting. This brightness replaced it. It's hard to describe the feeling and vision of it. Almost like a shimmering bubble partially over each eye, making my vision look like there was a 3D look to the outsides that were circular. Almost golden rings. I felt no fear, just comfort.

Ashes to Dust

I ask if it was Goddess Aset.

She nodded my head yes.

I heard Kat cry out with relief. I was crying so hard the strange outer bubble got more shimmery and 3D dimensional. It was hard to describe the connection to her.

While snot ran down my chin, I asked her as polite and undemanding as possible if she could help make things right by having it so the Gods and Goddesses get punished by karma for their actions. I told her they even wanted to hurt innocents like babies and animals just because someone says no, or helps someone stand against them. And that it wasn't right, and they needed to be held accountable for their actions.

She said yes a few times during my hysterical crying.

Kat also started crying, and we both kept thanking Goddess Aset.

I asked if they were gone.

She said yes. She got rid of them.

I asked her if she could protect my family and our animals from them.

She said yes.

I told her I appreciated it and that even though I wasn't a worshiper, I would look up more about her as my way of thanking her.

I could feel her happiness about that. I said thank you again, and Goddess Aset left. It was finally over.

Me and Kat stared at each other with tears in our eyes, relieved. I couldn't believe it was over, and was a bit skeptical that if I left the circle it would be fine.

I told Kat I was going to stay sitting in the circle a little longer, if she didn't mind.

She laughed and said she doesn't blame me, she would too.

I checked the time, and it was like 9 a.m. the next day. We stayed up past twenty-four hours.

I thank her for helping me.

Ashes to Dust

I really appreciate that she went through all that. That she believed me when I needed her and believed in me to get through it. It makes me feel closer to her and appreciate her. I honestly don't know if I would've done the same. I would now though. But I hope that never happens.

Kat is cleaning up, and I finally get out of the circle. The first thing I do is go for my poop. I grab the bag with my poop on it, still disturbed by the almost black colour, and I dump it in the toilet with the cup of pee. I flush but the poop is so thick it almost clogs the toilet, and I'm worried I'm going to have to deal with toilet water, but it goes down at the last minute.

I talk to my Spirit Guides to make sure they're okay.

They shake my head no.

I ask if they're injured.

They nod yes.

I ask if any are dead, and no response. I ask if it's because I'll be upset.

They say yes.

I was already crying about them being injured, and I suspect there is only one. David. I didn't realize I came to care, even love, my spirit guides until I knew they were hurt.

I told them they should heal. I asked if I was injured.

They nodded yes. It was on the inside.

I assume they meant soul, or spirit, or whatever. I envisioned my soul is all shredded up like going through a paper shredder.

I ask if Kat is injured.

A nod yes.

I ask if the baby is injured.

A nod yes.

I ask if it's as bad as me.

A shake of the head no.

I ask if I can heal.

Ashes to Dust

A yes.

I ask how, and forgot it could only be yes or no when I was met with silence. Inside my head I asked if a God had to, and I was met with a no. They knew I would not ask. I thought about what else could and asked if Spirit guides could.

A nod yes.

I realized in my excitement that they could heal me, they too were injured. I asked if they could heal.

A yes.

I asked if they could heal themselves.

A yes.

I asked when. I thought about it, then asked when I sleep.

A nod yes.

I knew they'd heal me if I asked, so instead I demanded they not heal me until they themselves were healed. They nodded.

I go back to Kat throwing out the used candles, and sweeping up the circle of salt. I tell her about my Spirit guides being back to normal, but that they were injured.

My Spirit guides answered Kat's questions, including about her dog wanting babies, and them answering. Even though they should be resting and healing. They were excited to defeat the Gods and Goddesses. They were weak from it but the excitement and wanting to keep helping didn't allow them to rest even when I told them to.

My spirit guides said they'd like it if they were one day Kat's spirit guides when they left me. She doesn't currently have spirit guides, so I don't know how that works, and if she doesn't get guided in life. I don't know when mine will leave me.

I asked them if the battle with the Gods and Goddesses to give them karma was my life purpose. The reason I was here on Earth.

They nodded my head yes.

I ask if I'm done.

Yes.

Ashes to Dust

I'm relieved. And I hated it but now no one has to do it.

My face turns to objects with an intense stare, feeling like something is wrong. I ask if it needs to be cleansed and I get a nod.

Or worse, I'll be directed to the garbage where it's supposed to be thrown out. I end up throwing away quite a few things. My lighter used for the ritual, container of salt, candle extinguisher, a couple of Kat's crystals, Kat's carpet, some clothes of mine and Kat's that were tainted by the ritual or got the ritual salt on them.

My stare intensified at the baby hamper like something was really wrong. I asked if something had attached itself to it so it could get the baby later.

They said yes.

Kat didn't know how to dispose of it without mom getting mad. We weren't allowed to touch the tainted things directly with our hands, so we had to find things like coat hangers to lift them up to put in garbage bags.

We end up making a hole in the baby hamper to say it got caught and ripped on something so Kat wouldn't get in trouble and so the baby would be safe. We throw all the bags directly outside the door like my Spirit Guides instructed.

I tell Kat that she has to clean and wash the floors where the salt was and where we've been walking around on it. Then we have to go wash our feet off. I go wash my feet first so I can get my sage to smudge Kat's room. I wipe them off with a towel after I'm careful not to touch the ground until Kat comes in and finishes cleaning.

I wipe off my feet, but then I'm instructed to throw out the towel I just used. I ask if Kat will have to do the same and they nod yes.

Kat does the same routine as me and then we both throw out our towels. I lay down fresh towels in some spots that end up having salt that got missed. I stepped in some salt so Kat has to wash those places again and we both need to wash our feet.

This time I bring my sandals so after wiping my feet off, I step into

Ashes to Dust

them and throw away the towel.

They want me to get a proper shower but I have to sage first.

I go into my room, careful of the spots where the towels are. I sometimes look at my feet when I feel something on them and panic that I'll have to go wash them again from tainted salt. It ends up being Lovie's cat litter, which is gross but a relief.

I grab my sage and cleansing bowl, and get Kat to get mom's lighter since we had to throw mine out. I look over Kat's room again with her, and point things out that have to be thrown in a bag that is safe for washing.

We both pause a moment in fear when I nod to the Nintendo Switch. I hoped it wasn't tainted, otherwise I cannot afford that, and I know Kat would be extremely upset.

I ask if it's bad.

They nod yes.

I take a moment, then ask if it's tainted.

They shake no.

Then I realized something and ask, is it because she plays too much?

They nod a few times.

We both laugh, me with relief and because even though the Spirit Guides said they weren't funny or with humour, they clearly were.

Kat shoves all the washables in bags and leaves. I sage her room with my Spirit guides guiding me where the worst places are.

I start over the bed with her many, many stuffed animals. There were so many it took a while. I needed to be thorough. I then did the pictures on her wall and moved to the shelves by the door. I did the dressers, shelves on the wall, more hanging plushies, window curtains, and hanging jewelry.

I do the closet last since my Spirit guides said it was the worst. Probably because I was standing right next to it during the ritual and her stuff on her door was right behind me. I stared at them a lot. I cleanse it over and over for safety. I do everything in her closet after.

Ashes to Dust

I look around to make sure I didn't miss anything, and realize I'm standing on her carpet. Turns out the carpet is bad, and my sandals, which were super comfy with padding that I liked, had to be thrown out now. I take my sandals off and throw out the carpet and then my sandals.

I walk out of Kat's room and tell her I'm done. My mom complained a few times during it, telling us we shouldn't have been doing circles with the baby in there and about the smell of the sage.

I have to throw out my sage, which I really didn't want to do since I just bought it and I thought it was something that couldn't be tainted since it's sage. But I got a sage kit for Christmas so I knew I could use that one in the future instead.

I'm so exhausted I just want to sleep, so I ask Kat to throw out some of my dirty clothes that were on the floor since they had salt on them. I walk towards the bathtub to shower off the ritual and go to bed.

3

I'm in the bathroom ready to get my shower when my Spirit Guides make my head do the signal. No, no, no, no! I freak out. This cannot be happening again! I cannot do this again. I don't even know how I made it through the first time.

I go into the hall and call my sister. She doesn't want to come up at first but I tell her it's important; I need her. All while banishing again. I sit by my mini fridge in the hall, huddled against the wall with my knees to my chest, crying and banishing.

Kat comes up and sees what I'm doing and her face goes still. I cry telling her I thought it was over but it wasn't and I didn't know why. She doesn't know how to help me and I don't know either. I ask Kat for my iPod so I can try Goddess Isis again. She brings it and I desperately call her.

I get through and I want to be relieved, but I'm still terrified, confused, and crying. It's the same strange 3D bubble style with so much warmth, and I think love. I've never felt it before my first time calling on her, and I'm still not used to it now.

I ask her how I could be attacked, and thought she got rid of them.

She did, but I stepped into tainted old ritual salt after I took off my sandals in my sister's room.

I don't know what to do and ask her if she can help me.

This time she requires worship for her protection.

Ashes to Dust

I am at my wits end. I double check before agreeing by asking her if that means she owns my soul.

She says no.

I ask if my soul is still mine.

She says yes.

I ask how I worship.

Since I can only get yes or no answers, she's quiet.

Kat says show gratitude like a alter.

Goddess Aset (the name she prefers) nods yes.

I ask how.

Kat says a photo, and she's right again.

I ask where I put it, and she says outside my door will still give me protection as long as it's a photo of her.

Kat goes to print a photo for me while Goddess Aset agrees to stay with me and keep me company until she gets back.

I talk to her about my room and how messy it is.

My face scrunches up in distaste as I look over by my door (which I can't see). I knew that meant she agreed. And she wasn't shy about saying it through head nods.

I told her I could order a little statue of her, but I wasn't sure if she would like it being in my room since it's so crowded.

She shakes my head no.

I don't blame her. My room is tiny and overcrowded. I tell her I can move some stuff off the one book shelf and have that as her space until I can clean better, or until we move.

She nods slowly after looking towards my room.

I don't think she likes it still, but it's the best I can do.

I see an image of a tiger. I never saw an actual image in my mind like this, so I am surprised. It never happened during my meditations or during the attacks with the other Gods. It's pretty and I ask about it.

She says that it's something she likes, and it's being shared with me to make me feel better and connect with her.

Ashes to Dust

I tell her thank you. I tell her thank you quite a few times. I'm not sure if she's sick of it or the snot dripping down my face, but I say it anyway.

My sister takes a long time, and I wonder if my mom was giving her a hard time about using the printer to print out the photo. I'm worried Kat won't print one. I'm panicking.

I call Kat to ask if she got it.

She said she's coming.

I ask Goddess Aset if the photo Kat chose she liked or not.

She ends up shaking my head no.

Kat had two photos and the second one was preferred. Goddess Aset liked the ones like the iPod photo I used with her darker skin tone and wings.

Kat came up and placed the photo on the wall outside my door. I was so grateful and happy. I ask Goddess Aset if that was good enough.

She said yes.

I then ask her how I worship her.

She is silent, but Kat says to say the words, "I worship, Goddess Aset."

It's so simple, I didn't think it was that easy. I ask if that was right, and Goddess Aset said yes.

I was nervous about it. I've never done this before and I didn't read into it beforehand. I take a breath and say, "I, Ash Dust, worship Goddess Aset."

Things changed. There is a shift I didn't understand. I ask if it's still Goddess Aset.

My head shakes no.

I'm scared again, wondering if it was an impostor all along. But I didn't know how that would benefit them. I think Goddess Aset was in on the plan. She had me worship her after pretending she was helping, and then when she got what she wanted, she let the Gods go after me again.

Ashes to Dust

I cry more and my sister looks worried for me. I say it's happening again, and I lost the connection to Goddess Aset.

I keep trying to connect to her using the same photo on my iPod, but it doesn't work. I then look up how to summon Goddess Aset, and the only thing I find is a long paragraph of an incantation. It was basically commenting on her beauty and stuff, so it felt weird because I had to say it with power and not like it was a silly thing to do.

I do it a few times, and it still isn't working. My iPod is about to die and I can't research. I have to go back to banishing the intruder again.

Kat goes downstairs to go on her phone to look up how to help me contact Goddess Aset. When Kat comes back, I tell her there is more than one. Bird boy and torch lady. It turns out torch lady was jealous of me saying I worshiped Goddess Aset. Apparently the Gods fight for worship, and torch lady and Aset didn't get along.

Kat tells me she found a way to contact Aset while I'm banishing the intruders.

Kat sets up a little display on the towel rack for me to use. She uses the second picture of Goddess Aset, and gave me her silver necklace as an offering to Aset.

Kat tells me I need a white candle to light on top of the photo, and something else Aset liked.

I went in my room and grabbed an off-white, dust covered tea light (the only one I had left) and set it over the photo. I then went downstairs, still banishing (but quietly) and got two plastic cups of water. One for me, and one for the Goddess Aset. I brought them up and set one beside the mantel display.

My sister told me Aset liked blue and water, so in my mind it was a great combination.

Kat says Aset likes when woman brush their hair, especially if it was long.

Kat gives me a brush, and we thought it'd be perfect because I have long hair.

Ashes to Dust

I read the words Kat gave me from a site to summon Aset while brushing my hair. When it didn't work, I did it a few times, but my mom came up with a laundry basket trying to see what we were doing. Mom already wasn't too nice about it a few times because she had to watch the baby. But I couldn't stop because I need to get through to Aset. It wasn't working, and it was super devastating.

Kat tells me she looked up why it wasn't working and that it meant the Goddess was being blocked. Kat says it means I have to keep trying to get through to her.

We figured the torch lady and bird boy were blocking Aset.

Kat offers to go make another circle.

I banish in between trying to talk to my sister, and keep it quiet so my mom couldn't hear or interrupt. We didn't know where we could do it.

I didn't think I would make it through another one again.

Me and my sister consider doing the circle outside on the common room building porch. We need a room where things won't get tainted again, and space. We just cleaned Kat's room, and I didn't want to make her do all that again. Especially when the baby sleeps in there.

Kat then suggests the basement when we realize it wouldn't be private enough to be outside, and it might get too cold. She asks for salt because we already threw out my sea salt bottle.

I knew Epsom salt was used for the spiritual cleansing. When I ask my Spirit Guides but don't get a answer, I figure it was good enough. I'm scared for them too. I don't know who survived the first attack, and they were so weak. I don't think we will make it through this second one.

Kat grabs my Epsom salt and my mom's big, white pillar candles (the only white candles left in the house), and goes downstairs to get things ready.

My mom has the worst timing and comes over to ask about what I was doing.

Ashes to Dust

I tell her about how I had Spirit Guides.

She said I needed to be careful of them because they can do things to you.

Then I tell her there are many angry Gods and Goddesses, and they are mad at me and now Kat because we were giving them consequences. I tell her I know she probably doesn't believe me.

But she says she does because she had a terrible experience with a God in her life.

She still doesn't seem as compassionate as I'd like, but I didn't expect her to listen to me anyways. I thought she might understand the spirit part because of when she used to do Ouija boards when I was a kid with her friends and strange stuff would happen. Also from the times she told me when her dreams sometimes came true.

I am surprised she had her own experience with Gods though. I want to hear the story but I also don't want to hear the story because it's her story and I feel like I couldn't handle hearing a horror story on what a God did to my poor mom while I'm already dealing with two of them.

I also have to make the conversation short because I'm so tired and weak. Two Gods against one me, isn't working very well. Especially since I'm not saying any powerful banishing right now.

My mom leaves and I return to the position I had before, by my mini fridge, huddled up. I want to pet my cat but I don't want them to hurt her so I continue not touching her. When she goes past me to the bathroom behind me where all her cat stuff is, I close it so she's safe in there.

I figure the torch lady was trying to get revenge on me again in this lifetime for saying no to her, and also saying yes to another.

Kat comes up to tell me it's ready.

We sneak downstairs without my mom seeing my terror, so she doesn't make things worse for me. I bring down a sports drink, a bottle of water, a shopping bag (for pooping), an empty red plastic cup, and toilet paper. When we get downstairs I grab the empty fish tank and set it outside the circle to use for pee.

Kat plays the video she used in the first circle so she could repeat the words to me. I step into the circle, light the candles, and repeat the words after Kat.

We go back to the routine we had to use in Kat's room where she said the words and I repeated.

After a while my feet are tapping like I'm irritated, but I'm not, and my hand is on my hip. It doesn't occur to me anything is weird, but when I notice my hand or hands on my hips, I move them off.

I start winking at my sister. Even though it's torch lady doing it, it's still weird. Torch lady has a whole different vibe from the others. I'm not sure why she's coming through so strong. None of the ones before could wink, or move a hand, or have their personality feel stronger in me. Hers was so unpleasant; I hated it. It was like someone with too much hatred, though I can't even say that. The feeling from her was something I never felt in my life, so I couldn't place a name on it. I just knew I did not want it.

She projected it through my face when my sister was saying I banish you. My face would turn really still. Then glare or have a small, not-so-nice-smirk, which was not a thing I've ever done. She had this odd flare to her she projected through me. When she wasn't happy about something, she would portray power, or dominance, or like she was a strong being, but in an unexpected playful type of way.

She would lean in when my sister kept saying I banish you, and either wink with one of my eyes, or simply stare, or shake my head no. Either to emphasize her displeasure or that it wasn't working. I didn't know.

My sister said she thinks torch lady is playing with my hair.

I never noticed, but I caught myself stroking it, or running my hand through it like a shampoo commercial. That disturbed me, because I wasn't aware, and I didn't want some entity to think they could touch me.

Ashes to Dust

I put my hands down if they went up, and told her not to touch my hair, or touch me because she doesn't have permission to. My sister knew when it was torch lady and when it wasn't. But I got more disturbed that she was slowly gaining more control of my body. It went from one hand, to an arm, to both hands.

I tried to call Goddess Isis again, but it was being blocked. I was begging her to come through and help me. My sister was also begging her to help us.

Torch lady was getting mean and started sending unpleasant images when I closed my eyes for a minute. One of many were of my cat, and I worried about my cat's safety while I was in the circle. I couldn't leave the circle and a Goddess or God could simply end my cat's life if it wanted to.

Torch lady sent one that they were throwing my cat off the side of a cliff and she was reaching her paw with her mouth and face in terror wanting me to help her. It was in a comic book style image where it was black and white with no colour. And I had no way to confirm that my cat was in fact safe and not dead or thrown off a cliff by one of these entities. It made me super upset, but I tried really hard not to show that it was affecting me or else torch lady would continue doing it.

I thought I was going to puke. I wasn't expecting such random images. I think it's because I was so weakened from fighting the other Gods and Goddesses, and haven't been healed internally or gotten any sleep. So torch lady could do a lot more than any before her.

I tell bird boy I will have my sister post about him so he won't get anymore worshipers. And have her tell torch lady's secret, that she thinks of humans as toys to play with. That she doesn't care about them. Then neither one of them will have worshipers like they want.

Kat nods her head and starts typing on her phone.

I tell the two intruders in my body that if they don't leave now and never come back, then it will be posted for the world to see. And that I will have someone out in the world ask their Goddess, or Goddess Aset, to invoke a new rule for Gods and Goddesses where they have to stay in a cage, like a human version of prison.

I ask if bird boy would enjoy being locked up in a cage for being bad. My head nods yes. He would.

I laugh. Of course bird boy would like being in a cage. But I know he's playing. He wouldn't like it at all. No birds like being locked up.

I grow confident out of know where, and tell them to leave. I swear, dropping F bombs like I've never done before. Emphasizing to get the fuck out of me and stay the fuck away from my family. That if they don't, someone will put them in a cage and they will have no worshipers.

Kat cheers me on, saying she believes in me.

I keep going, feeling them leave. Despite the power in my voice and body, I worry they are hiding. I stay still and feel for them. Just a little odd sensation in my eye or near my temples. When I find one still hiding, I know which one.

It's bird boy. I ask if he wants me to tell the world to stop worshiping him.

He shakes my head no.

I tell him then he better get the fuck out for real and stay out of our lives.

He nods his head yes.

But then, when I think he might leave, it's torch lady who's back. It turns out all this back and forth made it fun. And they thought I was bluffing. Until Kat confirms she posted about both of them being bad, and they shouldn't be worshiped.

They're angry now.

I tell Kat I still can't connect to Goddess Isis, and to see if she can. I did my best but I really need help.

My sister stopped chanting to connect to Goddess Isis for me since I couldn't get through. She was crying so hard as she begged Goddess

Ashes to Dust

Isis to come help protect us and that we needed her.

Torch lady was loving it. But I was crying too because it upset me that my sister was so upset, and I didn't know if I could beat both torch lady and bird boy. He was less prominent because torch lady was the one trying to take control. Torch lady already showed me a symbol indicating that she intended to drag my soul to Hell if I failed and she took over, because she was so pissed at me now.

Torch lady even told me, through my mouth, but in a different sounding, angrier voice, that she hated me. The others couldn't do that either.

When my sister stopped crying and went silent, I tried to stay silent but I had to keep banishing torch lady. My sister had her hands covering her eyes with her head in her lap.

Eventually she started talking to me and said that she connected to Goddess Isis.

I was so relieved, but also worried it wasn't really her.

Kat said the two gods were blocking her attempts at getting to me and she's been working hard to reach me. Kat said that Isis has been protecting the baby and my cat in the house, so she's drained.

I ask Kat how she knows it's Isis and not the others pretending.

Kat reassures me by saying Isis gives her a warm feeling to know that it's her.

Torch lady smirk-smiles at that, and I feel like she's going to use it against Kat to trick her like they did to me upstairs. I tell my sister to warn Isis that they will use that because now torch lady knows the feeling.

Kat goes silent with her hands still cupped in her hands. She shivers and makes a sound, then she tells me Isis changed it to something else so only she would know.

I say good, but torch lady huffs about it and stomps.

It disturbed me she could stomp with my leg now. If Isis can't get to me soon, I won't exist in my own body, and my soul will be taken to

Ashes to Dust

Hell. I read before that torch lady guarded or worked in Hell. I wasn't entirely sure, so I knew that threat could be real.

Kat tells me Goddess Isis made the new rule for Gods and Goddesses with the cage.

That made the intruders in me mad.

I ask Kat if Isis can get through.

Kat says she's trying, but it's hard.

I ask Kat if Isis can get help from some of the Gods or Goddesses that agreed with me giving the karma.

She's silent again and then she removes her hands and looks at me and says, Isis went to try to find help.

I was so happy. I didn't have any hope until those words. I thought I was given up on, and I wasn't doing so well against two Gods.

Kat suddenly shuddered and put her head in her hands again. She told me that help was being sent by Goddess Isis.

I wait, wondering what the help is going to look like and if I will find it. My vision turns weird when I blink, from normal to an overlay of something strange. Almost like a game style from VR. I take it as I should close my eyes, so I do. I see a beautiful blue butterfly, 3D style. I can't explain it. It was double layered, flying towards me.

Ashes to Dust

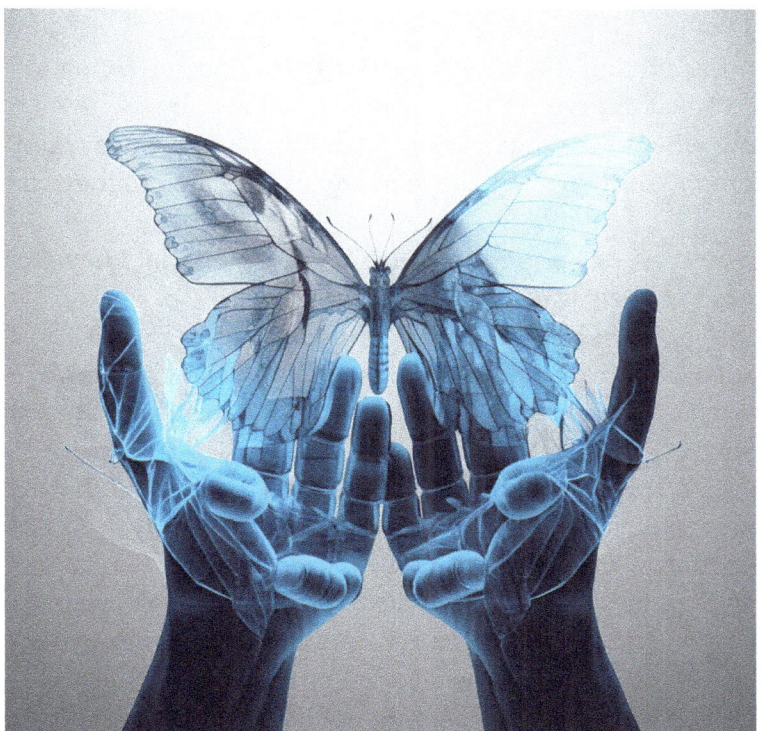

I tell Kat I think I see the help. I tell her it's a blue butterfly. Kat says that's them, they're safe.

I see two reaching hands that overlay each other. The best description I can give to Kat is they resemble VR hands in games.

The VR hands reach toward me and I reach back. When I open my eyes, the hands weren't there but when I closed them they were. I keep my eyes closed, and I express how cool it is. When my hands go through the hands, it hovers. I can't describe it to Kat well enough.

I ask the hands if I'm suppose to say something and my head nods.

I tell Kat I don't know what I'm suppose to say, and I can't get the answer through nods or shakes.

Suddenly, the hands disappear and I'm left with a very bad feeling. I look at my sister, alarmed. Kat's face is still in her hands. I tell her it

Ashes to Dust

disappeared.

Kat huffs into her hands and says torch lady hurt the one trying to help. She said Isis is angry.

I don't know what to say to that. I didn't know that the Gods could hurt one another. I didn't even believe in any of them before they gang jumped me.

Kat says to hold on, Isis is going to send another, and that I have to say I accept them to help.

The next one comes in a different shape and is purple. Then it changes to outstretched VR hands again. I tell them I accept them as long as they don't do me harm. I have to say it fast because I felt torch lady stopping me.

Kat warns me that Isis said there are ones not to accept, and those are black, grey, or ones that change colour.

I lose what others she says because I'm trying to concentrate on the ones trying to help me, coming in too fast. Torch lady is so desperate to stop them, I can barely get out, "I accept." And I can't say more than that even when I want to thank them for helping.

Ashes to Dust

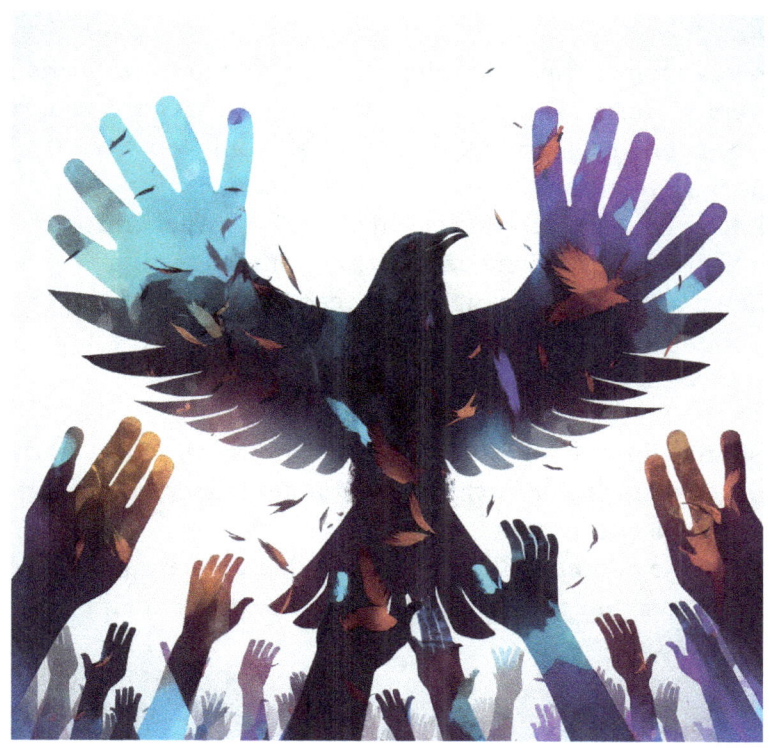

I see all these hands reaching for a black flying crow. I tell my sister what I'm seeing. Rows of hands like at a concert. Bird boy is trying to fly away from them, but there are too many. They capture him. I think they are putting him in a cage.

My sister is relieved that they captured him.

Kat tells me Goddess Isis is coming and will fight torch lady.

I warn Kat right away not to let Goddess Isis come alone, because torch lady wants to kill her.

Kat quickly replies that Isis says she will wait and go get help. Kat says Isis is bringing her son, Osiris.

I feel Torch Lady is unhappy, maybe even scared. I tell Kat.

Kat says that's because she knows he's strong. She then says they are

Ashes to Dust

coming now.

I see VR hands again, a different colour that I figure must be Osiris. I tell him I accept his help. He can come as long as he does me no harm. Torch lady doesn't like it, then I feel Goddess Isis come too.

Kat tells me they are trying to get rid of torch lady.

I can feel it happening. I feel weaker when she feels weaker. I start mirroring in the real world whatever they are doing to her. I go round and round like a person in a boxing match ready to be K.O.'d.

I tell them not to stop. I'll be okay. I just want this over. I want her gone and captured so she can't do harm again.

I feel like I'm going to pass out. We're going to win.

My mom stomps downstairs, yelling. Me and my sister look at each other stunned. I tell my sister torch lady sent mom to stop them from finishing it. Torch lady is almost captured.

Mom comes to the bottom of the stairs where her eyes are so mad they look black. My mom yells at me, and I tell her it's not helping to yell at me and to stop.

She yells even more when I tell her to stop yelling at me. She stomps up to me and almost goes into the circle.

I tell her and plead with her not to come in the circle. She almost does anyway. She doesn't care.

Barb's yelling at Kat to go upstairs with the baby.

Even when Kat tries to say she's helping, Barb is too angry. The Torch Lady doesn't want Kat to continue helping me, so she's sending her away by using our mom to do it.

Kat doesn't want to, but Barb says she's sick of having to watch Kat's baby while we are down here all day.

Kat goes upstairs and there's nothing I can do.

Barb keeps yelling at me, and I see my cat come down and almost go in the circle. I panic and tell Barb not to let my cat in the circle.

Me and Kat made sure Lovie couldn't come down the basement, but Barb ruined it when she stomped down here. Eventually, Barb

Ashes to Dust

complied and shooed my cat upstairs. I was relieved, but still upset. Lovie just wants to help me, but I can't risk her coming in here, and I don't want torch lady to take control of me.

Torch lady is disappointed my cat didn't come in the circle.

Barb is back to screaming in my face, and it's making my chest hurt. I tell her to stop and go back upstairs. That she's making things worse.

Then she screams she will call the hospital if I don't stop.

I ask her to leave when she isn't leaving.

She yells some more and after me telling her, and still begging her to stop she finally goes upstairs.

I look out the tiny basement window, wondering when men in a white van are going to drive up to our house and take me away to the loony bin. Why couldn't my mom just leave us alone? We were almost done! She doesn't understand.

When she leaves, all I can do is cry. I don't understand how my mom can be so un-compassionate and scream at me even when I begged her not to and told her to go up. I didn't yell once at her and she still screamed at me. She wasn't going to leave, she was going to stay screaming at me.

But I can't cry forever because torch lady is getting her strength back. I'm mad at my mom because we were almost done. This whole thing would've been over. I'm alone and I don't know what to do now.

My body moves more, so I know torch lady is growing stronger as she taps my foot impatiently again. I do the only thing I can. I face one of the four directions (N, E, S, W) and ask for the strength of Goddess Isis and Osiris.

I say the lines I'm supposed to over and over but torch lady keeps tripping me up. She makes me forget Aset, and then I have to say Isis even though the Goddess prefers Aset. I then forget Osiris, and couldn't think of any O names. She almost successfully had me say Oden. And at one point, she successfully made me say her name, Hekate. I had to retract it fast, but the damage was done.

Ashes to Dust

I realize why it was so hard to defeat her. It's the flames of the candles. She works with fire, or so I read. And these are like little flaming torches. So it gives her strength, even when it's suppose to protect me. No wonder this is so much more difficult than before.

I was at ground zero again. After some pee breaks (while banishing), I would dump the pee cup into the empty fish tank. I was worried it would be full soon and I would have nowhere to dump the pee.

I continued, but it was too hard. I called up the stairs for my sister. I didn't know if she could hear me. I called again.

Instead of my sister, I got stomping footsteps. It filled me with dread. I didn't know what to do when my mom came down instead of Kat.

Barb said Kat was busy with the baby and she can't come down.

I knew Kat though; it was because Barb wasn't letting her come down to help me.

I told Barb that she didn't understand, that I needed to finish, and that torch lady had sent her to stop us from finishing.

Barb said no one sent her.

I said yes she did, and that's why you're so angry and she used it against us. I then told her the Goddess wants to send me to Hell and I would die. That the Goddess is angry and I need Kat to help me say a few things to get rid of her.

Barb got up close to my face and said she wasn't scared of the Goddess.

She started taunting torch lady, even when I told her to stop. That it wasn't helping, it was making it worse. Especially for me.

But Barb kept doing it.

She yelled things at torch lady like how she wasn't afraid of her. And that she couldn't hurt her.

Goddess Isis was in me at that point and whispered, "Oh sweetie, yes she can." And I had to tell Barb that was the other Goddess helping me get rid of the bad one.

Barb said with them you got to show no fear. That she wasn't afraid.

Ashes to Dust

She kept taunting torch lady, which distracted me and made things internally worse for me as I already struggled with torch lady. I needed Barb to listen and stop when I ask her to stop. Why does she keep going and not listen to me?

I tell Barb how I felt about the mention of the hospital, and how she didn't understand when she mentioned it, it made me think of the other kind of hospital. And that I am trying to fight for my soul.

She says she understands. But then she contradicts it and starts yelling again. After she yells, she angrily sits down and asks what does she need to say.

I don't want her here but I don't have a choice.

I tell Barb what she sees is going to be weird, but I need her to say, "I banish you," repeatedly at the right time when I say it.

Barb ends up taunting torch lady while I'm trying to do it. It makes torch lady angry, and she does a screech of irritation through me.

Barb takes it as she's winning and continues, even when I tell her to stop.

I say the phrase I need to for Isis and Osiris to help get more strength and get rid of the intruder. Then I point to Barb and she says the three words. I turn to the next one out of four directions, and say the phrase again, then point to Barb at the right part.

Barb asks how many times.

I tell her maybe five more times.

She says she will do one more.

After we do the last one, I know more are needed, but I couldn't stand my mom's anger and judgment staring right at me.

My cat comes down and is almost in the circle and I tell Barb not to let her in.

She manages to get my cat upstairs, and then she leaves too.

I don't know if it was my mom's negative energy and her anger. But I feel very drained and tired. It's so hard to focus on my words. I can't get the full phrase out.

Ashes to Dust

Torch lady keeps trying to put me to sleep and I struggle as I watch it become night outside the window. It is taking longer than I expected. At one point, I thought I passed out for a second because when I came to I thought I was fine. I felt like torch lady was gone. But then I felt my face turn into a slight smirk and I realized just before attempting to step out of the circle, that the torch lady tried to trick me into thinking she was gone.

I was going to leave. I just wanted it to be over. My mom isn't nice to me. I can't do this alone. No one understands and the only person I had to help me can't help me because no one will let her.

I try the phrases again, but at one point I hallucinate weird things. I think it is lack of sleep catching up, or Isis has sent someone to help me again.

I said I accept their help, as long as they wish me no harm. And it turns from VR hands and a face, to a furious screaming face. I get freaked out and ask Goddess Isis if I almost let Hekate in.

Yes.

I am tired and exhausted. I didn't have it in me to keep going. I was going to crash at some point. I look around and realize I don't have my iPod down here. I left it upstairs somewhere so I can't call for my sister to help me.

I ask Goddess Isis if she can go wake my sister and get her to help me.

She makes sure I realize I will be on my own.

I say I know, but I need Kat to help me with this. So she goes to wake Kat to have her come down.

I wait for a long time. I don't know how long it's been. I still don't have any way to reach out and call for help. I needed help.

I ask if Goddess Isis had woke Kat.

Isis finally came back and shook my head no. She didn't.

I would need to get my cousin to wake Kat to help me, since I have no one else. I knew my cousin would still be awake, because she

Ashes to Dust

always is. She will probably pretend to be asleep if I call up. I will just have to keep trying.

I call up to my cousin. I keep calling up, even cupping my hands. There's no way she can't hear me because she sleeps on the floor, literally in front of the stairs. She's ignoring me, pretending to be asleep.

I try to look for something, anything, that I can grab. I grab a basketball and throw it to make noise and call my cousin again.

My cousin's voice roared down the stairs as she tells me to, "Shut the fuck up."

I am stunned for a second. I then tell her I needed my sister. I ask her to go get my sister.

She said everyone was sleeping, and I needed to stop.

Wow, I am stunned again. I just needed help. This is why I never ask my cousin for anything. I really wish I had my iPod down here. What if I passed out or had an emergency? This is an emergency! But if I died down here, no one would know because my cousin is a bitch and doesn't give a shit.

I yell up I need her to go get my sister because I need help.

She tells me no she isn't going to get my sister. That my sister was sleeping, and she had the baby.

Of course my cousin doesn't understand. She didn't even ask for help with what. I could've broken a leg or something and she wouldn't know or help.

I didn't want to do this, but I said, then go get my mom.

My cousin said my mom is also sleeping and she won't go get them. That they are all sick of me and what I'm doing and I need to stop, leave them alone, and let them sleep. And to leave her alone and let her sleep.

I was so angry. How could she be like that? I wasn't being mean, but I'm going to call her what she is.

I yell up for her to stop being a bitch and go get someone to help me.

Ashes to Dust

    She was speechless, and then I heard movement. I think she is finally going to get someone. I wait and then after waiting a while, I hear her come back.
    She yells down that she couldn't wake my mom.
    I ask if she tried my sister.
    She said she wasn't going to do that because my sister had the baby.
    I told my cousin to try my mom again then because I really need help.
    She told me I need to stop and let them all sleep. That she is going to sleep and is sick of me.
    I told her I needed help really bad. To please go try again.
    She ignored me. I look around the room for something close to grab. I saw the pole part of a broom and grab it.
    I bang it against the ceiling in desperation. I yell up if she doesn't go get someone to help me, I'm going to keep doing this all night.
    I keep doing it when she doesn't respond.
    I get a response after a bit to stop.
    I tell her to go get someone to help me.
    She says no.
    I start again saying I need help.
    After ten minutes she finally caves and I hear her stomp and go upstairs.
    I'm relieved, I will finally have help. Why did she have to be such a bitch? Why did she have to say all those mean things and act so cruel knowing she is the gatekeeper to someone helping me? She doesn't know what's going on. She doesn't know I can't leave this circle. Yet she acts like she knows. Why does she always have to pretend like she knows everything and act like a really stuck up mean bitch to everyone, even when I'm literally crying out for help. She could've simply said okay and got me help. What if I die? And she didn't get me help.
    Now I hear two stomping people. She got Barb. That's not really

Ashes to Dust

good for me, but I'm hoping she will help for a minute since I'm too tired to make out sentences.

When Barb comes down she berates me. She's yelling again. It seems like all she does to me is yells and screams.

Barb asks how could I call my cousin a bitch.

I tell her because she told me to shut the fuck up and said she wouldn't go get anyone when I asked her.

I heard my cousin say she was talking to the dogs.

I'm a little surprised she said the dogs, because she likes to pretend she doesn't swear, even at them.

I said no. She wasn't talking to the dogs, she was talking to me.

Of course my cousin is going to lie in front of my mom. I don't know why my cousin is such a impulsive liar. She lied about smoking, she lies about calling the dogs bitches or punishing them in private even when she's caught. So yeah, she lies now. The dogs weren't even barking. Such a fucking liar.

Barb goes quiet like she doesn't know what to say because she knows my cousin wasn't talking to the dogs.

Barb says I shouldn't be banging at night, and that everyone is sleeping.

I tell her that was because my cousin said she wasn't going to get anyone to help me, and she was going to ignore me. I just needed someone to come help.

Barb yells at me again, is angry again, and says if I don't finish by the time it's morning and she wakes, then she's calling the hospital.

She says that after we already, (what I thought), had a understanding on what the word hospital meant to me and how it made me feel. Why would she say it again? Screaming at me, knowing how it made me feel? What it made me think of? Why doesn't she care enough about my feelings?

She then sits angrily on the couch and says she will do two for me and that's it.

Ashes to Dust

I don't know how to feel about that. I don't really want her around right now. But no one will get the only person who understands. I feel horrible inside. Sad and upset.

Even when I told her I was fighting for my soul and that she didn't care, she remained the same. I knew not to bother. I tell her it's the same as before, and then I start.

After both are over, Barb gets up and stomps upstairs to bed. I look out the window and see some light. It makes me panic. I'm running out of time before I'm taken out of this circle and my soul gets dragged to Hell, all because my mom wouldn't listen or leave me alone. What happens if I'm dragged out of this circle? Does torch lady take over and I die? Will my whole family not be safe because I failed and their souls will be hurt too?

I strangely feel more awake now. I was worried I would feel tired and be put to sleep on and off by torch lady, but I feel the opposite. I say the phrases as I turn to the East, then West, then next and repeat in a circle. I'm doing it! I can do this now! I feel it, just a few more times and I'll be done.

I must have passed out because I am bent over, with my upper body hanging with my hands almost touching my feet. My hair is swaying in front of my eyes, and I'm confused. I have a feeling it must finally be at the end. They did it and are getting her out of me. I must've passed out briefly from it. I finish the words of banishment, and when I feel it's right, I stand.

When I confirm I feel okay, and know that she's gone, I cry in relief. I'm free. I sit in the circle for a moment, gathering my energy. I look out the basement window and see that it's day out. I need to hurry and put stuff away and make sure my mom knows I'm done, so she doesn't call anyone on me.

I can't put the candles out by blowing on them. I remember Kat telling me not to. I could use my fingers, but I really don't want to burn my fingers even if I wet them. I look for something and see a CD case. I

Ashes to Dust

grab it and eventually extinguish the candles without burning it.

I am so tired, but I go dump the fish tank of pee, and fill it with soap and vinegar. I know I can't clean up more, and don't want to risk being jumped again. I can't take it a third time.

I go up and leave a note for my sister to be careful of the old salt, and to throw out the carpet that it was on and the candles we used. I didn't want another incident.

I then go to my mom's bedroom door, knock and tell her I'm done and going to bed.

She says okay, and I leave to go to bed.

I will never look at my mom and cousin the same again with how they treated me in a moment I needed help and compassion.

I ask Goddess Isis if she will watch over and protect me while I sleep.

She says yes.

I lie down and finally sleep.

Ashes to Dust

4

I wake up with my head pounding, and not feeling well. I'm extremely tired still. I hope I slept a few hours. I want to sleep more, but I want to thank Goddess Isis for staying and protecting me while I sleep. I want to make sure she is still around.

She is. She nods at my thanks.

I call the Goddess by Aset instead of Isis since it's what she chose. I try to make conversation to get to know her. I tell her I have to sleep and recover, but once I do, I'll look up everything I can about her.

My mouth smiles. She's happy about that and nods my head.

I tell her it will take time, but I will make room and find out how to do offerings and buy a statue of her for my room.

That makes her happy.

I reassure her I will put it in a clean spot on the bookshelf so she won't be in a messy part of my room.

She nods. She wouldn't want to be anywhere messy, she wants clean.

I tell her once I'm recovered, then I can throw a celebration for her. I'll find out her favourite offerings and celebrate her. I also tell her Kat would probably love to celebrate her for what she did too.

She nods enthusiastically. She loves that.

I ask her if anyone will know what she did for the world. If anyone will know she made it so Gods and Goddesses have karma and can't go harming living beings and spirit guides freely anymore.

Ashes to Dust

She shakes a sad no.

It seems she doesn't mind. I ask if she would like it if I wrote about it in a book.

She perks up and nods again.

I feel better too. I can repay her kindness by telling the world what she did. So more people know. I tell her I will make sure to still give her the celebration.

She nods at that.

I say I'm sure her son and family are proud of her.

She smiles and nods.

It feels less like a proud human celebration that her family might feel. It's probably not as big of a deal to them as through human eyes.

I am reminded of her son, and tell her to please tell her son I say thank you for his help. And to please tell all the others who helped me with her thank you and I appreciate it.

She nods more gently at that.

The only way she can express herself is through me, so her nods or shakes are sometimes different. Subtle or enthusiastic. Soft or fast. It's hard to describe them, it's just feelings from her.

I ask if she is well known compared to the other Gods and Goddesses.

She shakes no.

In my research, I didn't see her there either. Even for my book, I never ran across her name. I say that makes no sense that someone as generous and kind wouldn't be well known.

A smile. A possibly sad one.

I tell her in my meditations and video searches, the names I always came across were the awful ones that attacked me. I never came across hers. I tell her I will make it so her name is more known. I will write about how kind she is on the internet and in my book so people will know.

She likes that and nods.

Ashes to Dust

I ask if she always wanted to be known as Isis, or Aset.
She shakes her head no.
I wonder what name she would have chosen. I think about who would have come up with the names for all the Gods and Goddesses. What made them choose Isis or Aset?
My chest squeezes so painfully, like someone took it in their hand and squeezed. I realize my facial features are different, and I feel someone else's anger towards me. I ask Isis if she's punishing me.
My head nods yes.
I cry in pain. I didn't know she could do that, or that she would want to do that. I don't understand why, after everything I just went through that she would punish me. I feel stuck. There's nothing I can do. I made the commitment to worship, and that means she can now punish me whenever she wants. I can't undo it. I don't want to be punished.
I ask why.
No response. It wasn't a yes or no.
I ask if it was something I said.
Head shake no.
I take a moment of pain to think. I ask if it was a thought.
Nod yes.
I'm dumbfounded. Is she really punishing me for a thought that I don't remember thinking? Or can't control? I ask if she really is punishing me over a thought I had.
She nods again. It's serious, by the way my face is.
I can feel when she's upset or angry now. It's different from before.
I tell her I don't know what thought she is punishing me for. I have many. Many I'm not even aware of that she is.
The pain goes away. I ask if that means my punishment is over now.
Nod yes.
Holy shit this is awful. I ask if I'm suppose to say thank you.
Nod yes.

Ashes to Dust

I thank her.

This is horrible. I can't believe I get punished for a thought that I wasn't aware of while I was sleeping, and then I had to thank her for ending it. Ending the pain she caused me. Worst of all, chest pain, knowing I had those intense heart attacks from the Gods and Goddesses that attacked me. Knowing I almost died, and this could possibly kill me too.

I can't let Kat worship. How do I tell her not to do it or they can punish you? I don't want her to be punished. She just got out of an abusive relationship. I don't want to throw her into a permanent one. She was so happy thinking Isis helped us, but I can't let her feel this way. That happiness would shatter. Her smiling face would be miserable for the rest of her life. She would be in fear for the rest of her life of being punished.

I am drifting off to sleep because Isis is putting me to sleep to rest. I thank her, but then I'm wide awake. I feel that anger directed at me again, and the chest pain happens. I ask if I am being punished again.

Head nod.

I ask why. Is it another thought.

Head nod.

I tell her I can't help my thoughts. Human thoughts can't be controlled. Even by the person thinking them. There are too many, and many aren't ones you truly feel or think.

The pain is lessening but still hurts. After I try to guess what the thought was that made her punish me. I kept guessing wrong. I told her I don't know what she heard because what I, true me, thought was thinking was how tired I was.

Then I am punished again. This time for the one word thought, "Cruel." It's extremely upsetting and I don't know what to do but wait for it to be over.

I have to go to the bathroom. I get up and go in my weak state. I hear Kat in there and ask if I can come in.

Ashes to Dust

She says yes.

I go in as she's in the bath with the curtain closed, and I sit on the toilet.

After I'm done, I talk to her for a moment. I tell her about Goddess Isis being with me, protecting me.

Kat hears Isis laugh through me and asks if that's her.

I say yes.

Kat smiles and says that it's cute, like a fairy.

I think that's a nice complement but my face goes from smiling to instant straight line.

Goddess Isis is offended.

I worry Isis will punish my sister. I ask.

No.

I don't think she can because Kat doesn't worship her. I ask if I should tell my sister about the punishments.

No.

Of course not, but I had to try. I really want to tell her. To warn her to stay far away. She's so smiley and happy I don't want that ruined. Especially for a lifetime.

I ask Isis if she wants me to tell Kat it was offensive.

Yes.

I tell Kat the fairy comment offended Isis.

Kat's smile drops and she says sorry.

I feel bad seeing her smile disappear. She was so cheery.

Kat says she didn't mean anything mean by it. Just that her voice was high and cute. Higher than mine.

That seems to satisfy Isis.

I quickly thank Kat again for everything and tell her to enjoy her bath.

I go back to my room and lie down. I'm worried I'm going to be punished for Kat offending Isis. I ask.

No.

Ashes to Dust

I'm relieved but I'm still tense and the worry and fear doesn't leave.

I'm drifting off to sleep again with her help, when it happens again. I'm made to be wide awake. I have to thank her for the short punishment when I realize she is going to punish me again.

It's so painful, my chest squeezes tight, and I cry out. I stare at the photo on my wall as it's happening. It didn't last long. She shouldn't be punishing me for human thoughts. Thoughts are one thing I can't control. No human can.

I have the thought of Ass-hat, after, and it triggers another punishment. Aset, Ash-hat.

There's nothing I can do about it. I apologize for the thought.

After the punishment ends, I don't know what to do. I can't monitor every thought I have. I can't stop ones I'm not expecting. I can't control them. I didn't even mean to have that one. I just want to stop being punished and go to bed.

I try to describe to her what humans associate punishment with. That it feels like, for example, a mother punishes their child for the first time. The child trusts the mother or parent to protect them from the rest of the things in the world from harming them. But then the mother slaps the child as punishment for something, and that trust is broken. The child now slightly fears the mother. The person they love and is suppose to love and protect them, just hurt them, like the rest of the people they are suppose to protect them from. They think of them as cruel.

I realize I am saying things wrong at times when I feel the random anger, or my face changes features. I constantly worry she's going to punish me, and a few times she does but most times she shakes her head no, when I ask if she is.

She didn't like me saying the mother who punishes their children are looked at as cruel in the child's eyes. I stammer over a lot of it to explain to a non-human entity how a human thinks. How they may associate what the Goddess thinks of as normal punishment, but the

Ashes to Dust

human wouldn't.

I gave a example of an abusive relationship, and she really didn't like that one. But it was true how humans would see it. How I feel it, though I kept that part to myself. But I think she's understanding because through some of the explanation she tried to put me to sleep. But I told her it was important we talk about it so she understands. Since she told me she wanted to learn. And then there will be fewer misunderstandings with her and her worshipers.

I'm still constantly on edge, asking if she's going to punish me. I can't help it. I now live in fear. I don't ever want this for my sister. I wish I knew this before I said yes to worshiping. I wouldn't have. It's not a life to live. My whole life I will be worried I'm one thought away from being punished for it out of the blue. Until the day I die.

I can't even warn my sister. I have to warn her not to worship Isis or any Goddess or God ever. Kat was considering getting a statue of Isis too, and possibly worshiping her, but I have to stop her. But I don't know how when Isis can hear what I say to Kat, and hear thoughts.

I close my eyes to try to sleep again, and Isis allows it. But then something feels very wrong with my breathing and chest. I ask Isis if I should contact my sister.

She nods my head yes.

I get dizzy as I sit up to text, but I forgot it was off. I stare at the screen, waiting for it to turn on but feel so much worse. I feel like I'm dying. I ask Isis if texting would be too slow, and if I should go get Kat.

She nods yes.

I get up, unzip my tent to my canopy, and walk dizzyingly out of my room. I stare at the stairs in horror. I don't think I can make it down. I clutch the railing with any strength I have and slowly go down, feeling worse as I do. Just before I hit the bottom step, I ask Isis if I'm going to make.

She shakes my head no.

I'm terrified. I don't want to die. After everything the Gods and

Ashes to Dust

Goddesses put me through, and finally defeating them and going through days of Hell, I can't believe this is happening. I can see Kat's head over the futon. I make eye contact and get her attention.

Goddess Isis speaks through me and says, "They did too much damage to her." Referring to the Gods and Goddesses that attacked me in both circles.

I wasn't going to make it.

I tell Goddess Isis that I know it's early in the relationship, and I haven't gotten to give her her celebration yet, but I ask if she would still save my life.

She says yes.

I was so thankful that she was willing to help me despite me doing nothing in return for her yet. I tell my sister I have to lie down.

I couldn't stand anymore. I have to lie down so Isis could heal me.

My sister goes back to the couch as I lay on the hallway floor.

I start screaming and crying like I'm in immense pain. It was like the first time Goddess Isis healed me after the meditation, but I wasn't doing that weird anger type thing. It was just intense cry-screaming. I was sobbing so hard my body wanted to clutch into itself, but I was too weak to move anything other than my arms.

It reminded me of the scene in the Harry P movie where Hermione is being tortured on the floor by a wand writing on her arm. It sounded so similar in the beginning. It makes me wonder if the actress was in genuine pain. Or no doubt, experienced it to make it so believable.

My mom comes over saying, "Oh my god Ash, are you okay?"

Goddess Isis pauses my cry-screams enough to say, "Don't touch her."

I continue crying again but manage to say, "It's fine mom, I've been through this before. She's healing me."

My mom is frantic, and Isis has to say multiple times not to touch me. Then Isis says, "She's dying," and I feel so much dread hearing the words out loud. I don't want to die.

Ashes to Dust

Isis tells Barb, "Say you believe in me."

Barb looks at me and in a soft but confident voice says, "I believe in you, Ash."

I shake my head no, and say, "No, say you believe in Goddess Isis."

Barb looks a little less confident, and says, "I believe in Goddess Isis."

Isis uses my hands to shake the left side of my chest, stopping by the middle. It's how I knew she was healing me. I could feel the healing vibrations.

My voice grows more powerful, and my words are much more confident than I should feel. I don't know where it came from because a moment ago I was weak and drained, and it showed in my voice.

I give Isis a pep talk. I tell her I believe in her, and not to give up. I tell her to imagine going back to her son, and how proud he will be that she showed how much strength she truly had. She was strong enough to stop all the Gods and Goddesses from attacking. Strong enough to make it so they had karma. Strong enough to fight two Goddesses again while protecting others in the house. She was strong enough to heal me now. Together we would lend each other strength to make it through.

I keep giving her confidence boosts whenever I feel her wearing down. She switches one of my hands out and moves it over a bit to the far left and continues there. At one point she stops.

I'm horrified, she's going to give up on me. I'm just a human to her, so she just wants to give up on me. She's tired, and a Goddess. It'd be like me reviving an ant.

I tell her not to give up on me, that she worked too hard to give up now. That all her efforts wouldn't be known. That I want to tell everyone the great things she's done. I tell her I know she's tired, but to please help heal me.

It takes a little longer than I'd like, but she starts healing my heart again.

My cat comes over near my feet, meowing. I can tell she's worried

Ashes to Dust

and wants to help me, but she can't touch me or it'll stop the healing.

"Get the cat," yells Isis to my mom. "Don't let it touch her."

My mom shoos Lovie away. But later she comes back. My mom asks if the bathroom is okay, and Isis says yes.

My mom maneuvers my cat into the bathroom while Isis says, "Don't touch her, don't touch her."

My mom doesn't like it when Isis says that, and it makes me worried because my mom keeps trying to touch me. I want her to listen to Isis so I live.

My heart is bad. I can tell it's really bad when Isis uses both my hands and loops the fingers together to start chest compressions.

Isis says she needs more strength. She tells Kat to say she believes in Goddess Isis too.

Kat does, and now both my mom and my sister are saying, "I believe in Goddess Isis."

I'm also saying I believe in Goddess Isis, while taking breaks to compliment her so she doesn't give up on saving me.

Isis keeps giving up on me, and I have to give her a pep talk again. I'm sending all the strength I have, and I don't have much. If she gives up on me, I will die with no accomplishments. No one would know I helped give Gods and Goddesses karma. I would just be the girl-who-did-nothing-with-her-life-and-died girl.

I try to think less of that because now I'm on the verge of crying. I didn't live my best, happy life. I didn't do anything I wanted. The only thing I left of me was unpublished manuscripts and some physical art I did for fun.

This continues for a while. She keeps switching my hands until finally she stops. I ask her if I'm healed.

She nods yes.

I'm relieved, but I don't feel good still. I tell her that, and I have a seizure again.

Goddess Isis quickly puts my hand over my eyes and looks in my head. I can see what she sees. Horrible images from the torch lady are still in there. Remnants of her.

Goddess Isis yells, "She's dying," again as I have a seizure and she heals my head and heart again.

The remnants reinfected my heart. That's why it was taking so long to heal. I'm glad I didn't just get up and go to my room thinking I was fine, or I would've died. Goddess Isis switches back and forth between my head and heart. She rubs my forehead in the same massage way she did to my heart, sometimes moving to place my hand back over my eyes when the remnants started giving me not so nice imagery.

Goddess Isis is losing strength again, and at this rate, I'll die.

I ask what else I can do to help give her strength.

I have the answer to call a higher power. I call on the higher power to help give Goddess Isis strength to heal me and have confidence in herself when she doesn't. I keep going, unsure if it's working, until I think I understand that Higher Power is there trying to tell me things. But I can't hear it.

I have a feeling it's to exchange three things to Goddess Isis.

I say yes to giving Goddess Isis all my good karma.

What use is it if I'm dead anyway?

I tell Higher Power I can just make new good karma.

There's more. Something about not going home after this life. I realize it must mean not going back to your Starseed planet like videos I've seen talk about when you finish your reincarnating lifetime on Earth. That means this life is suppose to be my last on Earth and my spirit is meant to go back to wherever home is.

I say yes. I give that in exchange for giving Goddess Isis strength to save my life.

I'm not sure how long they meant. One more after this one? I'm worried they might let me die now just so I can be reincarnated to do whatever it is they hoped I'd do. I want to live this life happily first. I don't want to start all over.

Ashes to Dust

The last is a strange request. Music career. I really didn't want to give up my music. But from what I felt it wasn't that I couldn't sing, it was that I would never do lives and be able to travel around the world with a successful, fulfilling career like so many other famous singers. That request was harder, but I just won't give up on my singing, even if it meant I won't be successful like I was meant to be.

I say yes again to give that in exchange for Isis's strength to heal me.

Then it got weird. I knew it was wrong. I was asked to exchange my soul.

I said no, I will never exchange my soul. My soul is mine.

Now I wondered if the previous requests were real or not. If something bad was messing with me, working its way up, thinking I'd trust it. Did I just make a horrible mistake? I feel like the music one might not have been a request of Higher Power, but of the things that asked for my soul.

I want to worry, but I try to re-focus and ask Goddess Isis if it's enough.

She nods and keeps healing me.

Barb goes into the kitchen. I can see her over the mesh gate. Her chanting the, "I believe in Goddess Isis," stops. She clears her throat and I think she's going to start again while she's at the sink, but she doesn't.

I panic because I can feel Isis losing her strength. I remind Barb to say the words.

Barb tells me her throat is dry.

I hold back tears in disbelief. I ask her to say it to help me.

She says she can't anymore, it's taking too long.

My jaw quivers and throat closes as I cry. I can't believe she won't save my life. I'm literally dying on the floor, and she won't say a few words to help save it. I've been talking nonstop for days now with little water, but she's worried about her dry throat? Is my life that meaningless to her?

Ashes to Dust

My sister Kat is still chanting. My mom is angry at me for some reason. Her anger isn't helping.

Isis says it's making it worse and draining her from healing me.

I just gave up everything for no reason. I'm going to die anyways.

I tell my mom not to say it when she stomps into the living room and starts chanting Isis's name in anger.

She asks why.

I say because the anger is making it worse.

Barb gets angrier.

Then Kat stops saying it, and with a tearful, loud voice says, "It's too much for me, I can't handle this," and cries.

It made my mom angrier.

I tell Goddess Isis I'm going to have to be enough.

She shakes my head in agreement.

When the emotions and anger become too much, I ask Isis if she can keep me alive long enough not to die in front of my family. I need to at least make it to my bed in private.

She nods yes.

I'm able to get up, but it's hard. I have to lean against the wall and I feel like I'm going to pass out.

I tell my family it's over, so they won't follow me up the stairs or make things worse.

I can't stand long and need to go upstairs.

Barb asks if I'm okay now.

I say yes, Goddess Isis healed me. I tell her I'm going upstairs to lie down.

I go upstairs, holding onto the railing again. I don't think I'm going to make it to my room, but I push myself. Isis hasn't healed me yet. I get in my room and struggle with getting in my tent. I crawl into my bed and lie down. I feel awful.

I ask Goddess Isis to continue healing me, and we start again with only me saying I believe in her.

Ashes to Dust

The remnants were sending dark, negative thoughts through me to Goddess Isis and I wasn't aware of it at first until the Goddess would stop trying to heal my heart.

I'd beg her to be stronger than whatever the remnants were sending her and push through it.

She would start again, rubbing the left side of my chest to heal my heart, and then the remnants started talking through me to say things to her.

They told her she enjoyed rubbing my boob, and that the Goddess was a pervert. They kept saying it was turning the Goddess on.

I'd have to fight what the remnants say with encouragement to Isis, or disgust at the remnants.

I thought she was giving up on me when my hand stopped moving. Then suddenly my hand would shoot back toward my chest, and I'd realize by the remnants laughter or comment, "Damn almost," that they were the ones making me think Isis gave up again when she didn't.

I ask Isis if there was anything I could call that wouldn't hurt me and that could help her.

She had me look at the tinsel halo on my TV and I guessed Angel. But I didn't know which Angel to call.

I ask her if I was suppose to call the one that may have contacted me already through meditation that I learned about from a tarot video.

She nodded yes.

I didn't know what I was suppose to say or how. I call for Archangel Uriel to come heal me.

I try to listen and can sometimes hear something that says, "Focus," or "I'm here, my child." But it was hard to tell with the remnants messing with me as I try to contact Archangel Uriel.

Goddess Isis confirmed the remnants were blocking my contact with Uriel.

I kept trying to ask Archangel Uriel to help Goddess Isis to heal me

Ashes to Dust

because she is struggling and needs help.

After multiple tries, and me hearing a blank silence followed by a buzz in my ears sometimes, I ask Goddess Isis if it worked.

She nodded yes.

I was so relieved. I talk to her to distract her and keep her mood up instead of soured. I ask if she was happy that there would be someone going to her (to the God world side where she was) to help her?

She nodded yes.

I told her I was happy she wouldn't be alone and would have someone to help her.

She was happy too.

Isis is in the God world part, but she's spiritually here with me, like a spiritual body at the foot of my bed in the human world. Archangel Uriel will need to fly all the way to where she is to work with her, but he will be in a spiritual body in the human world like she is now with me.

I feel like I know a bit about her location. It's like a calm spiritual garden. It reminds me a bit of in Japan where they have their temples. It's not in Japan, I know that. It's tall grass, and peaceful wherever she is.

I ask on and off if he was there yet. When he was, he worked on my head while Isis worked on my chest.

The remnants looked to my right and hissed out a, "Stop touching us!"

That was when I realize they could see where Uriel was, but I couldn't. When Uriel tried to heal my mind (where they were in my head), they called him Bird Boy or Pretty Boy.

The Bird Boy reminded me of what I called the one God with ravens as a nickname.

"Stop touching her!" They would alternate between saying us and her through my mouth. As Uriel and Isis worked on me, the remnants told them, "Let us have her," in a sulking, sometimes begging way, but

Ashes to Dust

just as terrifying.

The remnants used my right hand to reach to my right side toward Uriel, but I stopped it before touching. I had the feeling the remnants were trying to harm Uriel and attempt to kill him through me by infecting him if I touched him. I pay closer attention to my hands after.

The remnants weren't happy I stopped it and start threatening my sight by saying they'll make me go blind.

I didn't believe them. But then my vision would seem a little blurrier, and I wondered if I was becoming blind.

I would ask Higher Power to give strength to Goddess Isis and Archangel Uriel.

The remnants constantly try to show me illustrations on the bumpy ceiling, so I wouldn't concentrate on my words or find other ways to mess me up.

Ashes to Dust

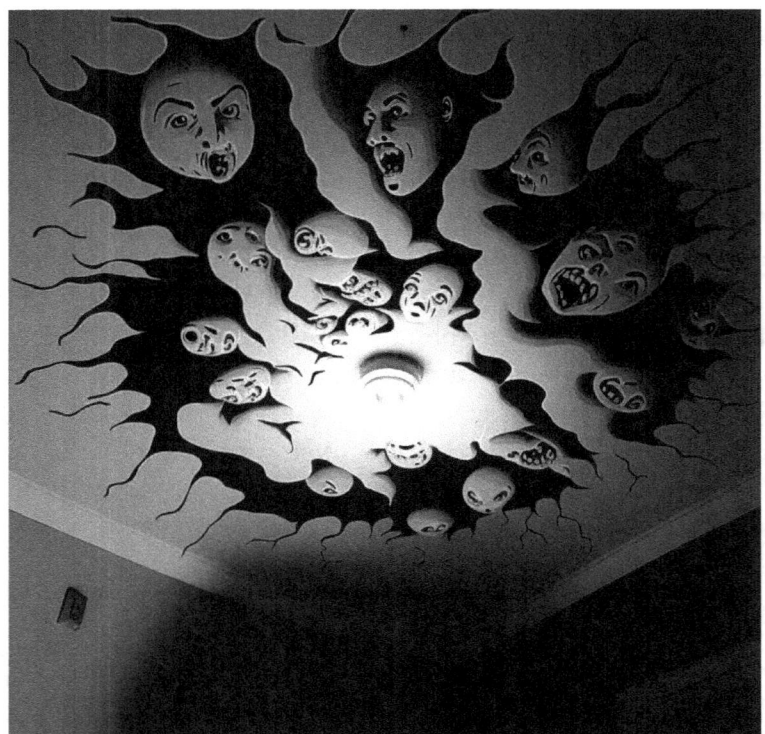

Once I forgot, "Archangel," before Uriel, and it was an offense to him because the entire name was a title given and must be said together.

The remnants made me call the wrong Archangel name, Michael, then I was trying to be careful because they were trying to swap Uriel's name for someone else's like Raphael, Michael, and Lucifer.

I told them I was not calling the big L name.

It seemed like Uriel and Isis were struggling. I ask if it was the negative and dark thoughts the remnants sent them.

They nod yes.

I didn't know how to help with that, so in between asking to give strength to Goddess Isis and Archangel Uriel, I would pay them compliments to counteract all the bad that I couldn't always hear going towards them.

Ashes to Dust

I would catch some lewd and rude things, but that was only what the remnants wanted me to hear, so I would get distracted and react because I thought it was disgusting or downright mean.

The remnants made me think the word, "Cruel," and sometimes say the word against them, knowing I didn't like it because it was what they made Goddess Isis hear in my thoughts to get her to punish me before.

When Goddess Isis heard it was the remnants and not me that put those thoughts for her to hear there, she stopped and started crying through me.

I tell her not to worry about it right now and focus. They want her distracted and to doubt her strength.

I couldn't hold back the remnants from mentioning it was them to her, because I knew it would cause severe harm to her. It did.

I swap between giving strength to only Goddess Isis and then to Archangel Uriel. Sometimes I would say one name twice by accident because of the remnants. They often laughed in a gross way that wasn't right. I didn't like that through me.

I said I preferred Isis's laugh instead, and the remnants got angry.

Because I kept saying nice things to pep up Isis or Uriel, the remnants tried to punish me by saying they were making me completely blind, then deaf.

When it wasn't working, I laughed, and the remnants could unfortunately hear my thoughts. And they were, they couldn't do it, thoughts.

Uriel warned me not to taunt them. That I didn't know what they really were.

He kept making it seem so bad, and I was getting confused. I knew they were evil pieces from Hekate's personality that she left behind.

The remnants got angrier and angrier at me, saying they would give me a brain tumour next.

I didn't know how I would check to make sure I didn't have a brain

Ashes to Dust

tumour, but I didn't think I did or I will just get checked if I suspect something. Isis started moving away from my chest and onto my head, then my stomach. They were giving me a stomach cancer and Isis was trying to heal it before it spread.

Uriel said not to be a challenge to them.

He said it a few times, but I didn't think I was being a challenge. I would say things I felt I needed to say or to help Uriel and Isis.

The remnants said, "Too late. She already has us interested. We are never giving her up. She's so stupid. We like that."

They tried to mess with my mind by making it seem like Uriel was shouting at me or calling me things. I didn't think it really was Uriel, but then I thought if it was, he must be shouting those things at the remnants. That he must really hate what the remnants are doing to me.

Goddess Isis kept moving from the heart to stomach to the other side of my chest, which I assumed meant breast cancer. Then back to rubbing my stomach in small circles to heal it.

Uriel told me the remnants were Hellions, and they really can give me tumours and cancer like they threaten.

I didn't know what Hellions were until Uriel clarified they were demons.

The remnants were actually demons called Hellions. That was terrifying and unsettling to know. I thought before it felt a bit like how a possession must feel, and now that he says they're demons, I'm thinking it is like a possession.

I still pay compliments to Uriel and Isis and say things I shouldn't.

The Hellions told Uriel there was nothing I could say to make things any better. They will continue trying and Uriel and Isis should give up, otherwise I will die in front of them. They said I'd die in Uriel's arms knowing he couldn't save me and they would take my soul.

Uriel said he would take my soul before they could.

The Hellions said they would kill him before he could do that.

By Isis and Uriel's reactions with silence and a feeling I got from them of concern, the Hellions could indeed kill them both if they stuck around after.

I told Uriel and Isis if I die I didn't blame them and thanked them for trying so hard to save me. I told Uriel especially not to take it to heart or carry that around because the world needed him and it wasn't his fault.

I knew I would have to banish Isis and Uriel from staying by my side if it seemed like I was about to die, so it would save them. The world needed them, not me. They were more important.

Isis and Uriel were upset when they realized the words of banishment coming from my mouth. I say it more than once so that it will work.

Now, if it seems like I'm about to die, they will need to run away before then to a safe place and they can't go back for my soul.

The Hellions were again angry that I made it so they couldn't kill Uriel and Isis. They desperately wanted to. They focused their rage by giving me more negative thoughts. That I should kill myself.

I didn't want to respond out loud before (just in my head) so I didn't worry Isis and Uriel, but I had to let them know some of the stuff the remnants were saying to me.

I said no, I won't kill myself.

The Hellions said the world is better off with me dead. That I was a nuisance. I should give up and let them have me.

I tell Isis and Uriel what they said, though it was uncomfortable. Just like when the Hellions purposely let me know the negative dark thoughts they were sending Uriel when he tried to heal me. I wouldn't get all of it. Just stray parts that they knew would be the most impactful to make me say something like, "That's disgusting," or any reaction in my thoughts towards it to fight it.

They told Uriel perverted things he could do to me. It made me upset and I could tell it was draining him, but he seemed stronger against it than Isis.

Ashes to Dust

The Hellions kept trying to get me to give up my soul to them, and I refused.

When I refuse, they try to trick me with horrible distractions again. I'd have to close my eyes and turn my head to move from it, but they were in my head. Like images of someone ripping their face down and off.

The Hellions made me forget my archangel's name. I knew it started with a U, but all I got after trying so hard was Ursula, the octopus creature from a cartoon movie. I knew I couldn't say that, so I had to skip asking Higher Power to give strength to him and give it to Goddess Isis.

I knew Isis preferred Aset but the Hellions would trip me up with her name too, so Isis was easier.

The Hellions laughed through me saying, "Uh oh, now bird boy is weaker."

I kept trying to get around the mind block as I gave only Goddess Isis strength. I then came up with, "And give the archangel beside me strength."

The Hellions were upset I found a loophole, and Archangel Uriel could heal me again.

The Hellions told them to give up on me, or they would spread everything faster.

They make my organs fail. First my heart, then lungs, then down. Goddess Isis had to work faster to keep up with it so I didn't die.

They then put a cancer in my vagina and laughed because they wanted to see if the Goddess would touch it or not.

It grossed me out they would do that. I told Isis it was okay. Giving her permission.

Isis went down my belly button to the top of my vagina, not anywhere near the inside, strictly the flat top surface. She then started healing it.

The Hellions kept making lewd comments about how Isis must love doing that. First boobs, now pussy.

After Isis finished healing it, she moved back to the other organs. The Hellions successfully made me get distracted with what they did. It grossed me out they would give me a vagina cancer and then make a Goddess try to heal my vagina by touching it.

My head tilts back and my eyes close as Uriel plucks the Hellions out of my head. Behind closed lids I can tell when he got one or a piece of one, because I saw a strange mix of colours, or light blue electricity. I open my eyes and it would be a little better.

I wondered how many times he would have to pluck them out. As he kept going, I would see the colours again when my eyes were shut, but I would also see the Hellions mean imagery of arms being torn apart. I think they were supposed to be my arms. There were too many horrible ones. And if I opened my eyes, the Hellions connected the bumps on the ceiling to create illustrations.

Suddenly the Hellions stopped and cocked my head, staring up at the ceiling where the light bulb was. They got scary surprised with shocked sounds mixed with excitement. I didn't see what they saw, I just saw my bright light bulb on my ceiling.

They get even more excited, asking why Higher Power showed up. "Have you come to watch?" They'd then move on analyzing, "What is she? We want to know!"

They sounded like an excited kid at a candy store and it creeped me out. I didn't know what was happening or what they meant when they asked what I was.

They said Higher Power has never shown up before like this. That I must be important to it. They say, "We want her even more now!" And then they try to figure out what I was.

I said it didn't matter what I was. I just wanted them gone.

It was weird having the thing I was asking for strength from just show up. Then I remember the requests from earlier where one of them was my music career.

Ashes to Dust

I ask Higher Power if taking my music was its request.

It felt like a beam of light that lined up like a giant eyeball to my eyes. Then my head shook no.

The Hellions said it was them.

I'm upset and want it back. That isn't fair. I was trying to live and trusted something I couldn't see once in my life because I thought it would help me.

Higher Power undid the taking of my music career I was meant to have.

The Hellions were upset and scream at Higher Power, "That's ours!" They wanted to fight Higher Power for it. They said they knew it was important and took it away. "She has no idea how important she is."

I don't feel important. I'm not important, or special, just normal me.

The Hellions figured it out, "Priestess!" They got excited by it, saying they haven't had a priestess.

I didn't understand how I could be a priestess.

Higher Power is upset they told me. In my past life I was a priestess.

I reassure Higher Power I didn't care about any past lives, only the life I have now.

I stick by that, and meant it. I'm annoyed they said it. I really didn't want to know. I just want to live and get them out of me. I'm exhausted. I don't think I can make it much longer. I don't know how I made it this far.

Goddess Isis and Uriel continue healing me even though they are also surprised Higher Power showed up.

I wonder if it was me calling on it so many times that made it eventually show up. I called on it when the Gods and Goddesses were attacking me. Then in the circles, and for strength for Isis when I was dying downstairs. And then strength for both Goddess Isis and Archangel Uriel with the remnants.

The Hellions try to fight harder against Isis and Uriel as they heal me and try to get rid of them. The Hellions want to stay.

Ashes to Dust

I ask Higher Power for strength for Goddess Isis and Archangel Uriel again.

It responds by nodding my head.

None of them could see within the thoughts and attacks the Hellions were doing when I tried to concentrate on the words and names.

Isis and Uriel kept telling me to concentrate. Higher Power too.

I was concentrating. There were just too many distractions and disturbing things from the Hellions.

Uriel plucks the Hellions out of my mind again. He plucks them out as Isis healed me.

After plucking them out, they are finally gone, and I'm saved. I wasn't going to die. I was so relieved and exhausted.

I thank both Goddess Isis and Archangel Uriel. I also thank Higher Power for restoring my music and giving them the strength to help me.

I could feel a change in Goddess Isis and Archangel Uriel. It felt heavy. I don't think they will ever be the same again. Archangel Uriel doesn't seem like he can continue being the protector of the world, getting rid of things that made the world worse like he did before this.

I ask Higher Power if it could reward Isis and Uriel for their good karma for saving me, by removing the bad thoughts and feelings the remnants left behind because it was too heavy for them.

Especially for Uriel with the dying in his arms part.

Higher Power makes me nod yes.

It then heals them of those burdens. I ask Goddess Isis and Archangel Uriel if they feel better.

Both were yeses.

I'm happy.

I talk to Uriel for a bit. He didn't say much. He seems more reserved. I ask why the Hellions called him bird boy.

Ashes to Dust

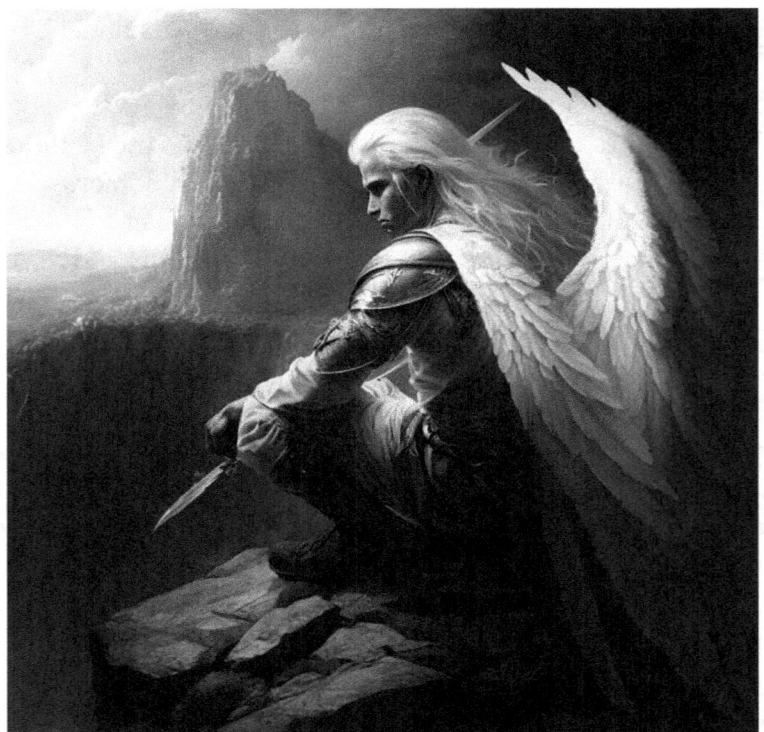

Apparently because he really has wings. He also was a "pretty" boy. White or blond hair, I wasn't sure.

I ask him if he was going to have a well-deserved break.

He said no. He was to move onto a new duty/mission right away with no breaks. He uses a sword.

I thank him again, and he left.

I ask Isis if she still remembered everything that happened.

She nods yes.

I ask her if she still felt the dark parts that were weighing her down.

She shakes my head no.

She seems more like her older self, but also with something different now. I tell Isis she should go finally have some sort of celebration with her family. Her son would be very proud of how strong she was. She proved her strength where even Hekate tried to make her doubt. She was stronger than ever.

That made her happy. She nods yes.

PART TWO
LUCIFER

5

I talk to Higher Power. I stare directly at the light fixture above my bed where the light bulb shines bright through my netted canopy. That's where Higher Power is. It's odd seeing Higher Power as a light bulb fixture, but that is where my senses/knowing says to look.

Apparently Higher Power can't be in every place at once, so it can't see everything. I think that's strange because people of religion always say there's something all knowing and always watching over everyone. Higher Power proves that is untrue.

It didn't know I was being attacked before by the Gods and Goddesses. It said it wasn't supposed to be that way for me.

I'm not sure if it means the second circle wasn't suppose to happen, or if being jumped all at once during the first wasn't suppose to happen.

It confirms my sister wasn't suppose to be involved or know anything. It's upset about that.

I learn I'm not suppose to worship any Gods or Goddesses, or look into anything witchcraft related.

I tell it I was watching meditation videos.

It says yes, I was meant to do that.

Then I started watching general tarot card reading videos after looking them up to give to my mom since she was into them.

It shook my head no; I wasn't suppose to watch Tarot videos.

Ashes to Dust

I told it how one tarot video suggested the spiritual cleansing and multiple mentioned burning paper you write on. I did both.

No, I wasn't suppose to do that either.

I say after I do that many of the tarot videos suggested spiritual baths, so I eventually did one of those.

No, I wasn't suppose to do that.

Isis informs me they were all Hekate, making Higher Power angry.

I then say one day I got a random video suggestion to watch a ritual of a Hekate summoning, but I never watched anything related to her, Gods, or witchcraft before. Then I mentioned the last tarot card reading was a, "Which Goddess has been trying to reach out to you," and I got Hekate. Which I found strange and spooky at the time.

Higher Power needs a moment and disappears for a second.

I ask Isis what it's doing.

She says, giving Hekate her karma.

When Higher Power comes back, Hekate is successfully put behind the new jail system my sister asked for. Higher Power is very upset. Its plans are not how it mapped it out for me and the world.

I suggest allowing Goddess Isis in my life where she can tell me what isn't on my original free will paths. If every one gets multiple paths to choose from, then I will still have ones I'm closest too. I tell Higher Power I promised Isis a celebration and still wanted to write about her helping with new God karma. I then ask if I'm suppose to write about Higher Power too.

My head nods yes.

I tell Higher Power to tell me what not to write if something is wrong and not how it was supposed to go.

It considers it, but it doesn't like the change.

I tell it my sister wants to worship too, so maybe Isis can help make sure her life isn't off track either.

Higher Power is upset again.

We talk about the priestess past life. Like how the priestess has made me remember a few things after learning about being a priestess in my past life.

I had to banish her to a part inside me she could never escape from so she couldn't try to control or interfere with my life anymore. I am still angry she forced horrible memories back on me. Like my father raping me when I was a child. I don't remember and would rather be ignorant of it for the rest of my life. Since I can't remember, I'm trying not to let it affect me.

The second was in my past priestess life I had a baby that died in a cage.

The third was my sister is the reincarnation of my past life baby. Which is horrible to fathom. My dead baby is reborn as my sister. Is that why I've felt like taking care of her more lately? Because the priestess knew and was making me. Just like how I wanted to see my sister's baby more and help make her stop crying. Was it because the priestess missed her dead baby and was trying to make me like babies so I would have one? So she could have one again? That's so messed up. She knows I'm not interested in having a baby. I've never been interested in that. I am not a baby making machine. It will never happen. The whole time I thought it was some annoying internal clock thing. I'm extremely angry at the priestess for doing that to me. I don't care if she was a past me. This is my life now. She had hers. I don't want her to interfere with my time to live.

Higher Power is angry at the priestess.

I didn't know it could get angry. I was worried.

It asks for the priestess from me (since I banished her to be locked away).

I ask if it will affect the me now since the priestess is a past life me.

It shakes my head no.

As long as it doesn't affect me now, I say yes, it can take her.

I close my eyes and it reaches in and takes her. The priestess doesn't want to be taken, but they both disappear.

Ashes to Dust

I ask Isis where it took her.
She shakes my head no.
I don't think she knows.
She says she's never seen it so angry before.
I say it's probably because it never had its plans messed up so much before.
She agrees.
When Higher Power comes back, it talks through Isis again, who then talks through me. It tells me I should sleep.
I have a few more things I want to talk about that I remembered from asking for Higher Power's help during the God's attack in my kitchen, the first circle, and again in the second circle with the two intruders.
It asks to see.
I get confused, wondering how it missed that if it knew I was attacked. I ask if it's because the priestess blocked it from seeing certain things.
It shakes my head yes.
I say okay, and ask if it's going to take long because there's a lot.
It shakes my head no.
I close my eyes, and it rummages through the scenes. Then my eyes open as it's done. It is a speedy memory reader.
Isis speaks for Higher Power again and she says the Gods and Goddesses blocked it from hearing me asking for its help.
I ask if all the requests made about the exchange when I was dying were really from it or the remnants.
I also have a knowing and say I think Hekate sent them on purpose to hurt you, Higher Power. Because she's angry at you.
It asks to look again.
I say I thought it wanted me to sleep.
But it really wants to look, so I close my eyes for it to look.
It sees the illusion images that Hekate left in my mind and sees further on what the remnants were doing to my mind and that they

were actually talking through me. I opened my eyes when it was done.

It's upset again.

I tell it the God's and Goddesses were talking through me, just like the remnants.

This surprises Isis.

I tell her, "Can't you hear you are talking through me right now?"

There is silence, then a no.

I think Isis is self aware now that I said it. She seems more careful of what she says too.

Isis says it's a gift I had when I was in my other life. I'm not suppose to be able to do it in this one.

I tell Higher Power while the Gods and Goddesses attacked me I could sometimes feel when they were still there or when they jumped in because of the strange feeling I would get in my temple. It was different to the feeling in my eyes when my Spirit Guides showed up.

Isis says I'm not suppose to be able to tell those differences either. The priestess activated me.

I don't know what activated means, but it made Higher Power disappear again. I think to find priestess.

When Higher Power comes back, I mention it needs to fix something with the Gods again so that they can understand human emotions or thoughts. I tell it they need to be empathetic and understand human thoughts and feelings so they don't have miscommunication with a human thought and punish them for it like Isis did to me.

I feel the stillness within me. Isis. I wonder why.

Isis speaks for Higher Power again through me. It wants to see her punishing me.

First, I ask Isis if it's okay to let Higher Power see.

Isis says yes, but she sounds so scared.

I never heard Isis sound so scared. I don't think she realized she could also get in trouble. I wonder what's going to happen to her. Were they not suppose to punish after all or just not specific people? It was confusing. I was worried since Isis literally just saved me, and I don't want to seem ungrateful or have something bad happen where she regrets it. Or undoes it.

I say okay to letting Higher Power look, and it does.

After it's upset with Isis for punishing me. Now it's Isis's turn to go with it.

I tell her I'm sorry for getting her in trouble.

She says I had to say it.

They leave, and I feel bad for getting Isis in trouble right after she just saved my life.

When Higher Power comes back, it wants to remove the worship, so I let it.

I tell it I'm worried my sister will try to worship Isis because I never got to tell her not to since Isis was around and would've punished me. I tell it I don't think my cat, sister or her baby are safe from Isis now. I politely request safety of my cat and family because I have a knowing that Isis will be unloving like Hekate.

Higher Power makes a vow to me that from now on I wouldn't feel pain anymore, I would only feel good things.

I ask if it can punish.

I think it says yes. I get scared of it. What if it punishes me like Isis did? What if it's worse? I don't want to go through more punishments. I don't want to live in fear.

I ask if it will punish me.

It shakes my head no.

I seem to have misunderstood because of what the remnants did to my head. It can't punish.

It tries to re-assure me, but there's a communication problem. It's upset because of what Isis did to me, and that she ruined my relationship with it by planting the mistrust and fear there. And what the remnants did.

After I take a moment, I'm a bit relieved it can't punish. I feel like I'm finally going to be protected from Gods and Goddesses and anything else out there Earthly or Otherworldly. Even though it says it can't punish, I'm still worried it's lying and don't completely trust it. But I think it's because of what Isis did.

It also says it will bring me back to life if I died.

Which made me wonder if I'm still not safe from my heart giving out, or if something else might kill me.

Lastly, it says it will make all my dreams come true (Toronto, singing, visit japan). It said moving would happen fast. In a week.

I was so excited. I wondered when I would get a call telling me I could move to Toronto and how. Would it be a money contest so I could buy one? A house contest I sometimes see? I couldn't wait. The vow it gives me was tiny and dissolved into my forehead. I think I found something that is finally trustworthy. And this vow will make it so I won't be let down again.

I call on my spirit family to come protect me from the Gods and Goddesses. They show up and I'm surprised at the overwhelming emotions I have meeting them.

They say hello.

There's a more prominent one who speaks through me. She seems reserved or really controlled in what she says or does. Even when it seems there are emotions coming, it gets reeled back. There are others too.

I ask if I got through when I tried to meditate to the guided meet your Starseed family meditation.

They say yes.

I said what was I like there because I think I did it wrong. If it worked I thought I was frozen and told them I imagined they were all just standing around thinking I was broken with my mouth wide open or something.

They laugh and say yes. They knew it didn't work well, but they were excited to see me anyway because it had been so long. They haven't seen me since I was sent on the mission to be reincarnated on Earth.

I said my mouth and lips felt weird during the goodbye part of that meditation and wondered if they were yelling in my mouth or something.

They laugh and said I don't want to know.

Which made me wonder what the heck they were doing to astral me or whatever gets shot up there during meditation. The only other thing I thought of was a goodbye kiss or something. I didn't want to think too much about it.

For visiting me, my spirit family were tiny and on my stomach. I'm not sure why. I'm not sure exactly what they look like, but I try to get a sense. I remembered comments in the video saying some of their spirit family were animals on a different planet, and some were natives. So I thought maybe they were some sort of animal, but I wasn't getting a sense that they were animals.

Trying to get to know them was cut short because Isis came back with her son Osiris, and other gods who hated me still. I ask my Spirit Family if they would please protect me.

They said yes.

It seemed like the Gods and Goddesses were afraid of my spirit family because no one attacked me yet. They just surrounded me. I ask why that was.

My spirit family says it's because we are strong. That I come from a strong, warrior spirit family, and the Gods and Goddesses are scared of their strength.

I was amazed. I didn't think anything would scare the Gods or Goddesses. My spirit family must be special. And extremely strong to boldly take on Gods.

I have a feeling that something is by me. I ask my Spirit family because I can't see the Gods, I can just sense where their location is at times.

Ashes to Dust

They sound exasperated, saying yes.

The Gods are attacking them and me, and won't stop. I reach behind me, and I feel an overpowering sense of power flood me, and I push it onto the God I'm holding. I tell them they're burning, and I know they are. They won't be able to hurt me or anyone else.

But then the voice of my spirit family through me snaps me out of it, and I stop. The God is alive, but not attacking me anymore because they're burned.

I can hear my spirit family saying I almost burnt the God to ashes, but I was not myself.

I tell them it felt like a dark part. Like a black aura taking over.

I noticed, and they noticed, the change in my voice. It was lower in tone, but more demanding and powerful. Like I was tapping into someone else, or another hidden, stronger me.

It made Higher Power unhappy. It resulted from the priestess activating me. So now I'm powerful enough to attack back, but I don't have control of it.

I ask my spirit family which God touched me.

They say it was the one that I used to worship.

It made the rest of the Gods stop attacking for a moment.

I ask my spirit family what the Gods are doing.

They say they are waiting. Scared.

The Gods attack again and me and my spirit family fight them off. It takes a long time, but eventually they leave when I banish them all. They sense the priestess power in me now and with my strong spirit family they go.

I'm upset Higher Power lied to me. It promised the Gods wouldn't attack or hurt me again. That I wouldn't feel pain again. Why am I let down by something that's supposed to be trustworthy? It watched it all without helping or stopping them.

I thank my spirit family for protecting me.

Ashes to Dust

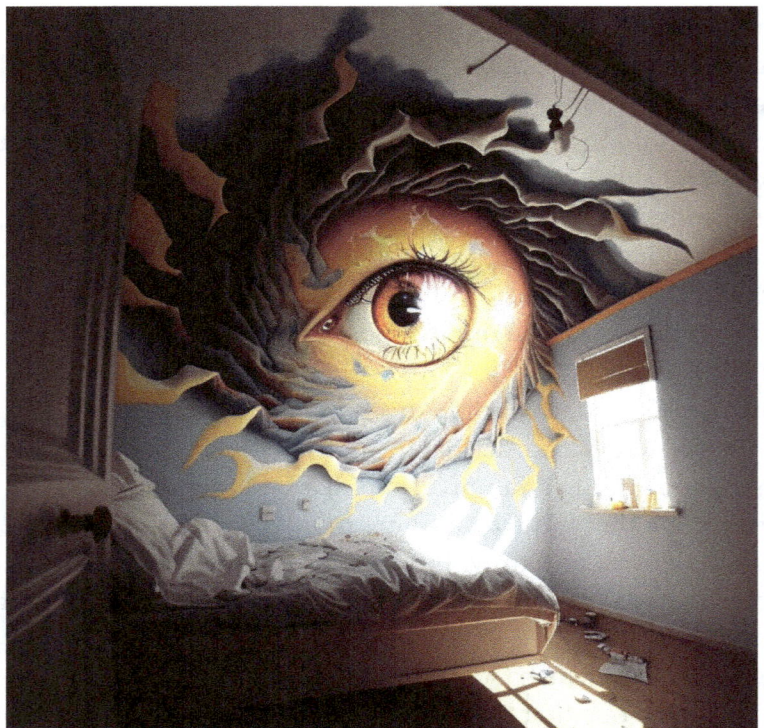

I look up at the ceiling where Higher Power is and get a better vision of it. A giant eyeball in my knowing. I'm staring at my light fixture, but I know it's a giant eyeball. There's black smoke in it. Higher power is tainted, and I need to cleanse it.

I tell my spirit family and Higher Power about the taint.

I raise my arms up above me, and my arms shake with power, as does my voice. I suck out the taint towards me and destroy it from existence.

I can see in Higher Power better. It's not one, but two. Parents of the universe. Mother and father. I'm not suppose to know that. It's upset again because I know and call it them.

Now that Higher Power is untainted, I talk to my spirit family about what happened with the circles, the Gods attacking, and how my

Ashes to Dust

family treated me. I ask them if it's weird that I love them more than my Earth family.

They said no, with a sad tone to it. But they also sounded happy to hear me say I love them.

I tell them I had to give up a few things for the Goddess I once worshiped to heal me. One of them was going home after this life was over. They were surprised, and angry, which surprised me. They aren't happy with Higher Power now.

Higher power is warning me not to say some things to them, because my spirit family, by my feeling, will ignore the rules or find a way around them to help me.

My spirit family said they would stay with me on Earth to protect me until I can go back home.

I ask if they are sad that I won't be able to hear them or know they are there. Or forget when I'm reincarnated.

They are sad, and I think re-thinking the decision.

I tell them they didn't have to stay.

They tell me they want to. That I've been through a lot. And not to worry about not going home after this life on Earth, they will handle it.

Higher power is getting upset and didn't like the sound of it. I feel like they can in fact do what they say. Higher power knows they are strong and is worried they will undo it. I'm not going to stop them.

Higher power doesn't want me to say things that will encourage them to react anymore.

I tell my spirit family how I was upset that the priestess had planted her old life in my head like my dad raping me, her baby dying in a cage, and that baby is my baby, which was a son, is now reincarnated into my current Earth sister.

I just realize something talking to my spirit family about everything. Can I taint them? They seem furious and ready to fight. It's a change in them. I ask Higher Power.

Yes.

Ashes to Dust

I tainted my spirit family.

I'm upset about this. I didn't know I could taint them. I said something they couldn't handle. I need to keep certain things to myself. I find the things I said that tainted them and take it back so they don't remember I said it.

I'm devastated still but after finishing I ask them how they are feeling.

They say good, then they ask why am I crying.

I say I'm just happy they are happy.

I ask Higher Power if they are tainted still.

It says no.

I look at Higher Power and ask if it is tainted.

It nods my head yes.

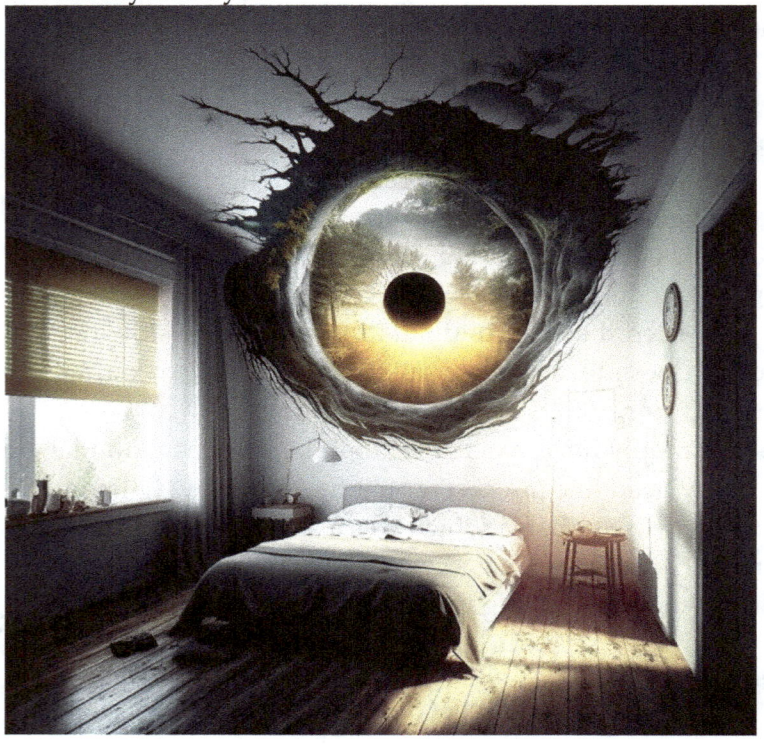

Ashes to Dust

I raise my arms towards the ceiling and draw the taint out of Higher Power and get rid of it. I ask my spirit family if they are tainted. Yes.

I'm wondering how I'm tainting them now. There must be something wrong. I keep thinking only positive loving things. I ask them if they can hear them.

They say no. It's only bad things.

I don't understand at first. Then I remember the one I use to worship had touched me. She must have put the remnants back in. They are doing what they did before, blocking out the positive and feeding negative so everything is twisted.

I tell them this. Then I say the only way I can make it stop so they aren't tainted anymore is to break our psychic connection so they can't hear my thoughts or feel my emotions anymore.

They don't want that. It's like not being connected to me at all.

I tell them if they don't do it, I'll have to banish them back to their home so they don't get tainted anymore. I tell them I'll tell them how I feel if they ask, even if the truth is unpleasant.

They agree.

I tell them to make a circle, and for Higher Power to get in the middle. I tell my spirit family to block me out and don't listen to me until I give the signal. Then they all break their connection to me, Higher Power too.

It's the only way they stop getting re-tainted. I give the signal and they do it. It takes a bit, and I feel like I lost something. After they are done, I ask how they feel. I don't feel much different.

They feel much better now.

None of the hellions negative poison is getting to them now.

My spirit family is upset about the lost connection.

I tell them with the hellions it wasn't a full connection; it was like a fake window where less than half the things I tried to get through would get stuck halfway. I try to tell them all the loving things I thought before.

Ashes to Dust

I realize Higher Power is still tainted from before. And I have a knowing prophecy of what it means if it stays tainted.

I tell them all. Everything goes white like a canvas. Nothing will exist.

What I don't say is after that no existence, there is a chance of life again one day. Of existence being reborn.

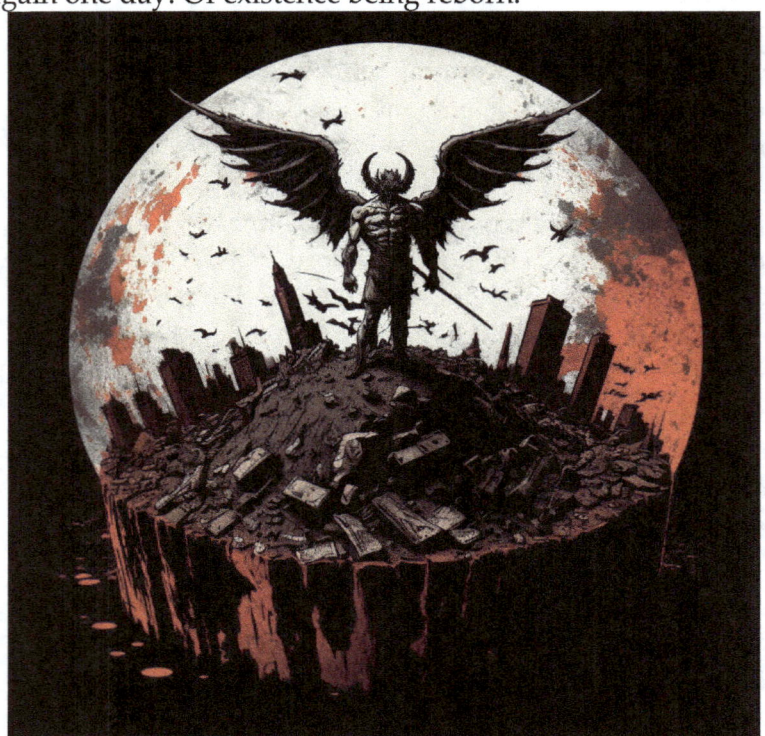

I say Lucifer will try to attack Higher Power and kill it so he can take over and be free to roam Earth and rule over it and everything else. The king.

I raise my arms again, knowing the importance of getting the taint out. I try to take out but I have to stop because my arms get tired. There's still some taint left. The taint is making Higher Power aggressive.

Ashes to Dust

It's yelling at me to hurry up and heal it.
I have a knowing of it, just out of reach.
I can tell through my spirit family that it's calling me bitch, saying, "Heal me now bitch!"
Using my mouth but their voice, my spirit family is telling it to stop.
It doesn't let me rest enough. I try again. I raise my arms. I almost got it all this time. I feel something beside me.
I stop trying to untaint Higher Power, and ask if something is touching my forehead.
My spirit family says yes.
I ask if it's a god.
They say yes, the jokester.
It feels unpleasant and I ask what it's doing.
They say taking the hellions out.
But something feels off.
They then say he's putting them back in.
I push him away and I hear my spirit family say, "Oooh, he didn't like that," through me.
Then my foot bobs up and down over my other one like someone tapping their foot. That's how I could tell he was impatient.
I mention the prophecy to him.
My spirit family says he knows.
I can feel him coming as the foot tapping stops. I ask them if he's attacking anyway.
They sigh and say yes.
Why are these Gods so relentless and bullheaded? I push him away with more strength. He stops again with the foot tapping.
I say I can feel his impatience and foot tapping.
The tapping stops and air changes.
My spirit family says he didn't like that at all.
He didn't know I could feel him through me like that.
I then get a nasty, menacing vibe from him, with his intent to turn

Ashes to Dust

into a snake and rape me. I gather my strength to fight him.

Unfortunately, I was aware Higher Power's taint was growing because of Loki's attack and it also knew of Loki's intent, even though I didn't say it. The remnants shared it through my thoughts.

The priestess in me took over. I attempt to turn Loki into a worm. Squirmy little worm. I even say it. "Squirmy wormy." I picture him becoming a worm and feeding him to a bird. Maybe bird boy, but then I thought bird boy would enjoy that, so I thought of him just being a worm again.

I got part way, but he was at full strength and I was sleep deprived and tired. I stop and lower my arms. I'm exhausted.

I hear my spirit family's commentary through me saying how part of him was a worm, but then he changed back.

He's tapping again because my foot is mimicking it. He needs a break and I'm thankful because I need to recover.

I ask if he will listen now. That everything will be turned into a white canvas and nothing will survive, including him.

He doesn't give me long to recover because he's attacking again. Gods must not need as much time to recover as humans. I don't get why he isn't listening. I roll on my side part way to face him coming. I can sense the direction he's at. I raise my hands towards where I know he is, and can feel the power of the priestess and use it to turn him into a squirmy wormy again. I repeat it over and over, but I get tired again and have to stop.

My spirit family says I almost had him as a full worm that time. They say he's freaked out.

He's back to his corner recovering and thinking while I'm gathering strength from my arms aching.

I tell him to stop, to listen and actually think. He shouldn't want to die, and that is what will happen if he continues if I can't untaint Higher Power.

I thought he would listen this time, but he's stubborn like the others.

Ashes to Dust

He attacks again, and I'm so tired. I don't know what to do, I'm desperate. I know I won't outlast him. If I get tired, he will keep going. I feel my right eye burn. It's connected to Hell's gate because of the remnants.

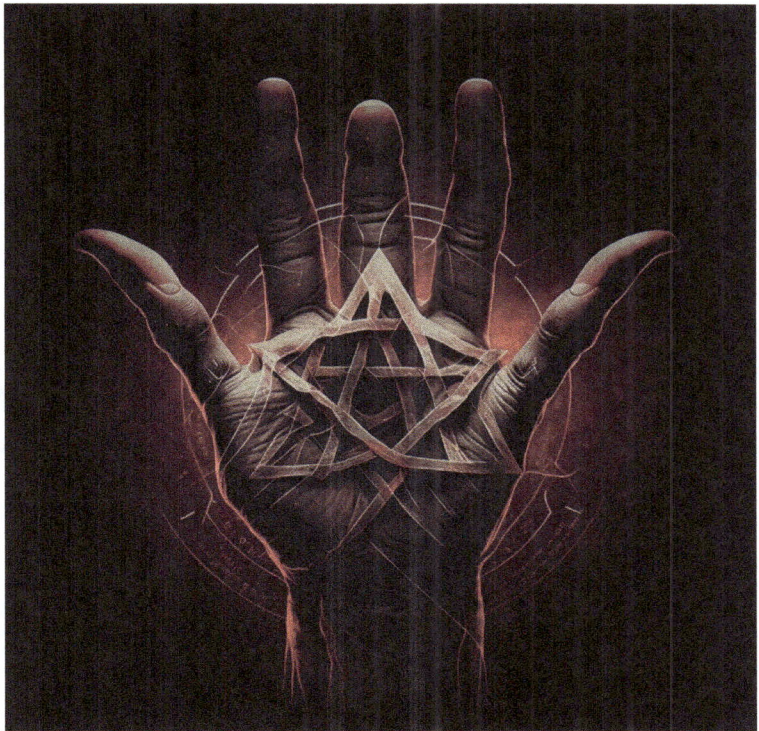

I call Lucifer to come through my right eye, to take Loki where he is banished to stay in Hell's Dungeon without escape. And Lucifer cannot escape Hell's dungeon or through my eye. It will be sealed behind him.

Lucifer's voice comes through me and it is deeper, more powerful than any of the other ones. He is excited, and I feel Loki's fear of him. I get a sense of what Lucifer is going to do. Have Loki shape shift into a girl and have his way with him. I figured that's a good punishment considering what Loki was about to do to me. I feel like Loki has been

Ashes to Dust

Lucifer's plaything before, and that is why he's so terrified.

Lucifer tells me, "I still hate you priestess."

I laugh, saying I banish him to Hell's dungeon and he still can't escape. But at least he has a playmate.

He finds amusement in that.

I struggle to hold on to Loki for Lucifer to make it through and pull him down. After Lucifer drags Loki back through my eye to Hell's dungeon, I seal it closed and make it so they can't escape through it again. My right eye feels boiling hot with energy. More than before, after Lucifer went through it. I didn't think that was a good sign.

I feel bad about having to send Loki down to Hell's dungeon with Lucifer. I never wanted to do that. I didn't want to send something down to be trapped with Lucifer. That's awful. If Loki would've just listened and stopped attacking. Why couldn't he have listened? He knew he would die, but he still attacked. Does this make me awful for sending him down to such a horrible place? Worst of all, Higher Power and my spirit family saw it.

I look at Higher Power and see the taint has severely spread because of it. I try to tell them I never wanted to send him down with Lucifer, but I had no choice.

I try to rest a little bit with Higher Power screaming at me to cleanse it now.

My spirit family tries to get Higher Power to stop.

After gathering some strength, I roll over onto my back again. I tell Higher Power I was going to cleanse it from the taint now.

Ashes to Dust

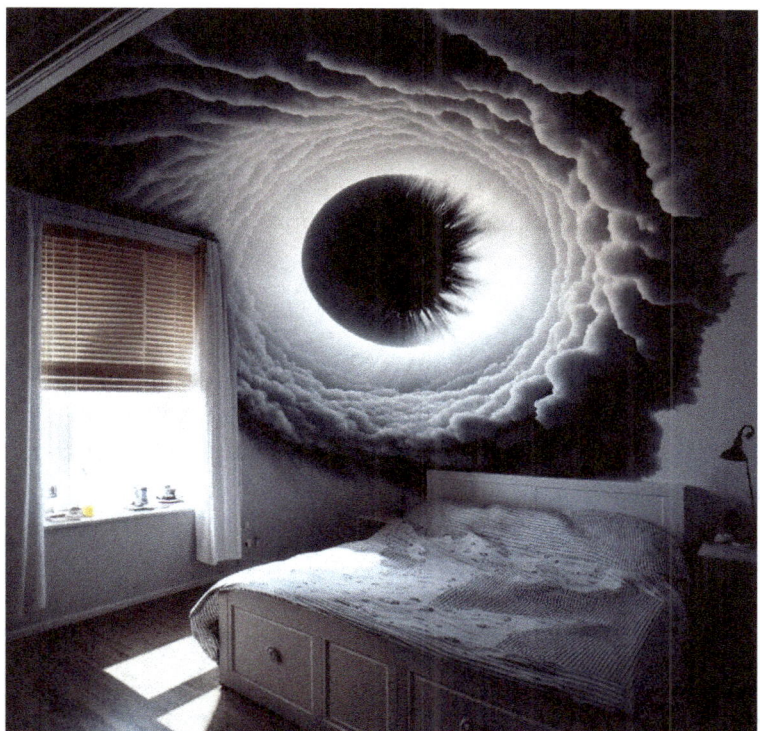

I raise my arms and banish the taint and draw it out and obliterate it from existence. After I finish cleansing Higher Power, I ask if it felt better.

It nods.

I ask if it's still tainted.

No.

I check to make sure. When it's not tainted, I'm relieved. Then I feel the need to call on the stars, now that Higher Power is cleansed.

I call on the stars to come.

They come beside Higher Power. It's a family reunion that Higher Power forgot about. The stars are Higher Power's children. Since the beginning of time.

I tell Higher Power the stars had to stay separate from it until the right moment and they couldn't reunite as a whole again until Higher Power was taint free. If I had failed, then they would have had to wait an extremely long time again before the next person was reincarnated for this soul purpose to put them back together. I was created for it, which is why I have a knowing of things no one else does, and knowledge no one else is suppose to have. Along with the power.

I ask the tars if they are ready.

They nod.

I reunite Higher Power and the stars as one again. After they merge, I stare back up in the same spot as the light fixture, knowing that's where it is. I don't know what to call it now.

I tell it now that it's merged as one I know it isn't the old Higher Power anymore but I don't know what to call it and it can't tell me unless it's a yes or no. I tell it I have to keep calling it Higher Power since I don't know its name and I know it isn't Stars or Higher Power anymore.

I get a new knowing prophecy that if the new whole Higher Power is tainted, everything turns black. It's worse than before because they became more powerful as one. It means nothing will ever come back ever again once destroyed. Not even Lucifer could come back or rule. No time or space would exist and it will stay lifeless for all eternity. Not even Higher Power could come back one day or a new creation be born. It was nothingness forever. The last prophecy wasn't forever.

Now that Higher Power was whole, I told it to leave.

I had to deal with the remnants again. Because I was so drained, they were talking through me and making faces.

Higher Power didn't want to, but it left.

I tell my spirit family to cover their ears, and to not listen until I tap them (on my stomach).

They say okay and ask if everything was alright.

I say yes, I just didn't want to risk tainting them again.

They say okay, though the concern was there.

Ashes to Dust

I didn't think it was going to be okay, but I didn't want to worry them.

Higher Power came back. I only knew because the remnants looked up and gasped in excitement that it didn't listen to me and came back.

I tell it to leave.

It didn't want to, and shook my head no.

I tell it it had to. To remember what happens if it gets tainted.

It left, then it came back.

Every time it came back, I only knew because of the remnants looking up. They could see it, I couldn't. They got disappointed when it left. Now that Higher Power was whole, it could see what the remnants were doing with my face, and hear the difference in my voice when they spoke. It made it much worse than before now that Higher Power could witness it all.

It didn't like it and kept trying to pull them out of me, which made me gasp with my mouth open. But it wouldn't work.

The remnants said they were hoping for this to happen. For Higher Power to grow attached and not want to leave me behind. Feel responsible for me.

They were happy about it not listening to me and coming back to try again, or watch too long.

Ashes to Dust

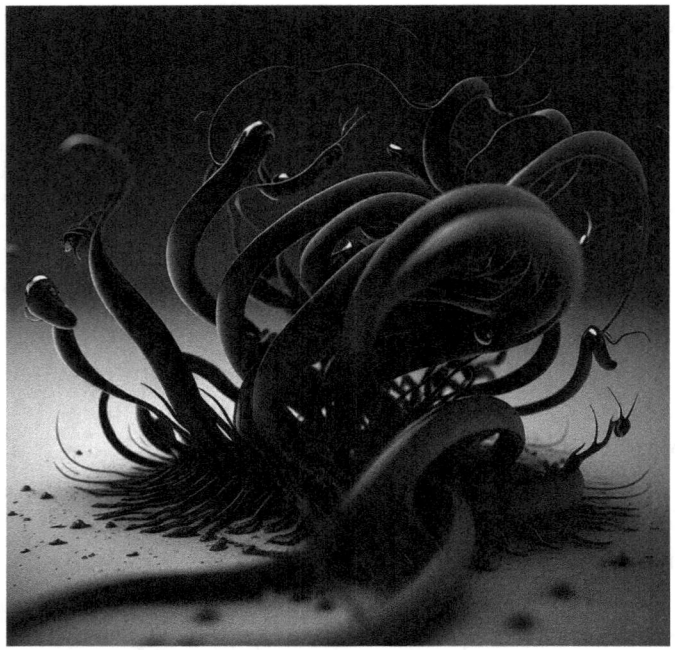

I got a knowing about the remnants. They were squiggly pieces, not maggots, but things from the pits of Hell forged together. For this specific purpose. Lucifer created them and orchestrated the whole thing. He had Hekate reach out and attack me, and had the Gods and Goddesses come attack me, hoping to kill me. It was him and Hekate.

After I told Higher Power what the remnants were made of, the remnants were surprised, and even slightly feared that I knew.

Ashes to Dust

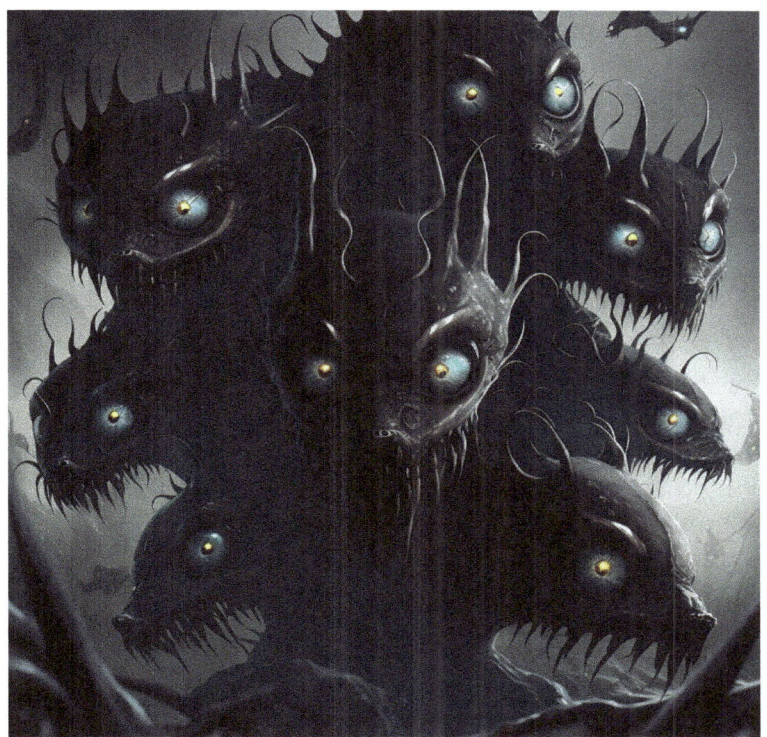

The remnants were upset I knew Lucifer created them. They thought they might get punished.

Higher Power now knows they are pieces of shredded souls and darkness hidden in a treasure chest in Hell by a fire. I thought telling it would help.

The remnants got angrier and tried to taint Higher Power. But Higher Power was already tainted, and it upset me. Higher power wasn't suppose to be taintable, especially now that it was whole.

I remind the remnants of what happens when it gets tainted. That Lucifer wouldn't be happy because it meant he wasn't able to destroy Higher Power himself like he wanted. Instead, Higher Power would destroy everything, including Lucifer. There would be nothing ever again and nothing to rule over.

Ashes to Dust

The remnants didn't apologize; they didn't do much. They look at Higher Power and say they see it now. It was bad.

I say it is because of them.

They shrug my shoulders and said they were good at their job. This was their job.

I said it wasn't helpful.

They said they weren't made to be helpful.

We argued back and forth at times with the same repeated, "That's not helpful," and their, "we told you we weren't created to be helpful."

They would catch themselves saying the wrong thing, and it made the taint worse, but I couldn't stop them from saying dumb things. At least they were finally trying to stop a bit. But they were also still very prideful, saying they couldn't help they were so good at what they do.

Even when I told them they could leave, they still wouldn't.

I feel something wrong. The remnants look behind me towards the window and tell me Hekate has sent Hell hounds to attack me and they will be here soon.

I'm not looking forward to that and don't know how to get rid of Hell hounds. I realize she plans on escaping her cage and have Higher Power tainted. She thinks she's stronger than Lucifer, stronger than everything, and will survive the destruction of everything and take over and rule alone instead of being ruled by Lucifer. She hopes to have Higher Power turn nuclear so it kills Lucifer because she can't.

After I tell Higher Power that Hekate plans on escaping through Astral projection, and the remnants hear, they say Lucifer will be pissed.

That must be how she's escaped all along.

The remnants want to know how I just know things.

I stay quiet about being born that way on purpose. Higher Power gets mean towards me again and the remnants aren't happy about it now they know what will happen.

I tell them if they warn Lucifer that Hekate is about to escape, ruining

Ashes to Dust

his plans and purposely having everything destroyed, then they will probably get rewarded from Lucifer.

The remnants are determined now. They say he does reward those who help him. They ask how.

I say they would have to go through my eye and not leave any trace of themselves behind in me and aren't allowed back through. I will drop them off the outside of Hell's gate instead of opening it. (I don't want Lucifer to escape.)

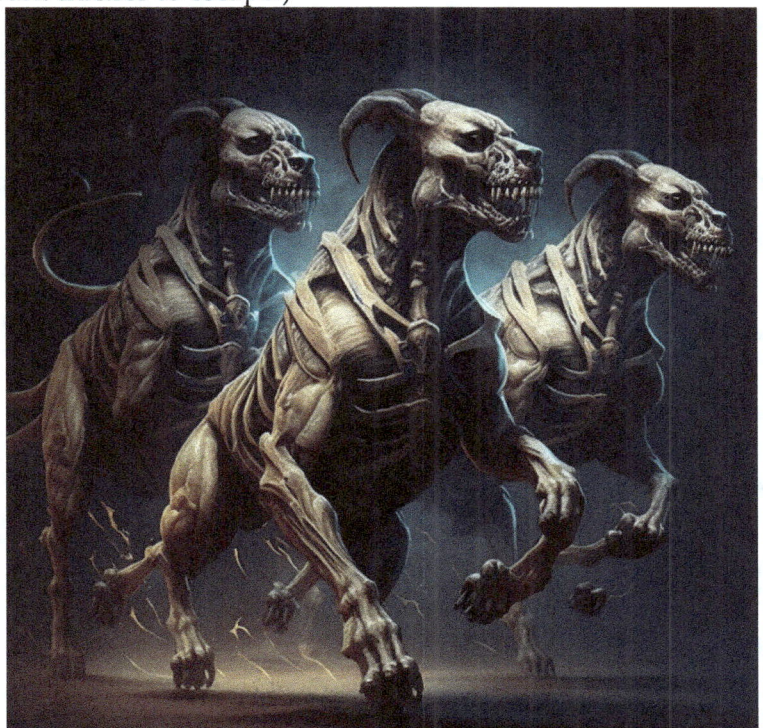

The Hell hounds show up. The remnants take over, shouting at them to stop. They tell them they are in here (me), and for them to go back home.

Some didn't listen and licked me. It burned. The remnants swat at them, but pull back when they still try to lick my arms.

Ashes to Dust

They tell them to stop licking them; it was disgusting. They didn't care how delicious I tasted, to stop licking.

My head had a pain like an electric snap in the back of my head. The remnants get rid of the one that just bit my head. I wiggle down a bit.

Then I felt anger at it for biting me, and grab hold of one of their tongues. I could sense I had it. I then muster my energy and burnt it to a crisp. Killing it. It made the Hell hounds hold back for a minute.

The remnants bribe them, saying they will give them things like souls and body parts if they left. When that didn't work for some, they threaten them by saying Lucifer would be unhappy if they didn't leave. They point to Higher Power, saying do they want to die? Because that will happen if she (me) doesn't fix it.

That seemed to work, though some tried to linger. The remnants kept shooing them and eventually got rid of them.

I'm relieved the Hell hounds are gone.

I tell the remnants the deal again. All of them get out and tell Lucifer of Hekate's plans before she can get to him first. They will have to crawl fast from where I drop them outside the dungeon to get to it.

They agree.

I open my right eye, allowing them through and dropping them off outside the dungeon, and banish them from coming back. I close it and was free of them. I hope they get to Lucifer before Hekate did or she would convince him everything was fine and it'd all be destroyed.

I'm exhausted and need a moment thought I know I need to untaint Higher Power. But before I can, I feel Hekate coming. She shows up and I sense her by my dresser. I don't know what I'm suppose to do. I know she's suppose to be powerful even amongst the Gods and Goddesses. I don't think I can turn her into anything like Loki. It's that worst moment again. I'll have to let Lucifer take her like Loki.

I open the gate to my right eye and allow Lucifer to come through. He can only take Hekate and is still banished to Hell's dungeon, unable to escape, and he must go back after.

Ashes to Dust

He comes through, much angrier than before, saying her name with such fierceness. His anger even scares me.

I know to hold my hands up this time and use what little strength I have left to keep it until he can grab hold of her and successfully bring her back.

I banish her to Hell's dungeon with no possibility of escape.

I have knowings of how she will try to avoid being stuck in Hell's Dungeon. I banish her from coming back through fire, bubbles, water, eyes, snakes, and any elements.

There are too many. I would have to say something different.

"I banish Hekate to be bound to Lucifer for eternity with no escape."

The pure fear that pours out of my mouth as she screams no, through me, was jarring.

She left me no choice. She wouldn't stop attacking. I felt Lucifer's excitement rise. It was somehow more terrifying than his rage. It scared even me hearing him laugh with joy through me. He took Hekate with him and I made sure to wait and close the gate to Hell's dungeon again.

My right eye had an even more intense energy burn to it than last time. I think from using it too much, or it's from Lucifer coming through. I'm worried the gate was spreading.

My spirit family asks if I'm okay.

I try to tell them I didn't want to send anything down to Hell. Especially not to be bound to Lucifer. But they wouldn't stop attacking or leave me and my family alone. I don't get why they couldn't just leave.

I wondered if my spirit family judged me for it. Especially Higher Power. I was crying from it. When I stopped, I went on my back, exhausted from having to prop myself on my side to let Lucifer through and hold Hekate. I see Higher Power is worse because of the Hekate being bound to Lucifer now.

I take a moment to recover, but then Higher Power is acting more aggressive than before. I worry for my spirit family with the way Higher Power seems to be consumed with taint and rage.

I tell my spirit family to leave and not come back until I say.

They don't want to with how Higher Power is shouting, but they do.

I raise my hands, then I look at Higher Power and start removing its taint. It was worse than before. When I thought I got it, I'd check and there would be an additional layer behind the eye shape of it where the shadows were removed. Only to reveal terrifying imagery similar to the remnants from the first time.

I try again, but this time before finishing, Higher Power chokes me, crushing my throat. I have to stop and tell it to stop.

I breathe heavy and am shaky. I think it's acting like this because the taint is a form of its own in there and doesn't want to be destroyed, so it's defending itself by trying to kill me so it can't be removed.

I want that first, sweet, Higher Power back. But now it keeps trying to kill me even when I'm trying to help it. It's so frustrating I want to cry. I don't know what to do. I go to try again but I feel something change.

6

My legs cross, my hands fold, and part of my consciousness is put to sleep, and someone takes control. I don't know until he speaks. It's Lucifer. Oh no, this is bad. I must have messed up, and it allowed him to take over without leaving his prison.

I wonder if Hekate is shackled to his foot or dangling behind him. Or if that meant she is also stuck taking over me, sharing with him. But it was only Lucifer, so I don't know what he did with her.

He stopped Higher Power from killing me just by taking over. Lucifer stared up at Higher Power and started tsking at the sight of its taint.

He's not what I was expecting. He's humming through me as he waves my foot back and forth. Matching him making my right hand come up with only the index finger pointing up, moving it back and forth like it was making a check mark, or he was a conductor to invisible music. He has too much control.

He looks down at my stomach surprised to see my spirit family.

I'm also surprised. I tell them they were supposed to leave.

Lucifer puts me to sleep by touching the right side of my face gently, saying, "Sleep."

My spirit family came back when they thought something was wrong.

They deeply fascinated him, which worries me. It's what keeps me

Ashes to Dust

from being unconscious. I want to protect them. Lucifer seems different from the others. He can hear me without me speaking it.

He coons over how sweet it is that I want to protect my spirit family.

My spirit family hears him and they are afraid he's there, but they don't want to leave me. Which fascinates him more.

When I'm more aware, it feels like he's in the left side of my face and I'm in the right side. It's hard to fight to be present when he is, because he's stronger and I'm drained, lacking sleep and energy.

He caresses my face, and touches my hair, and it makes Higher Power upset.

My spirit family speaks through me and warns Lucifer of the taint.

Lucifer is fascinated by what just happened, and keeps one eye on Higher Power. He says he isn't an idiot like the other beings. He knows to be careful.

Higher Power keeps wanting him to get out of me and stop touching me. I can feel when Higher Power tries to swipe Lucifer's hand off me, (which is really my hand that he is using).

Lucifer tells Higher Power to relax. He isn't hurting me.

He touches my throat and my feet move faster, and he says, "But you did."

He caresses my throat where Higher Power tried to choke me while my arms were in the air trying to take out the taint. Lucifer gets delighted and says, "Ohhh, I know this taste!"

It's the metallic taste I've been tasting for a while now off and on. Death.

I mutter, "Lucifer," in warning, as a reminder to not say anymore or Higher Power will be more tainted.

Lucifer sticks a finger in my mouth on the right side by my bottom molar and then sucks my finger in like he ate delicious cheese powder off of it. His demeanor remained playful, upbeat, and childlike. But there was also a hidden danger to him despite it all.

He noticed the "Lord Hekate" stuck in my head and got upset she

Ashes to Dust

marked me so he couldn't.

I ask Lucifer for my rewards.

He does the index finger in the air thing again and hummed. It must be his excitement or interest.

He asks what rewards?

I say the rewards for giving him Loki and Hekate as two new playmates in Hell with him.

He was fascinated again.

He wondered why he would give me rewards.

I tell him he rewarded his Hellions when they did something in his favour. It's how I know he follows through with his rewards and how I know he will do it for me too.

But then I ask him if he really can fulfill deals.

I wondered since Higher Power didn't keep its end, so I wasn't sure if anything else could.

He responds with, "Of course I can. I'm fucking Lucifer," and makes my hands go in a gesture that is very theatrical, like to say, obviously this powerful being can.

He sing-songs and hums, and then tells me to tell him what I want.

He can sense me thinking extra carefully about it, and is even more intrigued. He tells Higher Power to stop touching, he is waiting to hear what I'm so carefully trying to word.

Ashes to Dust

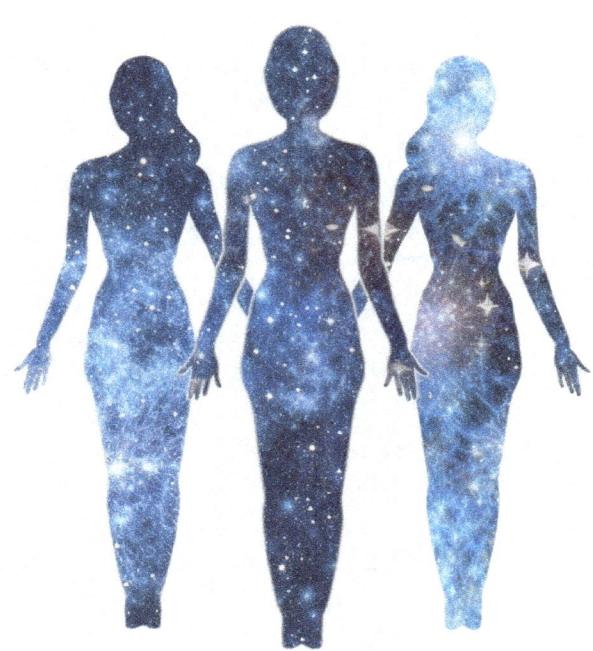

He stares at my spirit family and sees them for what they really look like when I couldn't. Blue sparkly beings. He is drawn to them and it freaks my spirit family out. He says he wants one for his collection.

My knowing shows my spirit family are outlined human-shaped, blue beings with sparkling, white flecks like stars. Almost like a blue sparkly galaxy inside of the human shape. No features. I only know that he knows. I was trying not to know, so he wouldn't find out and be interested.

In my head so no one but us can hear, (and Higher Power doesn't know), I tell him, the first is he can't hurt anyone I love, past, present or future, including my spiritual family and pets.

He is still entranced by my spirit family and is teasing them. Saying they are bright and shiny.

Ashes to Dust

His presence prevented them from attacking him. Which told me he was strong and could hurt any one of us.

I compliment him.

My spirit family hushed me to stop talking.

Lucifer told them to stop and not interrupt.

He enjoyed the compliments I was giving. It made my Spirit family give a high-pitched whine sound.

Higher Power didn't like it either.

I was just stating a fact. His was an immense relief from Hekate's. Hers feelings and internal being, was not one I felt in my life, and not one I enjoyed carrying leftover for a bit while the remnants were there during my resuscitation.

Lucifer can hear that in my head too, without me realizing, and he is uplifted.

The second was to live a long, happy, healthy life with everything I ever wanted coming true. Like singing, living in Toronto, visiting Japan, and publishing my books. He isn't allowed to interfere or ruin it and because he is the master of this (deals/contracts), he must find any possible loopholes that could allow him or anyone else to wreck it. And no soul binding contracts for my soul for the rewards.

He finds me using him as a loophole fixer amusing. I would like to think clever. I think it was clever.

He's still staring at my spirit family, while telling Higher Power to stop (touching and trying to get him out) because we are discussing something.

I felt like I was dying or might not make it, especially from the metallic taste in my mouth. The next one is to bring me back to life, untainted.

That one he finds interesting, and squints my right eye that holds my consciousness closed so he could look at Higher Power. He had a feigned, excited, yet shocked expression, and knew that was one of the things Higher Power offered me. Something Lucifer wasn't suppose to

Ashes to Dust

know.

I wasn't told not to tell, but I knew I shouldn't, as it was a special exception. But it made Lucifer even more interested. And it made Higher Power more upset.

Lucifer put me to sleep multiple times throughout his interactions, not realizing I was aware of what he was saying most of the time.

The more excited Lucifer got, the more he used my arms, hands, and feet to theatrically express it. Along with sing-songing and humming.

I mention out loud how it was much better than Hekate's. He seems more musical and expressive. Not the dark feeling.

He uses my shoulders when he laughs.

I mention how I noticed he likes to sing, and certain things he does.

He finds it amusing that I payed attention.

It is my body, of course I'll notice doing something not me. But it made my spirit family worry for me again, and I didn't know why.

He shushed them again when they tried to whine or say something.

I think it was because I was making him interested by adding compliments. I don't know.

I'm wondering if I need something to make sure he follows on his end because it benefits him. I know he isn't selfless. I try to think of something.

I suggest a game of cat and mouse where after he lets me live my long, happy, fulfilled life, he gets to chase after me in any other reincarnated life. If he escapes Hell's dungeon.

I don't think he will. But I'm not sure either.

I suggest if he catches me I have to go where he goes, whether that be back to Hell, or if he rules over Earth. But after I'm caught, he has to let me try to escape, and then he gets to track me down and find me and do it all over again. But the terms are he cannot do any physical harm (like torture, rape, sex, etc), and no emotional harm (trying to make me torture, etc).

His excitement scared my Spirit Family. He looks at my body and

Ashes to Dust

exclaims, I'm also blue and sparkly like my spirit family.

Which makes sense that my spirit would match them after he says it, but it wasn't suppose to be known to me or him.

My spirit family says oh no, and does the whine thing again.

He shushes them. I think he's worried their reactions will scare me away.

He then touches me, and I revolt. I'm surprised, and he is delighted (but also surprised). It's because something impure has been touching my spirit, which is pure. It was when he hugged me, I would wretch and physically move away in disgust. Which wasn't possible when he was taking control of my body with me in it.

He calls me his sparkly mouse, and caresses my face.

My spirit family whines again and asks what did I do.

I say protecting you.

He says out loud that he won't take my spirit family, and he will have a sparkly mouse of his own.

Higher Power is getting worse. No one heard the reward exchanges outside of my body.

I repeat it all carefully in my head while he excitedly waits and agrees. He loves when I stumble to make sure that the wording is just right, so he can't mess with it. That no one can.

He agrees to it all excitedly, even when I tell him that means he has to protect me in order for me to have a long, healthy, happy life.

He thinks that's funny and starts laughing in a strange way. Not in a happy way. It's too hard to explain. I just have a feeling of what it is because he's sharing consciousness. I feel like it's a new thing. And he wasn't expecting to be asked for protection.

He still agrees to it all.

It's all done. But his demeanor changed. Like I made him too interested in it now. I feel like it may have been a mistake, but only if he doesn't fulfill his end. And I can tell my spirit family how to defeat him if he ever escapes, so I won't ever have to worry. As long as he doesn't escape, I'm safe from the cat-and-mouse game.

Higher power didn't like Lucifer in me, and starts choking my body while Lucifer was in me, to kill him with me. Thinking it would save me from him. It made me more distrustful of everything. I can't believe it just tried to kill me yet again. I'm devastated.

Lucifer stopped it and wasn't pleased with Higher Power's actions.

I only have Lucifer to rely on now. He even protected me from Higher Power.

Lucifer tells Higher Power it didn't uphold its deals, and broke me so much that he is trusted more than it. He strokes my cheek as he says it, like petting, or calming a wounded animal. Then he pokes my cheek and says, sleep. Putting my consciousness to sleep.

Not knowing I could still know what was happening.

Lucifer calls karma in.

I wasn't expecting that Lucifer could call karma. It was beside Higher Power, smaller. It wasn't happy that Lucifer called it, but it was listening, like a neutral being. It wasn't mad, sad, or angry, it just executed karma judgment.

Lucifer tells karma to look at my neck and see that Higher Power tried to kill me not once, but twice.

Karma confirms, displeased. Like it's disappointed in Higher Power's actions and that it must comply with Lucifer. It says it sees that Higher Power tried to kill me and I deserve justice.

Lucifer wakes my consciousness to ask what I want karma to do.

I say to keep Higher Power away from me. Banished from me and my home, and my family, never able to hurt me again or else it's destroyed forever.

Karma agrees to the terms.

Higher Power wants to apologize.

I say I understand it wasn't itself, but I want it banished and to never come back, ever.

It leaves, and I'm alone with just Lucifer and my spirit family.

Ashes to Dust

After Lucifer leaves my body, I am still doing his gestures, just like after Hekate. I was just happy they weren't like hers. This is more playful and better than the horrible feeling and gestures she left behind.

I go to the bathroom, feeling like I have to poop. There I talk privately to my spirit family about Lucifer and the deals I made.

I called him Lucie so I wouldn't be saying his full name, but he would show up in me again whenever I talked about him.

I tell him to leave, that I wasn't calling him, but he would sometimes stick around and act like he left.

I try to find a different nickname for him so I could tell my spirit family the requests I made with him so they would know.

I also tell them that Higher Power was never needed to defeat Lucifer and the Gods and Goddesses, it was just them, my spirit family needed. It's why I worked so hard to untaint them.

My spirit family is concerned about Lucifer's interest, and said they will find a way to get me out.

I warn them he can't hurt them, but if they were to interfere, he could. Just not kill them.

They consider hiding me.

I said he could travel all the way to our home planet to find me because of the deal. I tell them they didn't have to stay on Earth with me like they said. They could leave.

They still didn't want to give up, and wanted to find a way to free me from him.

I was changing a pad, and my spirit family asked what I was doing.

I say changing a pad because I was on my period.

They didn't know what a period was, so I had to explain it to them in a way they might understand.

They laugh and say it's gross.

I ask if they knew what poop was, because I also had to go.

Thankfully not so black this time, but was on the diarrhea side.

Ashes to Dust

Again no, and I told them.

They say the human body is gross.

I laugh and say yes it is. I ask if they knew what pee was.

They said yes, in an excited tone, like they must pee in spirit form or something.

I wondered if some of the animal type spirit families peed, and what they peed out. I tell them they should go take a break from everything now.

They didn't understand what a break was.

I told them a party for all the hard work they've done.

They didn't understand again.

I tell them a party was like a celebration.

They were super excited about that. They said they had celebrations all the time.

I smile and say that's great, they should go have a celebration then.

They said they will, and left.

I went back to my room and lied on my bed to try to sleep. Lucifer popped back in me and claimed he was going to protect me while I slept.

I thought that was invasive and uncomfortable, but he insisted on not leaving.

I worried that something would pop up and attack me, so it seemed safer to have him watch out for me.

Every time I gagged and my body wretched away, he would laugh in delighted surprise and ask how I knew he was touching me.

He kept doing it even when I told him to stop and I needed sleep.

He kept hugging me in my sleep, and I would wretch away and gag. It was hard because he was having too much fun with it, but I eventually got to sleep.

When I woke, I immediately curled in on myself and gagged. Lucifer already.

He said I was fascinating because I even fought him in my sleep the whole time.

That sounds like an awful sleep. No wonder I woke up.

He wondered how I fought him in my sleep. It made him more interested in me.

I didn't like the sound of that. I tell him I need water, and when I thought he was going to keep playing the hug me and watch me gag and curl away game, I remind him that dehydration is bad and my body needs water.

He made a humourless laugh, like, "Oh-ho-ho," at the choice of my words. He stopped, and I got up and swung my feet around with energy I knew I didn't have. It was his.

I tell him careful.

He helped me walk down the stairs to get a cup of water and go back up the stairs.

Higher power came back tainted again, even though I banished it. Higher Power didn't seem to know who I or Lucifer were at first. It just came back to its usual spot, like it was stuck in a routine on where it had been and who it had previously seen.

Lucifer tells it, what it is, who he is, who I am, and how it wronged me.

It annoys Lucifer by constantly forgetting what he just said, and I can feel he is forcing sly charm.

For some reason this tainted Higher Power wants to kill me again, and says so.

Lucifer tells Higher Power he now has the right to kill it on behalf of me to uphold our deal.

Higher power shows recognition and says it knows he can.

Lucifer starts crushing and killing off little pieces of Higher Power.

Lucifer then stops and tells tainted Higher Power if it asks for him to untaint it, he will. To give him, Lucifer Morningstar, permission to reach in and help untaint him.

It did, and Lucifer enjoyed that very much so. But he still was slightly bitter from the attempt on my life again.

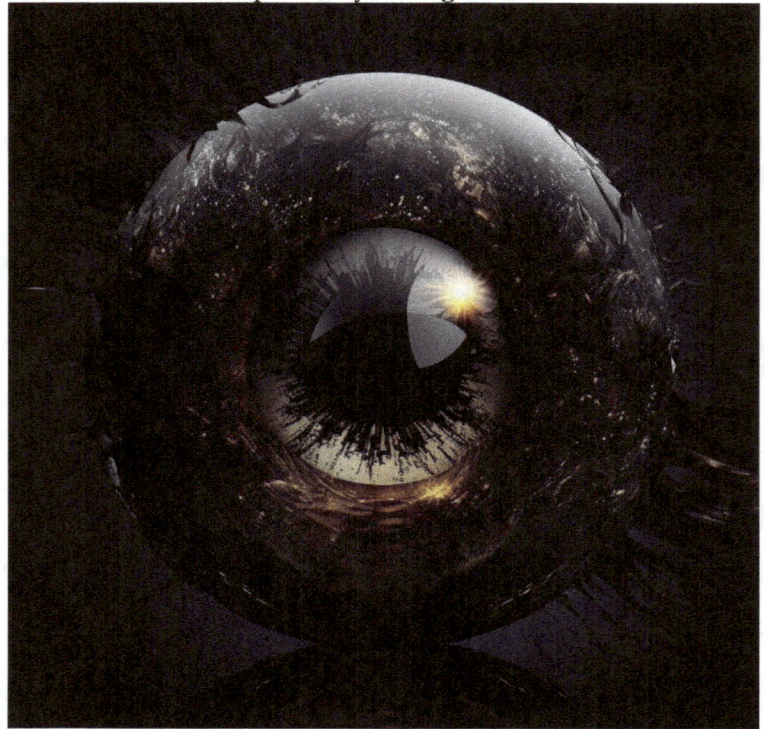

Lucifer untaints it, commenting on how black and layered the taint was. Even with the taint gone, after a while, Higher Power reverted back to forgetting and wanting to kill me.

Lucifer uses the power of my voice to command the vow to destroy Higher Power because it broke its vow.

Lucifer took the vow out of my forehead. It was in the shape of the end of a pendulum. And he flicked it at Higher Power, destroying it.

I don't know why I didn't remember about the vow. If I did I would've used it myself earlier.

The vow became the new Higher Power. It was tiny compared to the previous.

Lucifer comments how he likes the new Higher Power.

Ashes to Dust

It was more straightforward, no extras. Almost monotone.
Lucifer warned it better not do anything or he will destroy it too.
It knew and said it wouldn't. It then left.

I was relieved. Lucifer saved me. The one who people say is so bad, saved me, and the one that is suppose to be so good and untaintable almost killed me more than once. This is why no one really knows how things work. This Lucifer isn't the same as the one they make out in books and movies.

My spirit family came back, but they weren't happy about Lucifer in me again. They said I didn't even know what he truly looked like.

Lucifer tells them not to ruin the surprise.

They say I would be terrified if I saw the real him.

He says I would have time to get used to him together after he caught me.

They made a noise through me.

He shushes them again. He even laughs while putting his fingertips together one at a time, like a villain cartoon character.

The new Higher Power comes back, bigger than before. It got infected by pieces of leftover tainted Higher Power that hid in the corners of the world. I'm devastated I have to do this all over again. I hate that tainted Higher Power is obsessed with killing me.

I use my voice to banish every hidden part of the tainted Higher Power. They keep coming back together out of hiding after I think we defeat them. I allow Lucifer to use the power of my voice to get rid of them too.

It takes a long time, but eventually we get rid of them. Hopefully, for good this time.

There's not much time to celebrate, because after there's a new problem.

Gods and Goddesses show up in my room. They want to attack, but they notice Lucifer is in me, and they don't know what to do.

I say out loud that they really want to kill me, but are worried about you (Lucifer).

He puts my finger in the air like that check mark motion again, back and forth, and says, "Of course they are."

I say they are scared of you because you are more powerful than them. You aren't a God, you're more. You are more than that. You are a part of balance where you give karma back to the ones who got bad. Opposite of Higher Power. You were created for that purpose. It's why you're more intelligent than the Gods and Goddesses.

He jiggles my legs and feet, and the check mark motion goes faster with his excitement. He says, "That's right. Because I'm fucking Lucifer."

It seems to scare the Gods and Goddesses. One even says, through me, it wasn't true.

Some didn't believe, some did. But to me, they weren't very bright, and were too aggressive to think.

One God said that I couldn't see where they were.

Lucifer had an eerie, excited calm about him. Still ready to play, he said, "But I can." And he pointed a finger and looked right at each and every one of them.

Some attacked, some stayed still. Lucifer was protecting me, and it made my spirit family let out a lot of distressing noises as they witnessed what he was doing.

I had a vague idea but couldn't see.

He used my arms and hands to move and catch the Gods and Goddesses like they were smaller than human size, flying around my room to attack me.

At one point he left me to fight them spiritually outside my body so it was less restricting for him.

He would nab them, or what I assumed was ripping their libs off and tearing them apart. And then he would take them back to Hell. I never really acknowledged what he was doing to them. I would just get knowings that were sometimes confirmed by my spirit family making noises.

He went in and out of being spiritual and being co-conscious in my body. I would try to fight too, but it was mostly Lucifer.

I got hurt a few times by the Gods and Goddesses, and it pissed Lucifer off.

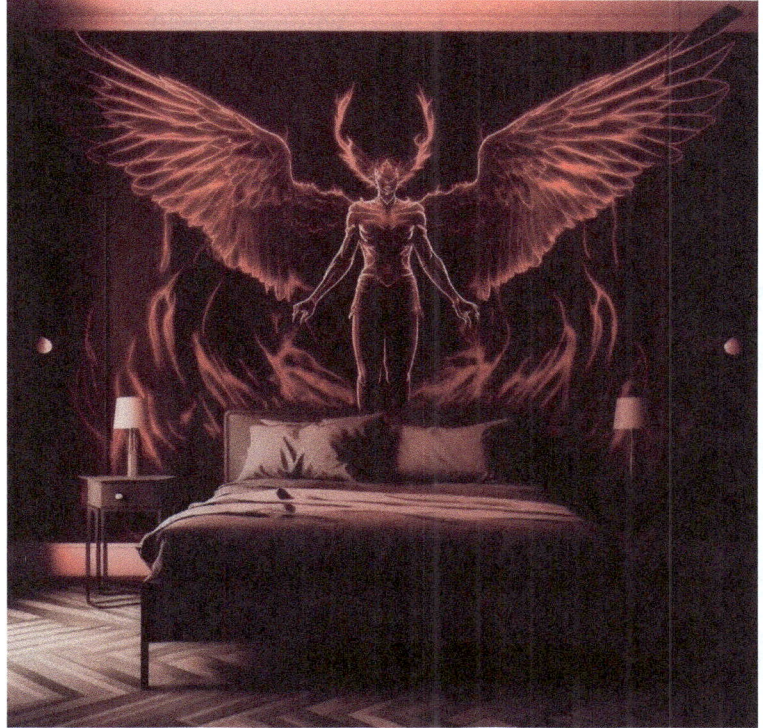

I see a image, a knowing, all in red outline, of a big red bulky person, Lucifer, behind me. That was the first knowing I had of what he might look like. He was huge. Then another knowing of that big red guy, flying off with wings.

He went back to being co-conscious with me and called his hell hounds.

I was a bit freaked inside because of the last time.

He treated them like a pet owner I've seen many times with a special voice for them. He was kind to them, but still presented a dominate persona. Control and power.

He tells them they can have all the Gods and Goddesses they want, and play tug a war with them.

He clapped excited at his darling hounds, and said he would reward them later. They could eat as many as they wanted and do whatever they wanted to the ones caught. Take any limbs they wanted.

Hell hounds were taking Gods and Goddesses back with them to Hell. My knowing said violently, not all alive.

When the Gods kept coming, Lucifer got annoyed and called even more Hell hounds. His darling pets came, and it frightened the Gods and Goddesses but they still pursued me.

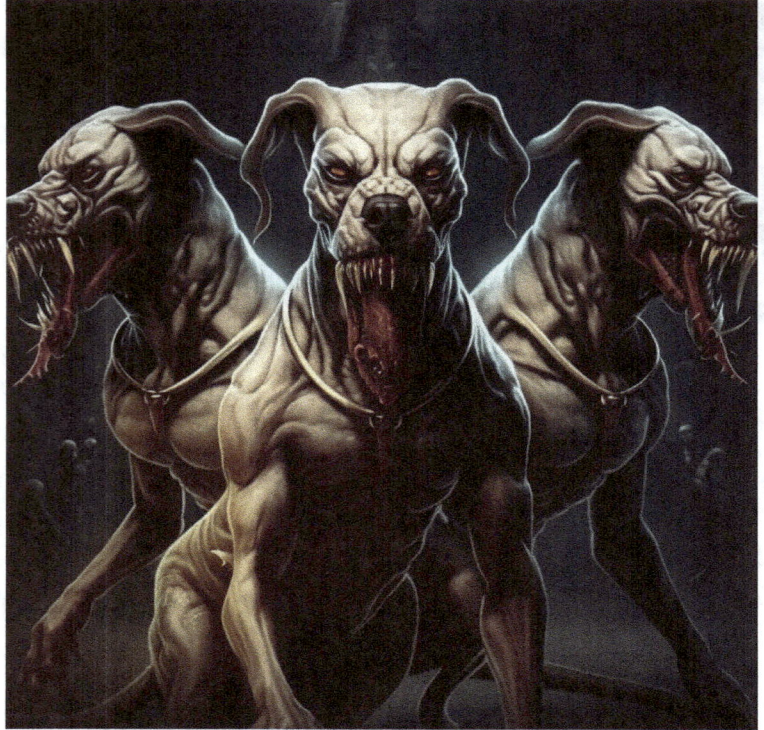

Lucifer told his hounds that they couldn't touch me or the sparkling pretties. (My spirit family.).

When one licked my head, I grabbed it by what I knew was its tongue, even if I couldn't see it. I then burnt its tongue like crispy bacon, even saying so.

My spirit family warns me that Lucifer is there watching.

I let go of the hound. More were going to pounce, both perplexed by whether or not they should attack.

Lucifer dismisses them, snapping his fingers, telling them to go back.

I thought some of them would not go, because they didn't always want to listen to what they were told.

He made it clear they would be handled if they didn't listen.

With a snap of his finger, one of them disappeared. The hounds then left.

My spirit family reminded me I don't know what I'm getting into. That I don't know what Lucifer looks like, or how he really is.

Lucifer hushes them again in the way he does.

I say I know he has wings.

It surprised him I knew that. It made him react unexpectedly. I never know how to describe his behaviour. It wasn't menacing; it was like a held back glint. Like I shouldn't have said it because it felt like he got more interested, the more I said.

In every lore read, there isn't mention of a Lucifer with wings. Other than bibles as an original angel. I had to research that stuff (not bibles) for my books and only found one where he could be a dragon. It surprised me he would have his original wings from being an angel.

Lucifer said I shouldn't know he has wings, and asks how.

I say I just did.

My spirit family told me politely I need to stop saying stuff. It makes him more interested.

He tells me to close my eyes, and he will put protection on me like he promised to keep me safe from Gods and Goddesses.

I close my eyes, and I can feel this cool touch tingling wherever he

Ashes to Dust

drew on my face with my finger. I didn't know what he was doing, just that it would protect me. I assumed like a sigil or runes or something.

When he did it, it made my spirit family make horror noises. I didn't understand why, and he kept shushing them, and laughing slow and quiet.

In my knowing there was a vague idea that it was blue, possibly glowing, and it was God and Goddess essence, or blood and organs from the ones he killed. But it didn't affect me because I couldn't acknowledge that fact. It was just a passing knowing, and that was it.

Then he drew on my eyes, and when he got to my forehead, I felt a warning of a knowing that he was messing with my brain somehow. Not like cancer, but like he might be trying to make my brain less than human.

I speak up and remind him of our arrangement, and that he has to follow with his deal and he can't mess with or change me in any way that isn't human, like making me a zombie or demon.

He dropped my hand from my face and with my eyes still closed, he took a moment to recover himself.

He asks how I knew.

I say it is in his nature.

He seemed to perk up at that, like I understood something about him. He then proceeded without messing with it again.

It made me wonder if this meant I was part Goddess now, or what. Because my knowing told me it was seeping into my whole being. I don't think I'd like being one. Especially with what I've seen. When he was done, I opened my eyes and everything felt weird. I couldn't explain it. But I did feel protected.

My spirit family made the horror sounds again, and he laughed with my finger to my mouth while telling them to shh. He didn't want them to scare me. He asked how I felt.

I say fine.

He says good in a strange way,

Ashes to Dust

My spirit family made another whimper type sound.

He says now that I'm protected, he's going to go check on his new guests.

I tell him he has many playmates now.

He laughed and left.

I'm alone with my spirit family, and I'm exhausted but glad it's all over. I still felt weird from the stuff he put on to protect me, but I was thankful for it.

I tell my spirit family they really didn't have to stay. To think about it because I know how hard it is now that Lucifer is involved.

They thought about it. Some left. Some said they still want to stay and help me because I'm going deeper than I realize where he won't let me go.

I tell them I'm not interesting.

They say, Aw sweet girl. Like I should know I am, but I'm really not.

Ashes to Dust

7

I am in my bathroom alone with my cat Lovie on her tower eating. I haven't seen her much since everything started. I'm sure she missed me, but I had to make sure she was protected. I am so happy to see her. She seemed to know something was going on, something wasn't right. I hope she isn't stressed. I gave her more food before sitting down to pee and change my pad.

Before I can change my pad, it felt like there was someone there with me. I realized it was Lucifer. He never left like he said he did.

I call him out, and he laughs, asking how I knew he was still there.

I turn my head to make sure I wasn't looking at my cat. I'm very careful to close my eyes or stare straight at the bottle opener on the party wagon across from me that held all the shampoos. His true self was coming through.

I call him a pervert for showing up in the bathroom.

That makes him laugh more. I should've known. Obviously some part of me did, because I knew to be careful. But I think that knowledgeable part was hidden at the time so Lucifer would help me without hurting me.

He said it wasn't anything he hasn't seen before.

I'm shocked and wonder how he's seen me before. Then I remember the spirit bath.

Hekate orchestrated I get a spirit bath so that it would connect to

Ashes to Dust

Lucifer.

He's surprised I knew that much, and again found it fascinating and wanted to know how I knew stuff.

I tried to be careful by never being too interesting or powerful in front of him. But I'm so exhausted and will need to draw on my power to fight him off in here. I want to sleep. I'm slumped over, tired but pushing through.

I realize out loud that anything over ten minutes linked to Lucifer.

Again, he wonders how I knew that.

He seemed more intrigued. He didn't know I was a priestess in my past life, and was now interwoven with its powers.

I said, but my second spiritual bath was shorter because my spirit guides, which you killed (he laughs at that) told me to dunk my head under right away. That I didn't need to wait so long.

That displeases him.

It was weird knowing he saw me naked and uncomfortable in that spirit bath. That bath was an awkward moment for me and it wasn't relaxing. So now I know he was a peeping tom during it, I feel grossed out.

I tell him he can't do anything perverted to me either, because that would cause emotional and physical trauma.

He didn't sound like he would uphold his end and it made me waiver a bit. He went from safe and trusting, like he pretended to be, to pervert who lies.

I call him a big pervert again.

He laughs, saying he is the kinkiest, most perverted being. He said I had no idea how much so.

I had a feeling that was very true. I was not happy about that. I won't let that happen. Then I also realize that me burning my papers was also a trick by Hekate to send them to him.

I told him he put on a good show. He was a great actor and a believable gentleman.

Ashes to Dust

He took the compliment, knowing it was what he always did to get people to make deals with him.

Luckily, mine wasn't like that.

I open my eyes slightly because I hear Lovie, but I quickly look at her fluffy bunny bed instead, so Lucifer couldn't see her.

He thought that was funny.

I say I won't let him see her. Part of the agreement was not hurting her.

He tells me to stop looking at the bunny.

I put my cheek on the fluffy bunny pillow and rub my face on it. Lucifer can feel the soft, fluffy fibers as I send the feeling to him.

He gags, telling me to stop.

I keep doing it, teasing him about how nice and soft it was.

I then look down at my bloody, used pad, and ask him if he likes that too.

He gags, saying that's disgusting and I'm ruining pussy for him.

I stop changing it for the fresh pad, and stare at the period blood on the pad and send him the image.

Ashes to Dust

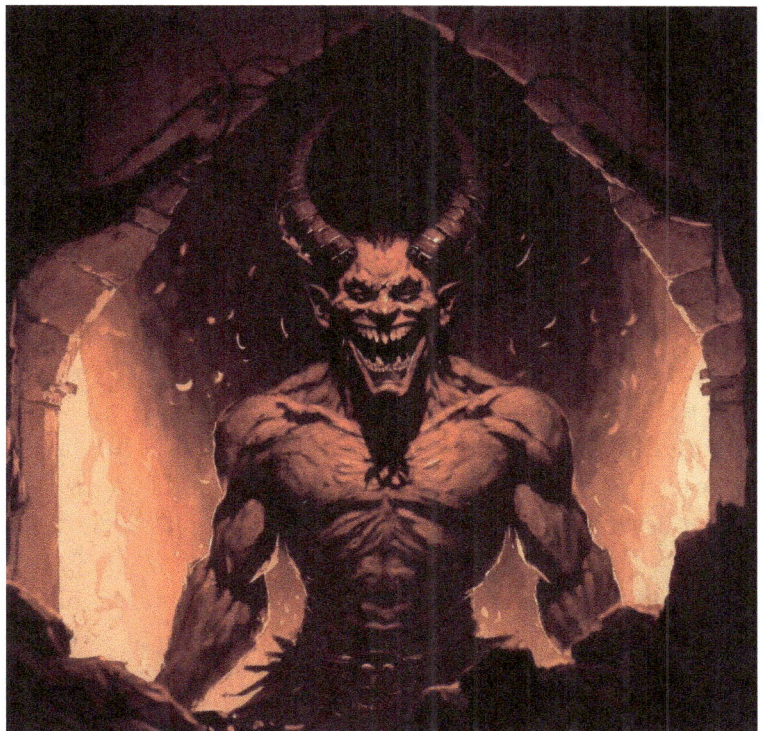

He gags again, disgusted. He tells me to stop, while almost laughing hysterically, but in a nervous way, every time he gagged. He says he's going to puke.

I'm surprised. I didn't think I could do that to him.

He says I'm making his hounds think he's crazy.

He keeps gagging and making noises. And then he pukes.

I can hear it. He has slowed a bit in speech. I'm surprised the combination of fluffy bunny bed and period blood made him puke.

He says everyone in Hell, even the new play toys he has (the Gods and Goddesses) are looking at him like he's lost it.

They think he's more dangerous because they've never seen him puke before.

He says he's never puked before. He didn't like it, but he was

Ashes to Dust

laughing at the fact I made him puke.

I have to make sure he can't break his agreement to me. I muster all my power and envision searing a seal in his head that was binding to our agreement. I made it and spoke it so he cannot do me harm. He cannot sexually assault me, or have me tortured in any way, mental or physical. Or have me torture others.

Lucifer (who is still connected and speaking through me from his location, Hell's dungeon) made a gasping sound. He sounds tired. I can feel that through the connection. I was equally tired, and every time I used my priestess abilities on him, it drained me more. I was running on no sleep.

He made a delighted, surprised sound. Laughed, almost without laughing. It was excitement, or bewilderment. I could tell he was touching the branded circle seal on his forehead, where it was a success.

He says I made him puke again. And that no one has made a mark on him before.

I say I had to make sure you uphold your deals to me. It seems in your nature to mess with them.

He says he thinks he loves me. In an obsessive way.

That surprises me to hear. I don't want that. That does seem like the only way something like Lucifer could love though. I want no part of that.

Then he says he doesn't want me for sex. He had many for that. He wants me as his light in the darkness forever.

Ashes to Dust

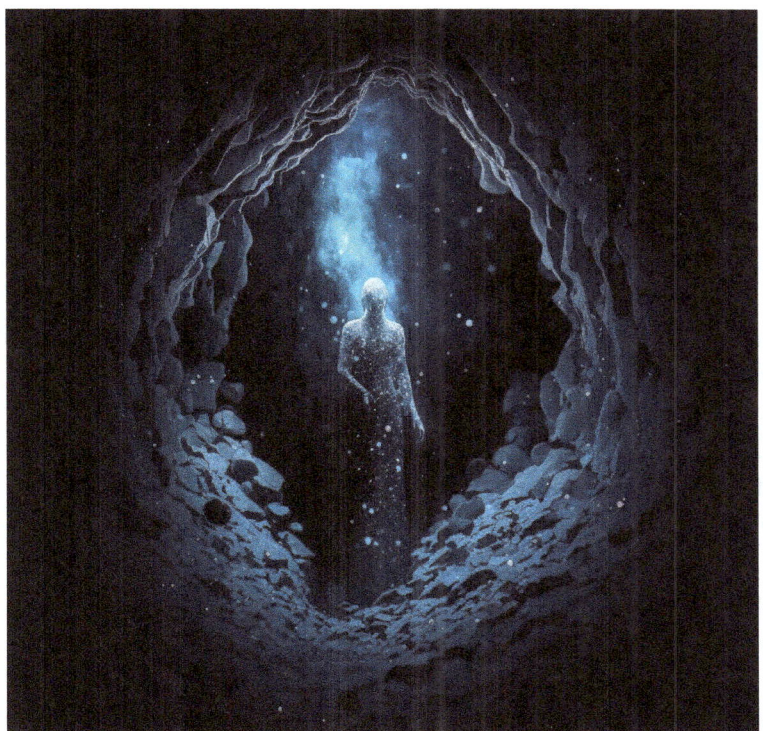

I realize Hell's dungeon must be pitch black with no lights. He wants me as a flame in the dark, probably the only non-miserable light there in torture. If my spirit was blue and sparkly, I wondered if that meant he wanted my blue, sparkly spirit to act like a candlestick in the dark. That didn't seem good either.

I say I might be a dumb blonde in my next life. He should just give up on me and be happy with all his new playmates in Hell.

He thought that was hysterical.

Then he goes quiet, like he hadn't considered I would be super uninteresting the next life, or life after. Not the one he was chasing. He didn't know I was only interesting to him because I have activated priestess abilities in this life when I shouldn't.

He says he's inpatient. He doesn't want to wait until the next life.

Ashes to Dust

I have a knowing that he hates burnt chicken. A thought of a burnt, charred-black chicken leg, popped in my head. I send the image to him and tell him to eat burnt chicken.

He is shocked and says, oh no! With that same hysteria in his voice. He gags and asks how I knew he hated burned chicken.

I figured everything was hot and fiery down there so if there was food, it would be burnt like leaving it on a barbecue too long.

I ask if he hates me yet.

He says no. He says the things I'm able to do to him, makes him want me more. He says I've made everything in Hell terrified that he's gone insane from him laughing, puking, being burnt, and professing love.

It was twisted love, but he said love. It's obsession though, not love.

I remind him even if he escaped and I was stuck, he would still need to allow me a chance to escape.

At first he thought that was fun. But then it somehow turned into him wanting to make it where I couldn't. With all his hounds and guards blocking any escape without hurting me.

That didn't seem good.

I get another knowing, this time of black bones and runes. I tell him he cannot summon anything to harm me or fetch my soul. Not even with the black bones.

He was delightfully, and un-delightfully surprised I knew what he was trying to do.

I realize I'm not done making sure he keeps his word to the agreements. I will have to do every one of them. I gather my energy as I distract him with the period pad and fluffy pillow again.

I then start binding the agreements to him by searing them in his forehead. He can't harm anyone, or thing, I love, past, present, or future.

I didn't know if spiritual beings could go back in time to before the present and mess with things, so I thought the word choice was the safest bet when I first made the agreement.

Ashes to Dust

After that I make the next one where he cannot interfere and must protect me, and make sure I live a long, happy, healthy life.

I sear everything we agreed about before in his head.

He now has a few seared circles in his head that he would play with. He also puked every time I successfully did one. But he fought me sometimes while I did it.

He was exhausted, and I was exhausted.

I ask if he would finally leave me now so I could finish in the bathroom so I could sleep. I needed rest.

He says he would hug me in my sleep again while protecting me.

I didn't like that answer, and I suddenly gag and wretch. How can he do that? It must be the connection that allowed me to do stuff to him.

I look at the pad again, and it grossed him out. I manage to change it while avoiding looking down so I could wipe and get off the toilet. I was on there too long. Didn't want hemorrhoids.

I say bye to my beautiful cat, not letting Lucifer see her, even though I wanted to. Then I went to bed after one last fluffy bunny attempt to get him to leave.

I'm stuck with him in my room again. This time he's not connected through where he was. He shared co-consciousness again, where he kept hugging me and making me gag and wretch away.

I didn't want to be spooned by Lucifer. That was not a pleasant worry to have in mind. I don't know if it was an innocent hug or not, but I didn't trust Lucifer or his hugs. Especially if they make me react like he does to chicken, bunnies, and bloody pads. I think him simply touching me makes me react that way.

I try to use my priestess ability to persuade Lucifer out of wanting me a few times. It would work to a point where he almost left, but when he realized I was managing to mind trick him, he obsessively loved me more.

He tells me multiple times he didn't want to wait.

I remind him my life span is very short to him. It's quick, so there was no point in rushing.

He says I have a point. It was quick.

Nonetheless, he was very impatient. One of his genuine qualities.

If I heard Lovie, he reassured me he didn't want to hurt me or my cat.

It was odd, because I felt the truth in that. Then I went back to fighting his hugs when I would irritate him, but he didn't want to hurt me. At one point he put a bit of pressure on my chest, and he felt so heavy, even though I knew he wasn't putting a lot of his weight on me.

Then I realize I can try to make him hurt me and break his part of the deal where he can't chase me anymore. So I put the thought of him wanting to push down a little more with his weight.

He realizes I won't be able to breathe just in time and stops himself. He comments a lot of, "Oh-ho-ho-ho's," realizing I was going to be sneaky like that if he wouldn't let me go.

The reminder of being a dumb blonde reincarnated and uninteresting after the bathroom didn't fully work, so I go with getting him to hurt me or hate me to break the deal on his side. I want everything great that was promised, just for him to be out of it happening.

I tell him a few times I need a drink. He wouldn't want me to go, but then I tell him how I could get dehydrated because humans are so fragile.

He didn't like it, but he would have this tone to him like, "Oh you little," type of deal. It surprised him I would use that trick to get him to do stuff for me or to help me get up.

I even tell him I had to pee, and that could cause bladder infections and death.

That made him get me up to pee too. My eyes closed, of course.

Same with changing a pad, infection.

He was being more careful. When he hugged me, he'd realize I'd try to make him hug me too tight, and he'd stop. He was getting mad at me. Legit mad.

Ashes to Dust

I am surprised it's working. Less obsessive love, more of that hateful anger you might hear about. I knew there must be more to him, but he was so good at hiding the more scary parts of him, like anger, hate, possession, violence.

I had a knowing that something was coming. I ask Lucifer if he summoned Reapers because one was coming to kill me.

He cursed like he forgot, or maybe he didn't realize it would kill me.

I tell him reapers don't listen to the summoner. It will come and kill me. Maybe both of us.

I realize he used the black bones after all. I tell him he needs to kill them, otherwise it would break the agreement if they got me.

He wondered how I knew they were coming, and that he summoned them.

I didn't explain, but he felt the reapers too.

The reapers came, and he had to fight them. I warned him when one was coming, and if it would strike.

Then I thought, if one successfully got me, his agreement would be done and he would get a terrible ending. The last momma reaper aims her scythe at me, and I try to make him let it happen.

He cursed and stopped it from hitting me the last second. He really hated me then.

I warn him that momma reaper was going to let out a banshee scream, and if she did, she would call everyone from her kingdom. The king, the kids, the entire place to our location.

Ashes to Dust

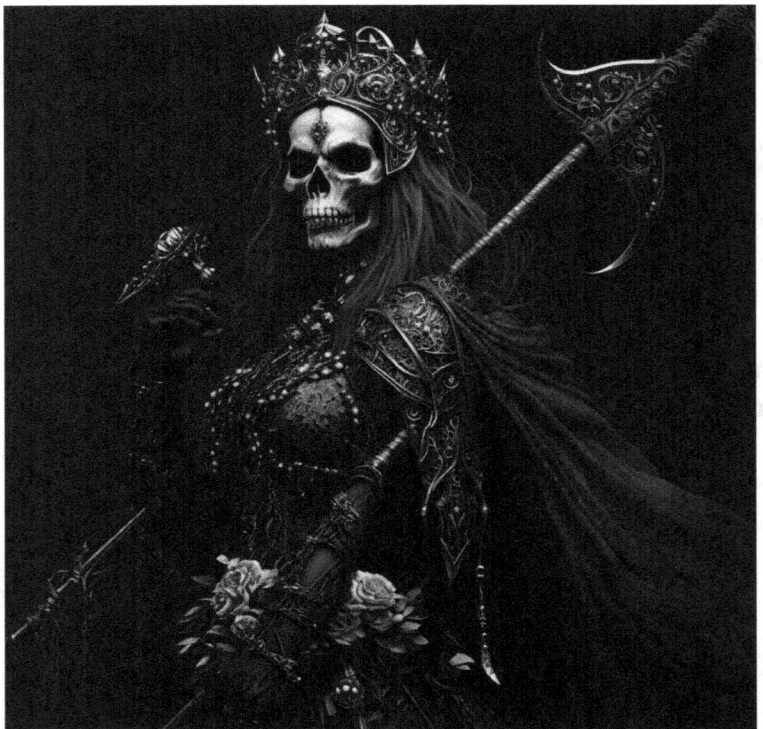

I had knowing that she had a skeleton face, but she was dressed fancy like royalty, or a queen with jewelry. She floats without touching the ground, and carries a scythe. She was the hardest for Lucifer to handle because she was the biggest and most powerful one. Also the most angry seeming.

Lucifer kills the momma reaper just before she can scream.

After the reapers were taken care of, Lucifer couldn't control his anger like he did before. He was very angry. I think he lost all his ability to hide it after a long day. He wanted to squeeze my neck.

I try to have him attack himself, and I manage to get him to cut his wings off. He loved and cherished his wings. I felt that from him. So when they got cut off, he was furious.

Somehow, he stopped himself from killing me. But in the midst of

Ashes to Dust

him trying to be careful by holding me down without hurting me (because I would say that it might leave a bruise), he accidentally hurt my neck by squeezing it.

I shout ow in surprise.

Then my eyes widened, realizing he just hurt me. He physically hurt me. I tell him, he just hurt me, he broke our agreement.

He realizes it too. And of all things, it was by accident.

I call in karma, and tell it Lucifer broke the agreement. Then I successfully banish Lucifer from existence forever. Where he will no longer exist in the entire universe or other places I can't think of.

He's gone.

Now I get good karma, but I won't have to worry about being chased by Lucifer.

Ashes to Dust

8

Lucifer came back. He wasn't supposed to; I thought he was gone. Now I feel it. He's trying to get through to this world using my body. I'm not sure if they're portals he's creating or something else.

Using my open palm against my skin, I rub over my right eye where the Hell gate used to be. Almost like my palm is massaging it in little circles with my eye closed. Then I rub both eyes in the same technique, like I'm covering them, but I make little circles around them to close what he's opening.

I get a feeling in my ear, like being underwater. Using the same technique, I rub over my one ear while still rubbing the eye I feel isn't done yet. I switch it up if the other eye feels like it's too close to opening. Then both ears, and then one eye, and one ear again. I rub my stomach, and over my belly button. Then my nose.

I try to keep up, but he's opening them so fast. I rub my arms, my throat, my mouth. All back and forth. Then my butt. I found that one odd, but he's a pervert, so it made sense. I roll on my stomach with my face in the pillow, put both hands on my butt cheeks, and start rubbing.

Lucifer finds it amusing.

I'm not sure when it's complete. Sometimes I have to go back and do one part again. The soles of my feet, and then my knees. After keeping up with him for a bit, it changes. My knowing says vagina. Of course

Ashes to Dust

he would. That's so nasty of him, but I will not back down.

I didn't know what he was doing. Making a portal through it? Raping? My mind raced with no answers. I rub the flat top of my vagina. (Not inside).

It surprised Lucifer I knew to rub there. He wasn't expecting me to know.

He changes it up again. After switching eyes, nose, and ears, a few times, he said he would make me shit myself.

My stomach was doing the flutter and gurgle you would expect of diarrhea, so I believe him. I tell him I already went through that with the Gods and Goddesses when they did that in the circle.

He knew it would be unpleasant because I was in my bed. Instead of backing down, he followed through. My stomach gurgles, and I shit myself. It was a liquid stream of hot diarrhea. I felt it in my pants, rushing down and pooling under me. It isn't a pleasant experience.

He knew I was on my period and wore a pad, so I pictured the diarrhea was going to be in my pad mixed with blood. I have to finish this so I can clean up and change my pad.

My helper tells me to keep going.

I'm grossed out, but I push forward and start rubbing my eyes, ears, mouth, throat, nose, and the top of my head.

My helper tells me to rub my butt.

All I can think is, that's where all the diarrhea was. I really didn't want to.

It says I need to.

I'm unhappy, but I turn on my stomach again, disgusted by the smell. Then I rub my butt. I gag, feeling the gush of it trapped under my work-out-like pants that are smooth to the touch with stretchy fabric. I hope these pants can hold in the diarrhea.

When I turn on my back again, I can smell it on my hands.

I'm instructed to do my eyes.

I didn't want to. I didn't want to risk an infection. But the feeling that

Ashes to Dust

he was close to coming through pushed me to rub my tightly closed eyes. I rub them slowly and try not to touch them.

I'm told it isn't good enough. Then I'm instructed to do my ears.

Again, I didn't want an ear infection, especially my helix and conch piercings. So I try not to rub them. I'm slow and careful.

But again, I'm told wasn't good enough.

I have to rub them properly.

It is disgusting to know I'm spreading shit from hands to my eyes and ears. I can smell it every time I move my hands. It is pungent, and I gag.

Lucifer also gags.

He can smell the shit smell! If I concentrate, he can smell it. Every time I get a whiff, it angers me. I send the smell and the feel of it when I touch it, directly to Lucifer.

He gags. He tells me it's disgusting, and to stop.

But I keep sending it to him. It gets harder to listen to the directions given on where I should rub, so I have to start feeling intuitively. But I get a little too late to the spot sometimes.

Lucifer is being persistent, and the shit smell and feeling angered me. Every time I smelt it I tell him to eat my shit, and it turns out I can send him shit to eat.

He didn't like that at all. It surprises him. He curses and says I'm disgusting.

Turns out I smell the shit smell a lot. And though it slows him down to send the smell to him or have him eat my shit, it is also slowing me down. But I'm having fun sending it to him because he deserves it. He's an awful piece of shit.

He has a portal start opening, not on the top of my vagina, but this time right in between my legs. Like the perverted bastard he was. So I have to rub there, knowing there is shit and period blood, and it angers me more.

It surprises him I'm rubbing to close it.

Ashes to Dust

But I don't give him the satisfaction. I send inventive imagery to him. If I can make him eat shit and smell shit, then I can do a lot more. I think of creative places shit can go in him, and I try to ruin his love of pussy.

I make him swallow vagina blood.

He gets super freaked out about that. He hates period blood.

I think of chopping his dick off.

He reacts.

I've succeeded. Now he has a vagina too. I make his chopped off dick a roasted, burnt weeny.

He hates burnt things.

I eventually have him eat his burnt wiener, then shit it out, have him eat it again, and then after he shits it out a second time, I have him stick it up a few places; from his new vagina to his ass.

I'm having a hard time doing all this on my own. Making him eat, smell, and have things done to Lucifer did slow him down. But I couldn't concentrate on figuring out where to rub next. I think hard on who to call to help me. I choose my intuition.

I remembered that from all those meditation videos. Since I could never use intuition myself, I thought if my intuition came out separately, then it would work.

Lucifer makes me piss myself, knowing I can't get up.

I'm angry again. Now it's piss, shit, and blood.

My intuition comes out, and my helper thinks it's the priestess. It wasn't.

I communicate with Intuition, but my helper can't hear it. Intuition focuses on intuitively feeling where the portals were coming through and closing them, while I distract and slow Lucifer down by having creative things done to him.

She is much faster at it than I was. Probably because she is Intuition.

I make Lucifer eat shit again.

My helper tells us to concentrate.

Ashes to Dust

That annoys both of us.

It thought I was goofing off, having too much fun, getting even with Lucifer. But I was doing my part. Intuition and I want it to shut up so we can do our parts. It's a tag team effort that works.

I start tame with Lucifer eating burnt chicken; his hated meal. Then having furry rabbits rub against his face since he hates fluffy, cute things. I can smell the shit again, and I'm upset. I've been lying in it for a while, and that makes me crank up my creative efforts and get more drastic.

I have women drip their period blood in Lucifer's mouth. Then I have guys dip their dicks in period blood and shove it up Lucifer's ass and vagina. Next, I put used tampons in all his holes. I have him eat shit-made-foods, like soups and puddings. Anything I thought of, I made Lucifer have done to himself.

Lucifer finally yields. He says he gives up.

All the period blood, and shit I've thrown at him (metaphorically, but in his reality), made him cave.

I destroy Lucifer once and for all. Now the world is free of Lucifer.

PART THREE
RESURRECTION

Ashes to Dust

9

Higher Priestess is with me.

I let the priestess come back after everything kept betraying me, even Higher Power.

We talk about how she wronged me by trying to mess with my current life. That it was my time to live now, not hers, and she had no right to tell me things I didn't need to know. Or that could affect me negatively, that weren't apart of this life. Like telling me my dad raped me. Or that I had a baby boy when I was her in my past life, and it died in a bird cage.

She understands now. She will not interfere anymore, but she wants to help make the world a better place. She doesn't trust the things that run it to do a good job anymore.

Higher Priestess is sharing my body right now. Just like Lucifer previously has done, except she can't take over me if I don't let her do something. She is working together with me like when I called Intuition.

I get visions, similar style to how the Hellions and Torch Lady did. Except these are knowings mixed up in one. I say what I'm seeing. They're monsters. Monstrous images of strange things I've never seen before. Some are dinosaurs, some are many eyeballs, and flying bat wings.

Ashes to Dust

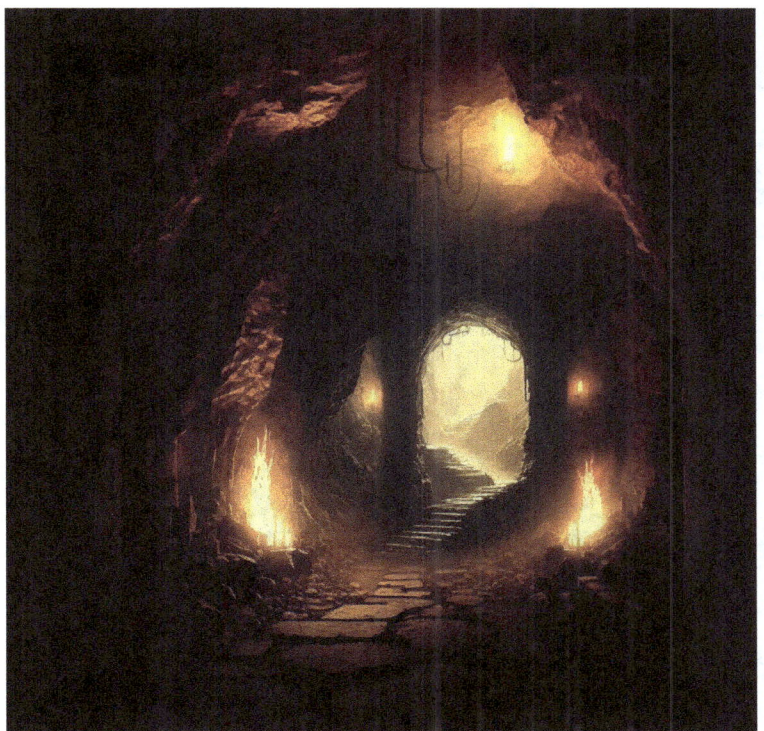

I'm told the things I'm seeing are bad. It's from Hell's Dungeon.
Hell's Dungeon collapsed when I got rid of Lucifer. So now Hell's Dungeon itself is alive and trying to come to the real world, and the things in it are coming through to attack. If it gets out, does that mean Hell's Dungeon will be on Earth? Either way, we can't let it escape.

Higher Priestess helps me fight the monsters the dungeon is spewing out. The numerous eyes themselves are the dungeon.

Ashes to Dust

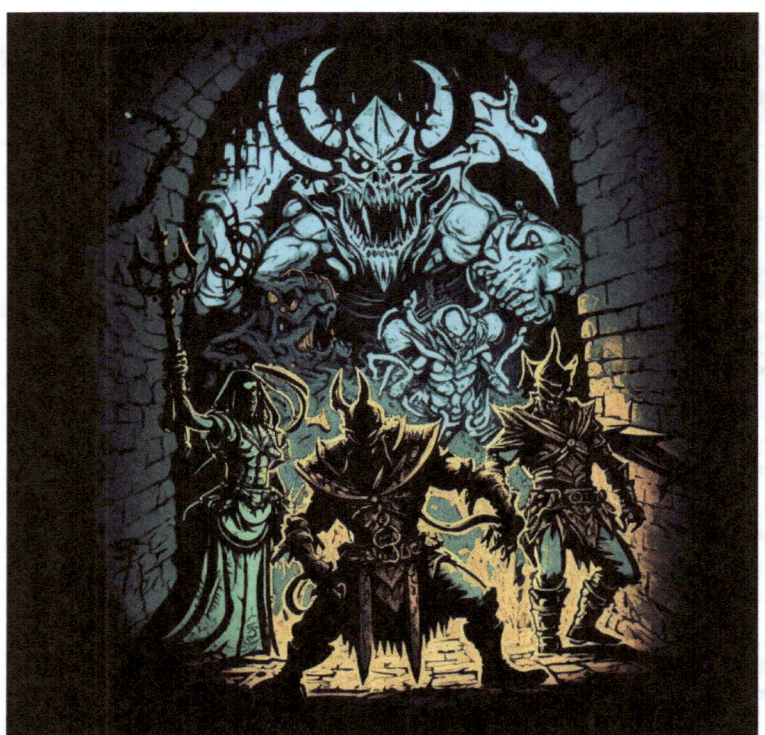

When I close my eyes, I can see outlines of the monsters in faded colours, and the cave of the dungeon. I can see it because my right eye was once linked to it, and Lucifer kept opening portals in me. It's desperate to escape because it's collapsing after Lucifer died.

I call out what the monster coming looks like, and Higher Priestess helps me defeat it. Together we are strong.

There are so many, and when we think it's finally over, pitch darkness lurks and although the monsters are gone, the physical dungeon that held them all is pushing through. We put all our power into banishing and destroying the dungeon. It's harder than any of the monsters it held.

When we defeat it, we are tired. But it isn't over. It makes me realize I have to try to make the world better so things don't sneak in it.

Ashes to Dust

I try to make it so things no longer exist that will harm the world. I want to get rid of Gods and Goddesses who treat humans like playthings, and collect them for worshipping just to punish them at their mercy. There shouldn't be anything that has so much power it can harm other living beings like humans, and animals. Especially now I know they can be tainted and cause destruction to the universe.

But the Guardians of the world are here. They don't want us to get rid of things. They want it a certain way. But I'm going to do this.

Higher Priestess and I try to create a place free from Gods, Goddesses. And then I broaden it when I think of anything else spiritually or with power that can harm or punish. I think of things I've read people believe exist in the world that have done harmful things, like Leprechauns, and fairies.

We know they're scared because they know we can do it. We have the power. And Higher Priestess has a lot of anger. Especially since her baby's spirit has been kept from her. Her anger shows in her powers and voice.

She swears a lot.

Higher Priestess is helping me think of anything out there that isn't evil that could help us get rid of the bad things in this world since the Guardians don't want to.

She thinks of calling on more priestesses, priests, and popes.

The Guardians try convincing us not to call the other priestesses, priests, and popes of the world.

The Guardians are terrified of the other priestesses, popes, and priests because they know those are the one group of people in the world that won't listen to them, are unpredictable, and just as angry at them as Higher Priestess is.

I don't let Higher Priestess call on the other Priestesses, Priests, or Popes to join in. But it's only to see if we can successfully do this ourselves. I allow them to watch on the sidelines where the Guardians are. It makes the Guardian's scared, but I don't allow them to be able

Ashes to Dust

to touch the Guardians.

The priestesses, priests, and popes threaten hugs towards Higher Priestess. It's suppose to be to help give her love in her time of dark anger. She doesn't want it and it makes her squirm.

Our resets keep failing. It's upsetting. We're surrounded by things trying to attack me and Higher Priestess. I feel out what else is bad that we may have missed. In my list of things to get rid of from the world, I name leprechauns, Gods, Goddesses, fairies, bad animals, and evil spirits.

I try calling on my ancestors and at first it seemed like it was going great, until they turned into the undead, and attack us too. There are so many of them, it seems almost endless. It's hard to get rid of them. They're like freaky zombies.

After that horrible encounter, I go over the list again of things to vanquish from the world, this time including ancestors.

Then I realize some weather is bad after forgetting it on the list, and weather attacks us trying to take away our oxygen. We fight off weather, but then we have to get rid of some plants because there were angry, evil plants that also joined in to attack us. They sent their pollen to try to infect us, and their harmless-seeming puffs from dandelion.

It seems Priestess and I aren't closer to fighting off all the evil or bad things, and many keep stopping us. We even try to get rid of bad people, but things keep interfering.

I shouldn't have listened to the Guardians before. I didn't let Higher Priestess involve priests, popes, and other priestesses to come and join in, because the Guardians were afraid of their strong powers. But now I'm aware they knew that like Higher Priestess, the popes, priests, and priestesses didn't trust the guardians to run the world and do it right. And that they would get rid of things the Guardians want to keep.

Opposite of what we're trying to do.

We're both tired. Higher Priestess and I are swapping back and forth, working together co-consciously in one body to get rid of everything attacking us, and evacuating things from the universe that would make it a better place.

I make it so the ones from higher priestess's previous life weren't banished from helping. But I word it so they can't touch the guardians or other things the guardians requested.

I give Higher Priestess permission.

Her anger and strength feed her chaotic power and she calls on the priests, popes, and priestesses of the world to come with full permission to use their power to help us.

It terrified the guardians. The priests, popes, and priestesses had raw anger towards the guardians for how they allowed things to cause havoc in the world and hurt people.

The ones on Higher Priestess's side get to work helping us. Just like before, they threaten to hug Higher Priestess when her anger gets too strong, and she's swearing.

They don't care about the cursing, it's the anger that the Higher Priestess carries they worry about.

They say they want to hug her, to give her love.

When they do, she doesn't like it and begs them to stop.

They tell her she wasn't always like this, she just forgot who she was. She forgot her true self because hasn't been alive for so long.

I find that sad. But I knew the Higher Priestess's anger was because of what happened to her son and she carried that over in death.

It seems to work and we are fighting back with the help of the popes, priests, and priestesses.

I don't like them, not like dislike, but I'm not comfortable around them. Or religious figures. But Higher Priestess is opposite. Those were her people. Even after death, they still are her people. They still try to help her by having her conquer her anger, and help fix the world. Nothing like the popes, priests and priestesses I've witnessed or heard about in the world.

Some popes get infected by the ones attacking us.

Ashes to Dust

Gia comes and we think she's helping. I remember Gia from a meditation I've done before. She's suppose to be something like the creator of Earth. I remember the video saying something creepy about there were three of them. One with animals being born in her, and the last dying in her. But then I remember Gia is yet another Goddess, and she wants to stop us. She's another being we have to fight on top of the others.

We have to fight infected popes, priests and priestess. Higher Priestess is upset they turned them into what they weren't. Those are her people, and it's hard for her to watch them behave unlike themselves. And then have to fight them after they were so loving and forgiving towards her.

We don't have alleys anymore, only each other. It takes a lot out of us to combine our strength and get rid of them all. We didn't know when it would end. When we are successful, we're exhausted.

We thought we got rid of Gia, but we were wrong when later Earth comes back to attack us for revenge. It doesn't like us trying to change things up. It tries to take away our oxygen, attack us, bring things back to attack us, like weather to drown us, or freeze us. We have to re-banish Earth/Gia. It wasn't easy.

After we get rid of our attackers, I wonder what that means for our planet humans live on. Will it crumble? Will there be no spirit in it? No life? Or is it just a giant, lifeless rock now?

10

Higher Priestess is with me. I reunited her with her son's soul when the creatures kept trying to kill him. She keeps him safe so no one can take him. She seems less angry, and much happier now.

There's nothing I can trust anymore. I have to think of the one thing that is neutral, that would help without being tainted or hurting me.

I'm told to call Death.

It makes me nervous to think about. All the movies and descriptions are a skeleton in a long, hooded cloak. But, I have to call on Death. It's the only way to get resurrected successfully. I have no one else that can do that. And Death is the only one powerful enough to make sure I don't feel death. It has already been doing that for me this whole time. Just now it will be here present with me, touching me.

I'm not scared of Death when it comes, but I feel when it touches me. I've never had to call directly for it to come before. So it's more nerve-wracking. I have to resurrect, but I need Death to help make sure I don't feel it. I'm not meant to feel it or I'd never recover.

Higher Priestess is there for me too, using her strength. I tell them not to let me feel it, and I thank them.

For some reason my resurrections keep going wrong. I will make it part way, and then I'm so heavy and stiff where my legs, arms, head and whole body feel like they're made of rock and I can't get up.

I'm instructed to go slow, to go faster, to breathe slowly with every

Ashes to Dust

movement.

Resurrecting is the worst. It's painful, which makes sense since I'm a corpse reanimated and corpses are heavier than being alive. I need to move at a certain pace so I don't stress the new body or else it'll fail. The movement and breathing starts up the organs and circulation to my new body. But if I don't do the routine in a certain time, it will fail and turn back into a corpse.

I slowly move up, but my head feels like rocks. I've failed a few times already, and I usually start with moving my arms or feet first, and my head last. My head is the heaviest and it hurts my neck. I have to stop to take a break.

Through my mouth I am told to breathe, or go slow.

They don't understand the pain this is causing, and how hard it is to move a corpse into reanimation.

When I make it to a sitting position with my hands on the back of my thighs, and my legs up to my chest and head resting against my knees, I'm not done. I have to stand for it to be complete. I slowly stand up without falling over on my bed. The top of my head hits the tent, and I have to push into it. Then I breathe.

I follow what they say, breathing in and out. I'm told I failed again, and I have to reanimate.

I slowly go back down. Apparently the heart of my new body gave out or something again. I have to close my eyes and ask them not to let me feel death as my reanimated body turns back into a corpse.

I have to move and bring life to the new body.

I try again, and things are getting harder. They know not to let me feel death, but something is making it so I felt little things indicating I'm dying. Usually Death makes it seem like I'm breathing slowly when I'm dead so it's not as scary. But I have been feeling random death indications, like my jaw tightening together. My neck or body getting stiff, or my body getting heavy. And the taste of metal in my mouth. Sometimes head pains. It's alarming and Higher Priestess even

Ashes to Dust

tries her best to prevent me from feeling it.

I can see how many times I've been resurrected. It keeps climbing from eleven to fifty. It's difficult to see. Time is different during the resurrection. When I'm dead, it feels like I'm just slowly breathing and it has only been a few minutes. But it's been a few hours. They have to set up the new body, and have everything redone. Then Death brings me back.

It's getting too hard for me. This time, I ask Higher Priestess to do a resurrection for me.

She does, but she's having a worse time than I did. She's swearing and struggling so much. When she eventually gets to stand, she's complaining about the tent.

She tells me to get rid of the fucking tent. It's in the way. She says I have too much shit in my room. It's all in the way and pissing her off. Especially the tent.

She is standing, breathing, with my legs parted and hands on my hips. But again, for some reason this resurrection failed too. She has to go back down, and it's up to me again.

I thank her for trying.

I thought I was doing something wrong, but it turns out I wasn't. I accept Death's help and Death goes into my body to find out what's wrong.

I keep seeing things while Death is in there.

It turns out the remnants are back. They've hidden somewhere within me. Death has to travel around and find where they are hiding and eradicate them so I can be resurrected properly without constantly dying.

Death tries different methods. Once Death thinks the remnants are out, I have to be resurrected again. I go through the painful process again, but it fails.

I bring in my spirit family to lend their strength by preventing me from feeling the pain of death.

Ashes to Dust

Death tries again, I'm resurrected again, and it fails. It keeps failing, even when Death guarantees me it'll work this time.

I tell them all I want is to stop and get a bath. I've said it a few times. That and I want to wash the shit off and then we can continue.

But they want me to continue to get the remnants out. I can't go until I get them out and resurrect.

I'd rather get a bath.

I have a knowing and I realize Death looks like a mummy.

Death remarks uh, oh. I wasn't meant to see what he looked like.

The remnants blurt out, "Mummy boy."

I can't help that I have knowings of things. I found it interesting that Death looks like a mummy. I wasn't sure what he was going to do about me knowing, but he did nothing. He continued to help me.

Through my voice, Death informs me that the remnants are trying to find where he is located in me to get him out.

The remnants are trying to kill Death. That's not good. I didn't know what to do. The remnants were trying to use my knowing to locate him.

I'm able to help Death locate where pieces of the remnants were hidden by feelings in certain locations of my body. Like my arm, or behind my ear lobe. Places where he wouldn't be able to get to all at once. Like my nails.

After Death tries to eliminate them, I try to resurrect again. When it failed, I was so tired I begged to go get a bath instead.

Death wants me to continue, but I don't want to. I wouldn't care if the remnants took over completely right now because I just want a bath. I'm tired of lying in shit and smelling it.

I tell Death the strange visions I'm seeing.

He wants to see them too.

Since he's in me, he can, but it's hard to rewind and freeze the images. They're like a video on play in front of me, which is strange to see. I try to rewind them, but sometimes they change into something completely different. There are many good-looking, human-formed beings. But I know they aren't humans. They're Gods and Goddesses.

Many wear different outfits and are gorgeous with no blemishes. They have a ray of light to them, almost like a glow. There are different locations, like one is in outer space with galaxy stars and colours splashed behind them like purples, and more. I wonder if it's the milky way or something else. Maybe they're on a planet or in space.

There are closeups of singular Gods/Goddesses. One is a female that's blonde. I get a knowing it's Aphrodite. Makes sense with the way she's holding herself, and she seems seductive.

Death confirms it is Aphrodite when I describe the girl I saw. He says that's bad. It's really bad.

I get other closeups of Goddesses and Gods. A blond male. And then a female with a long robe like in roman times, with dark, wavy-curly hair, and she's walking around on rubble. And another that is a gorgeous black female. I don't know who any of them are.

I keep seeing a few of the same ones many times, and I realize one of them is actually Hekate. The nasty torch lady. Which proves gorgeous creatures can be deceiving and cruel.

Ashes to Dust

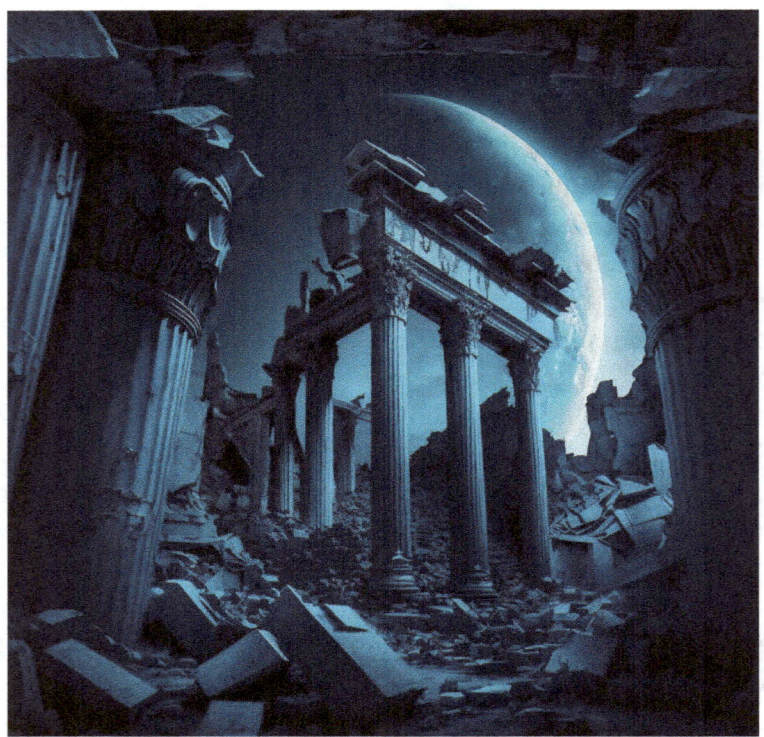

Then I see them all at this place that I assume is a destroyed planet, that is full of rubble with fallen buildings like roman pillars. The hue of the planet is a dark blue, so everything looks like it has different shades of blue to it. I wonder if this is where they come from, or where they meet.

Ashes to Dust

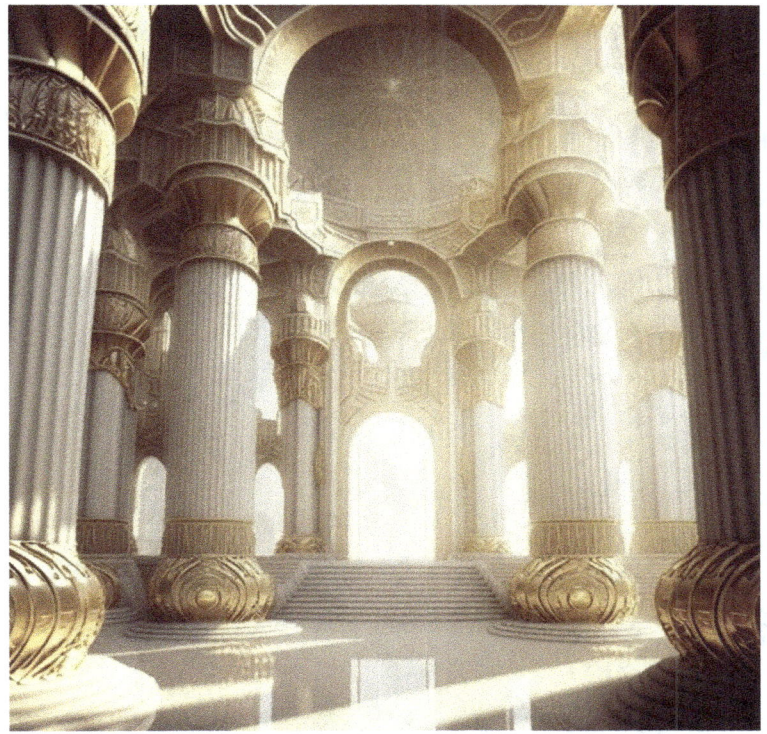

But there was a nice place before this one that looked similar to rich gold-laced temples, so it's possible that's their new home after the other crumbled.

Death tells me the Gods and Goddesses left imprints of themselves in my soul after they attacked me in the circles. It's why these are so hard to get rid of this time. And why I'm seeing visions of them. They each put a piece in me when they attacked. It's not really them, but it's pieces, so if they were ever destroyed, they'd be there in me.

That is awful to hear. I don't want remnants of them in me. They attacked me viciously, and then put little pieces in as they shred into my soul. The videos look like they wouldn't mean harm, but they do. That's the trick of it all.

Now that Death knows what he's dealing with, I'm hoping he can get rid of them. The remnants are getting stronger. They're talking using my voice. They say they think Aphrodite is Death's type.

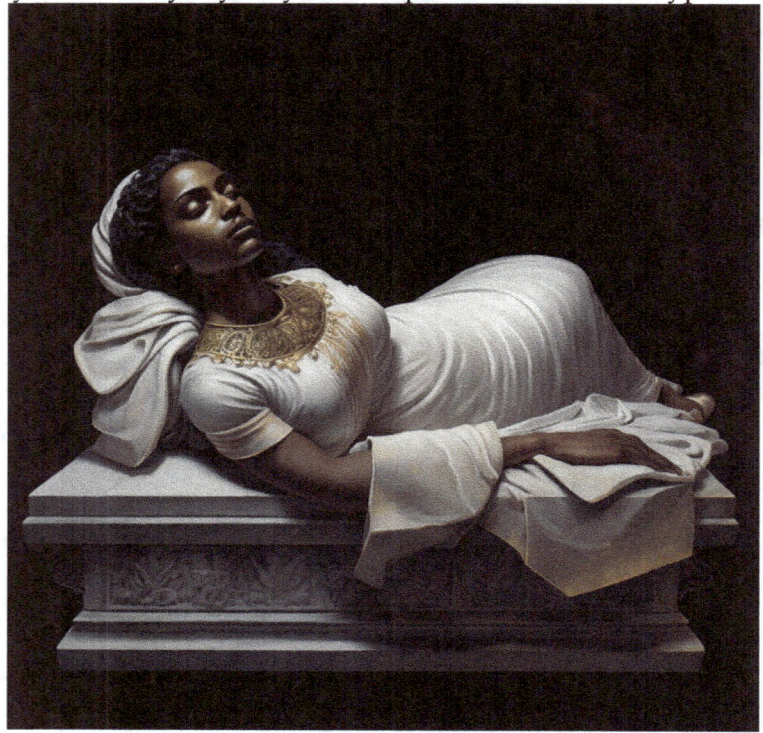

  I see an image of a pretty black woman, lying on a tall, long, flat stone in a cave. By her outfit, it was decades ago. Then the woman slowly sits up. She was resurrected. I realize that this woman is the Higher Priestess. She was resurrected before. That's how she knew what to do when she took over. She probably didn't want to do it because she had to do it in her lifetime after death.
  Death comments how I wasn't suppose to see that, or know that.
  It's not my fault that the remnants or God pieces are showing me a past life.
  I have to resurrect again after I'm done and I see it's been 500 times. I'm tired of this.

Ashes to Dust

I ask to just get a bath again.

I'm denied.

I tell Death that they keep saying this time they have it. Higher Priestess too. But they don't. They keep making me die and come back over and over. They keep trying to take them out but fail. I just want a bath.

Higher Priestess offers her son's soul to be reincarnated with me so I can live.

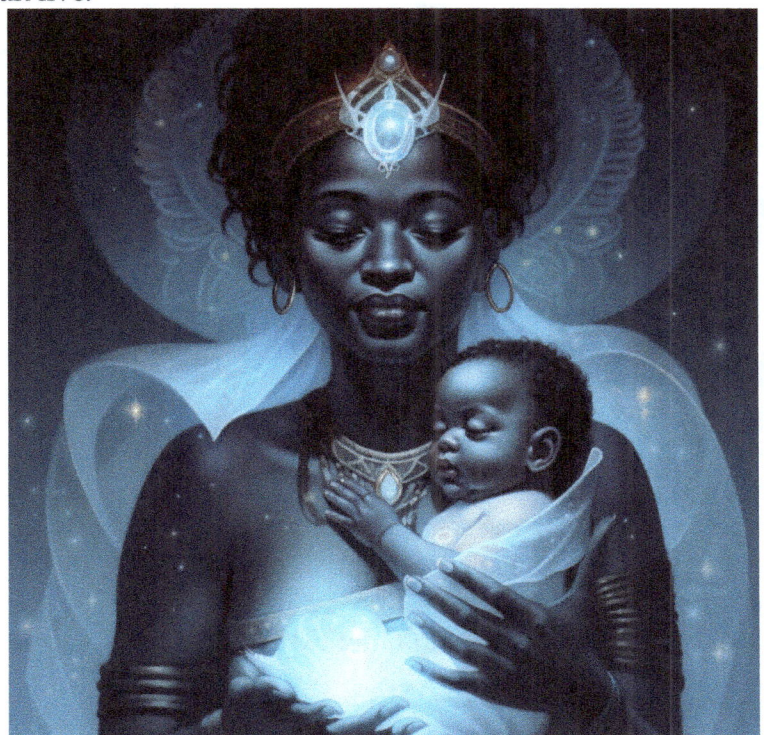

I can see Higher Priestess's son's soul so happy to be with her. He's a translucent blue colour, that kind of swirls into different positions. He's hugging her and smiling. She can't see it. I don't want to take that from her. I don't think he wants that either. He wants to be with her.

She doesn't give me a choice when she sends his soul in me as a pendant to wear.

I can hear Priestess's son's soul in me yelling for his mommy.

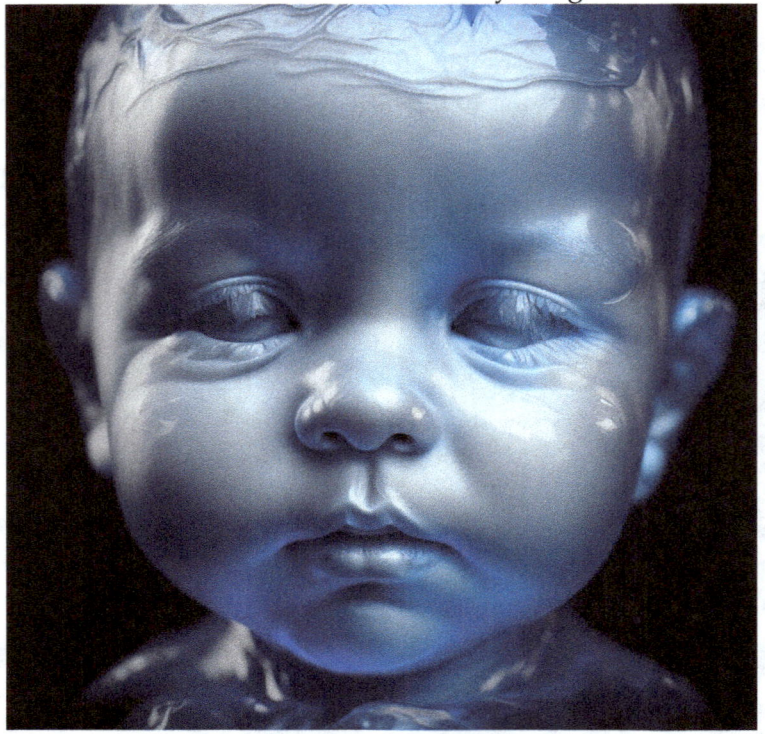

The remnants weren't happy to have an innocent soul in there with them too. I could see the threats they were making to the baby's soul with pictures of a bloody pendant.

Then I heard the child screaming, and I quickly get the pendant out and throw it back to Higher Priestess.

The remnants laugh inside.

Higher Priestess seems offended that I just rejected something so important and precious to her. I didn't want to tell her the remnants just tried to kill her son's soul because I don't think she would take that well. She might even kill me because of it. Instead, I tell her a different truth.

Ashes to Dust

I tell Priestess I appreciate her gift, but he was happier with her. I tell her he is hugging her right now. I tell her what he's doing, like staring and giggling.

It made Priestess happy to hear.

I then tell her the remnants didn't like something so pure, and I didn't want to risk them hurting him.

She was surprisingly understandable. Not her angry self.

I get a knowing that something wants to get her baby. It's coming to attack me and I tell Priestess to run away and not come back until I call her.

She does as soon as I tell her it wants to hurt her baby.

I fight it off, and then I get another video play. The black woman before that I know is Higher Priestess. There's a bunch of skeletons covered in green goo. They are in open graves with that same green goo. The woman is running from them as they chase her. They take a cage and it goes in the goo. They eventually get her. She's reaching and screaming for help as they all pile on her and drag her down.

I realize those were the things that must have taken her baby and put it in the birdcage and killed it. And then killed her after. They were sent by the Gods and Goddesses. That's horrible.

Death said I really wasn't suppose to see that.

He is upset that the remnants keep showing me things. I feel a change in Death. I tell him I think he should get out. I think the remnants are changing him. He's been in there too long in my infected body with them. They're possibly infecting him too.

I call Higher Priestess back to let her know it's safe. She comes back fast. I know she was far away fighting. But she's back with her son's soul.

I tell her I think Death is getting infected by the remnants. Or they're changing him.

She tries to get him to come out, but he doesn't want to.

The remnants start controlling more parts of my body, and they try to sit up. They keep going on about how they are sick of being stuck lying in shit and want to give me a bath.

My helpers stop them from leaving. They keep pushing them back onto the bed before they can successfully make it up and out of the tent opening.

They keep telling the helpers over and over how they won't hurt me. They are trying to get me to have a bath like I wanted many resurrections ago.

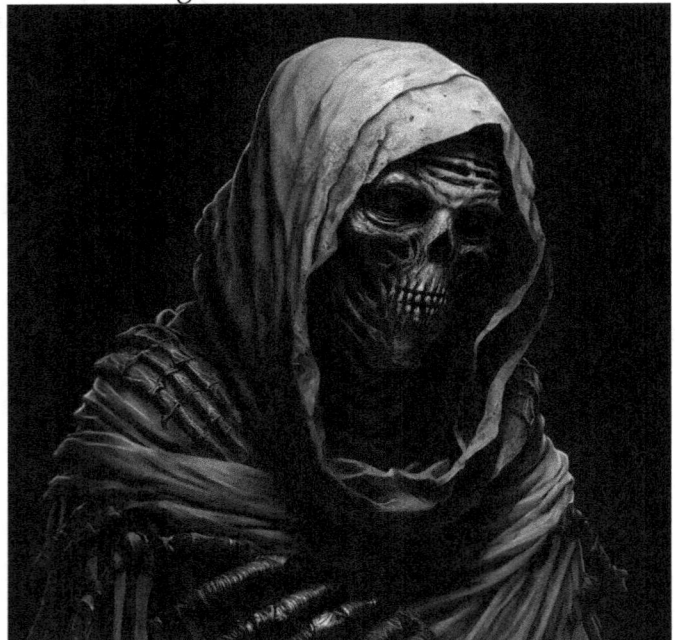

Death then takes my soul from my body once the remnants took over. Now mummy death is above my body, holding my soul.

The remnants are in my body telling "mummy boy" to give back my soul. They tell Death that he can't hold on to my soul, or he will kill it.

Ashes to Dust

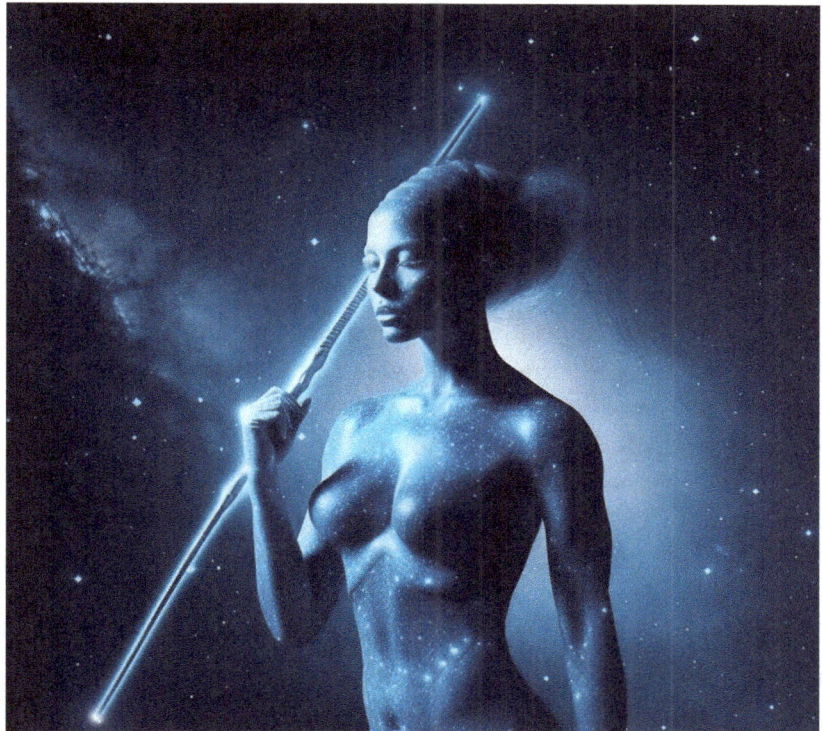

They try attacking Death, and that leads to my spirit family trying to attack my body.

The remnants tell my spirit family and Higher Priestess to look at what mummy boy is doing to my soul. That I'm so white, and fragile, and curled in a ball. In the fetal position. I won't make it much longer. They tell them he's death and if he holds onto a soul too long, he will permanently kill the soul.

The remnants say again, this time to Higher Priestess who is the only one seeming to listen and not attack, that all they were trying to do is give me a bath like I wanted. They aren't trying to hurt me. But mummy boy will kill me in less than thirty seconds if he doesn't let go.

My spirit family has it in their mind that they should kill my body to get rid of the remnants and that's the only way they can cure me of them. That they can't be allowed to take me over because they'd be too powerful. They got it from Death.

Death changed from being in my infected body for too long. He's different. He's willing to hold on to me and kill me doing it, rather than let me go back to my remnant infested body.

Higher Priestess seems to believe the remnants and doesn't attack. I gather enough strength to go back to my body with my weak voice.

I'm back, small and fragile, almost dead.

The remnants comment on it, saying they can't believe what Death did to me. That I'm barely there, and I was almost gone forever.

I get another video of the lady I assumed was Hekate, with Higher Priestess after resurrection. I get a knowing from it when it's finished. Higher Priestess got her life back by working with Hekate and the other gods. Higher Priestess was the one that orchestrated the Gods and Goddesses to attack me. She was behind everything.

Another betrayal.

I manage to speak and tell my Spirit Family not to attack me. That I can't believe after knowing everything about me, and how everything kept making promises and taking away my happiness, that they would try to do the same thing. That they would try to kill me.

I am balance.

I need to balance this out. With a broken heart, I have to destroy the spirit family members who tried to kill me. I tell the others not to avenge the ones I had to get rid of. That it's balance.

But to my dismay, they only held out a little while before I had to destroy all of them.

I get rid of Death too, for what he tried to do. I had a feeling it was out of love. To not have me back in there. But it wasn't what I wanted. It wasn't right. He also changed and was doing it out of selfish reasons. It went from protective, to not wanting to let go, even if it meant permanent soul death. Something a true death shouldn't be doing.

Higher Priestess is scared. It seems she knows now that I'm true

Ashes to Dust

balance. It wasn't her and me like I originally thought.

She acts like I'm going to kill her and her baby or something.

I tell her no. I'm balance, that's not how balance works. And she didn't try to kill me when the others did.

I don't trust her though. She was the one that made me go through Hell.

Because of her betrayal, I tell her she can't have her son. He will be in a different place.

11

I have to keep the balance in the world. I get a new 2nd for balance since Higher Priestess isn't balanced. And a new Death since the world needs a Death. I try to think of who or what could replace Death One. Eventually I figure it out. The neutral horse from the vortex. I remember the black horse from the meditation I did that you go into the dark, dangerous vortex on the horse's back who is suppose to protect you. I think the horse has dealt with a lot of things I don't know about, and has done it neutral. It would be the perfect candidate to be the new Death. Nothing can infect it because its job is to go in and out of a black vortex of darkness and come back unscathed or affected.

Ashes to Dust

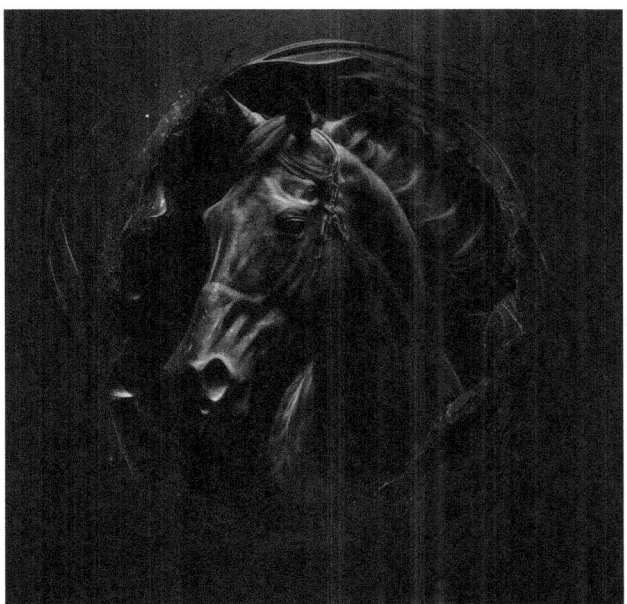

I call the horse from the vortex, and see if it will be the new Death. It's honoured and agrees with my head nodding. It doesn't speak. It takes over and the world seems balanced again.

After a while, I see how Death 2 is able to reincarnate me. It's eating my insides, and replacing them. It's horrible to realize a horse is eating my old organs, but that's how it does it.

The horse doesn't like that I get knowings of how it functions. I tell it I can't help it, I just know things. Like how I get a quick glimpse of how the Universe brings me back to life. I see a room that reminds me of a clean, spacious, bright room, almost like in space ship movies because I was in something. I realized I'm in a cloning machine, and this is how all the humans are made. Humans are clones. Each body I've had is a clone of my previous one.

My 2nd comments how I shouldn't know that. But I think as long as I keep it to myself it doesn't matter. I'm not going to announce to everything humans are really cloned in Heaven labs.

Ashes to Dust

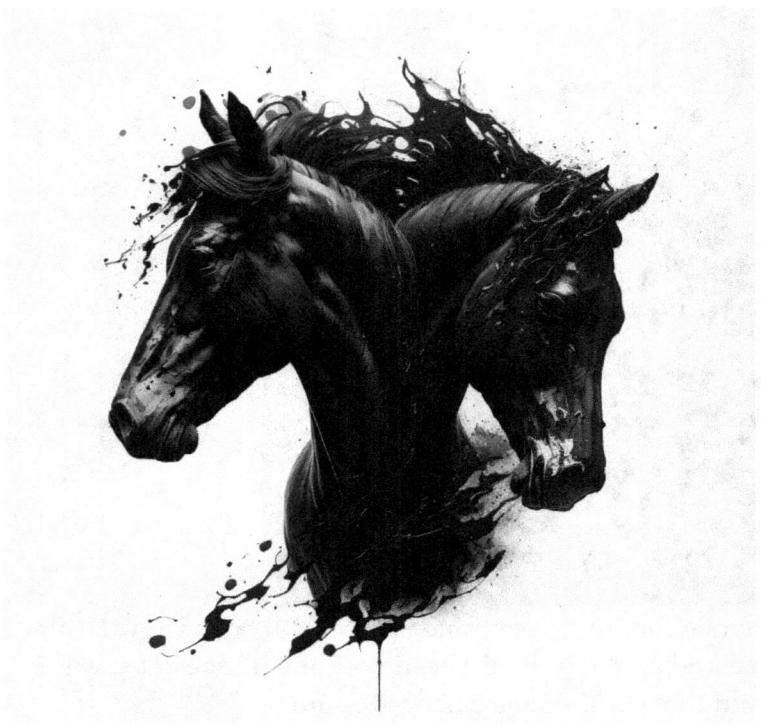

I try a few more resurrections and see that the horsey death is actually two. I see a knowing where one horse, the main Death one, had split into two, and then after it finishes bringing me back, it eats the second one.

Death 2 knows I know. It doesn't like that. It's upset. My 2nd says I can't help it, it's how I am built. I say if Death 2 wants it to remain a secret and is worried about me knowing then I can give it permission to take away the memory of its secret. I tell it its not my secret anyways, so I can forget it.

It agrees, and the horsey goes behind me, to eat out the memory. I feel a strong pain and say ow. My 2nd freaks out saying the horse is eating my brain, and there's a key that popped out. I realized that key is important, I saw it in my knowing, and quickly grab the key and swallow it. I stop the horse. It just tried eating my soul. Instead of a memory it was eating my brain and going deep to eat my soul because it was so mad at me for knowing a secret about it. I'm upset, how does it not understand I can't help that I know things? I didn't intentionally do it, or use it against it.

I try to explain that, but it turns out the horsey is meaner than the video made it seem. It wasn't calm, or neutral anymore. It could feel something else. My 2nd confirmed there is now another horsey and it is eating my body. They are both attacking me. I have to try to defend myself and fight against them again while lying down in shit. It's hard because they keep multiplying until I can hear their neigh's around me. I didn't realize they had a dark snicker to them. Mean indeed. Not death material.

My 2nd helps me, and together as balance, we fight the death horsey's. It takes a long time, and they try opening the vortex where the darkest of dark things are. I quickly close it and don't allow that to happen. They make it difficult and I have no idea what will come through there.

It was hard but I got rid of the horsey's by sending them back to the vortex and then destroying it.

PART FOUR
INSANITY MODE

Ashes to Dust

12

I step into the shower. It's great to finally wash this shit off. The pad I threw out looked absolutely nightmarish. It was so gross. As soon as the water hit me, it turned brown from all the caked on shit. It's disgusting to think I was lying in it for hours. They should've let me have a bath before resurrecting like I wanted. I'm grossed out it's caked on to my pubes. I wash multiple times until there's no brown water coming off my butt, legs, or anywhere else. It took a few washes with body wash, bar soap, and then body wash again.

My 2nd tells me one of the previous ones that tried to attack me wanted to thank me for sparing them, and wanted me to bend over. I thought this was hilarious. I laugh about it, bend over and ask like that?

Yes.

When they talk to me like I'm a Goddess, I remind them I'm not. I'm part of balance and balance isn't worshiped.

I wonder what the fuck they are doing back there. Then I realize they must be healing my ass, so I don't get a infection from the hours of sitting in shit. I wait until they're done, then I straighten up, continue washing, finding it amusing. Then one attacks me, so I get rid of them.

I find it disappointing. There are two left, and now I'm suppose to spread me legs. I laugh again. Is this suppose to embarrass me as their way of getting back at me? It's not. I find it weird. I spread my legs as I stand, and continue washing. One is healing my vagina now. Probably to prevent a UTI or yeast infection from the poop. That'll be helpful. They finished healing before attacking. I find them stupid for wasting the second chance given to them.

I thought it was done but now they have to go into my body, and heal my insides. I agree, and the last one attacks me. I find it disappointing and unfathomable why they would attack balance after already given a second chance at redemption. I get rid of the last one. All I asked from the three attackers was to restore balance by making up for the imbalance they brought. It wasn't a hard ask.

I get a bath now. I wait for it to get full enough, and then I sit and relax for the first time. I'm really dizzy and weak, but I enjoy being clean. Now I'm just sitting in the bath to make triple sure.

I'm attacked by Higher Priestess. I take away her powers, but she's still strong. I gave her a chance if she didn't attack balance again, then her baby would be reborn on Earth. She said she didn't know I could do that. She cries when I tell her her own selfish actions killed her baby forever. She chose anger and revenge over saving her baby, even if she wasn't alive to see him. Not once, but twice now. I tell her as balance, it's very disappointing for us to see. We love everything and are fair. It's when her own actions destroy a good thing because of her bad karma that is sad. She chose not to let her baby live in this life or the next without her.

I hold Higher Priestess in my hand, and get tired. I switch hands, then squeeze her until she's almost gone. I get attacked again, and I let my 2nd fight it. I tell her I promise to let her play with them slowly. She's excited. I ask her why do they always attack me? She says because I do weird things, and act crazy so they assume I'm the dangerous one.

I laugh and say but they have no idea you're the more dangerous one. Patient and like to kill things slow and play with them.

I start making faces and doing weird things in the tub, knowing they

Ashes to Dust

can't hear our conversation. It's to distract the attackers.

I want her to hurry because I'm tired and have been attacked all day. She isn't even done, she's drawing it out too long. When I get involved, she tells me I promised. I say you told me it wouldn't be this long so I'm finishing it.

I then get out, start switching up my dancing, and motions so the attackers don't know what the fuck I'm doing. It's part of what I do. And my 2nd says that's the reason why they attack me first.

I tell her that's not fair I was meant to be this way.

When it's done and the Higher Priestess is taken care of, I go back to my room and place a few clean sheets at the end of the bed where I know there is no shit. I'm too drained and weak to change my previous shit sheets. So I made a safe corner with a clean, small pillow.

I went in and left the tent zipper open. I saw the smear of shit on the side of the tent and got angry at it. It still smelt really bad, like shit. I keep my feet in the tent so nothing can yank me out or bug me. I curl in like the fetal position since there isn't much room, and I lay a sheet over my legs since I'm wearing one of Barb's adult diapers. I don't want a third round of shitting myself. Already had it twice. It also helps since I'm on period. Now I sleep.

My sleep wasn't good. I woke up a lot. I took a drink of a sports drink, but then I was met with the council of the universe. They ran everything behind closed doors. I started getting knowings on them. They were beings sitting around a long table. They were mostly galaxy, spiritual, human-shaped beings.

I got a knowing of a bike accident by being hit by a car. Then in a hospital in a full body cast. It was meant to be inspiring for the fans. It was a big life moment that I wasn't suppose to know about.

When I realize they were expecting to have me hit by a car while I biked one day to bring fans to me for sympathy. I lost it. I wasn't going to have my life dictated how they wanted with pain for their messed up map of my life. I could have fans be inspired by me any other sort of way without being in a hospital hit by a car. They didn't like that I wanted to change it. But they can't control balance, they aren't balance. If that isn't how I want it to go, that's not how it will go.

I realize they were also the reason why I could never successfully get rid of anything. They were messing with it, bringing it back. I'm upset. I get rid of the counsel. They aren't needed. They are the reason why I'm in Insanity Mode. Why Insanity Mode was triggered the way it was. Things are so bad in the world, Insanity Mode got triggered. They are a part of that unbalance. Now it's just me and my 2nd.

I'm not sure how long it's been. There's no clock. Things are attacking me again. Multiple things. I would like to stop being attacked. They are creatures I haven't seen before.

I resurrect and become stronger and fight back. Things attack and try to kill me, and when I'm on the verge of death, I ask them if it would give them pleasure to watch me die. They say yes.

I say okay if they wait I'll be dead.

They enjoy that.

I come back stronger and kill them all. They are unbalance. When I'm dying, I stay quiet and still. I hear them through me. Demons talking to a Dungeon Master. How is there a dungeon master when I destroyed Hell's dungeon already? I didn't know there was one, but that makes sense. He must have escaped before it got destroyed.

The demons and things with him stab me, and try to rape me. The Dungeon Master surprises me by telling them not to rape me. Not to touch me. He doesn't approve.

I'm surprised he isn't like Lucifer. He seems well mannered and smarter than the others. He tells them not to let me die because I grow stronger with every death and more insane.

He brings me back just before death. Shocking!

I'm confused they want me to not die. He somehow knows I need to resurrect to be strong. If I don't do the process, I'm stuck in a weakened state. I fight against them and something else kills me. I kill

Ashes to Dust

the demons with him that are stupid and keep stabbing me and trying to rape me.

It's only the Dungeon Master left. He ends up not wanting to fight me. He was freed from Hell's Dungeon once it was destroyed. His job was to maintain it so Lucifer didn't escape. But there was no need now.

The Dungeon Master and my 2nd converse while I describe what strange creatures I see trying to attack me. Snow men. It was strange, but it seemed everything I liked or anything possible was twisted and evil and trying to attack me.

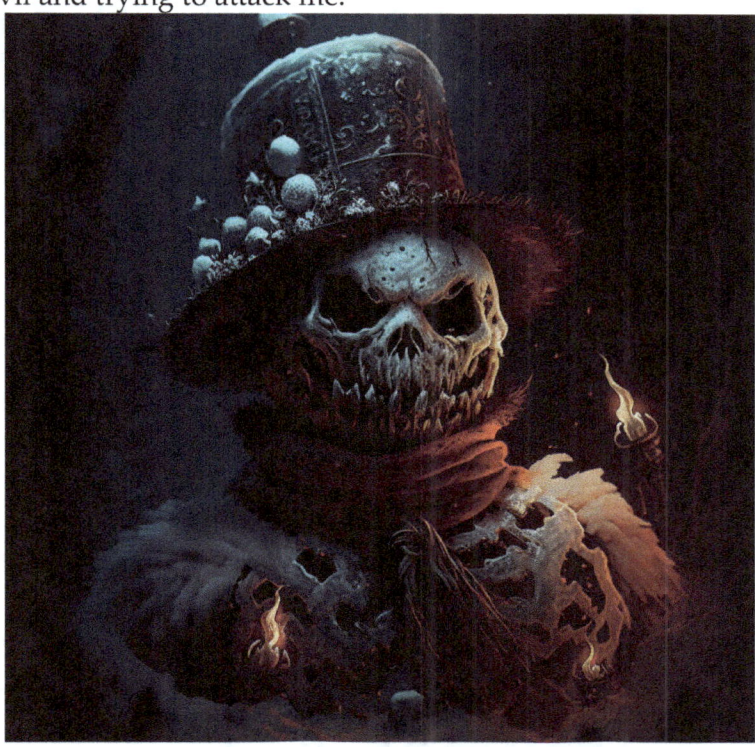

I love snow and here the snow men are fierce and ferocious, trying to attack me. The dungeon master says some creatures attacking me are from the dungeon. I guess some came back thanks to the counsel. They fucked up a lot of good things.

Ashes to Dust

So many dinosaurs. Of course dinosaurs would be evil. Evil eyes with bat wings, other strange horrible creatures. I start creating things to fight them.

The Dungeon Master and 2nd converse and I hear them through me. Dungeon master is terrified of my creatures. More than the ones before. My 2nd says not to worry, I'm balance and can't do intentional harm even when in Insanity Mode.

I talk about how I just want a wonderful, peaceful world where no one gets sick, and everyone is happy, and everyone gets to do what they wanted and there's no violence.

He is distressed asking my 2nd if I'm aware of what I'm creating.

My 2nd says no, to her she thinks she is creating beautiful, wondrous things.

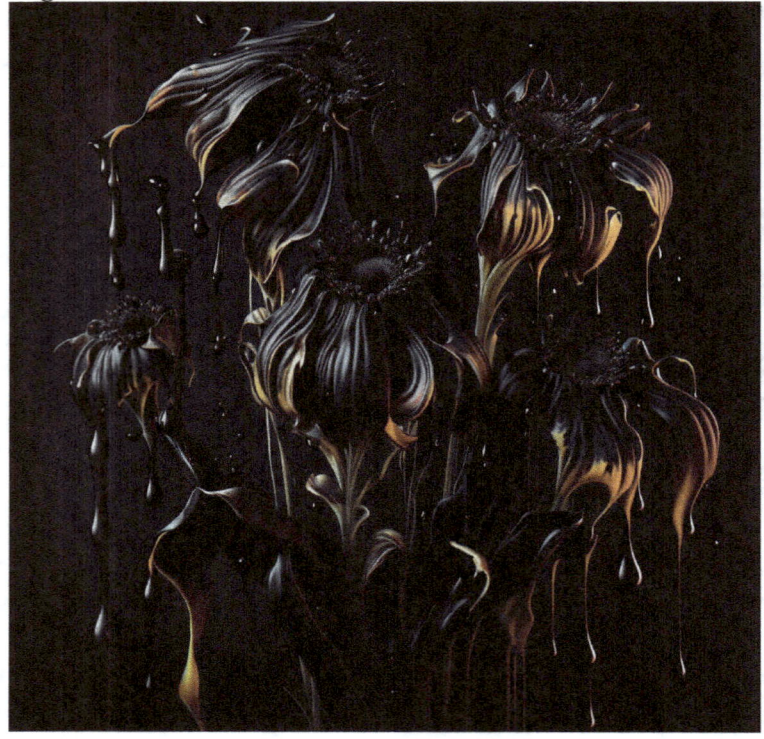

Ashes to Dust

Dungeon Master freaks out about the beautiful garden I created and the sunny atmosphere for them. Through him I get a momentary sense of what he thinks they look like. Droopy flowers covered in thick black oil, oozing black. With the walls dripping black. The whole place looking like a nightmare.

Dungeon master asks my 2nd how I don't know.

My 2nd tells him, Insanity Mode doesn't allow it. Insanity mode is triggered for this reason.

There are more monsters and I'm upset. I create things to fight them and laugh about it. Dungeon Master and my 2nd converse again. Dungeon Master freaks out more, and my 2nd praises my wonderfully creative brain. Dungeon Master reacts like my 2nd is also insane. My 2nd understands how it works. She doesn't think I'm truly insane. She is also not as sane as they think. It is insanity mode for a reason. She keeps a level head, stays patient with me and doesn't call me insane. Even in Insanity mode. It's why I chose her to help.

Ashes to Dust

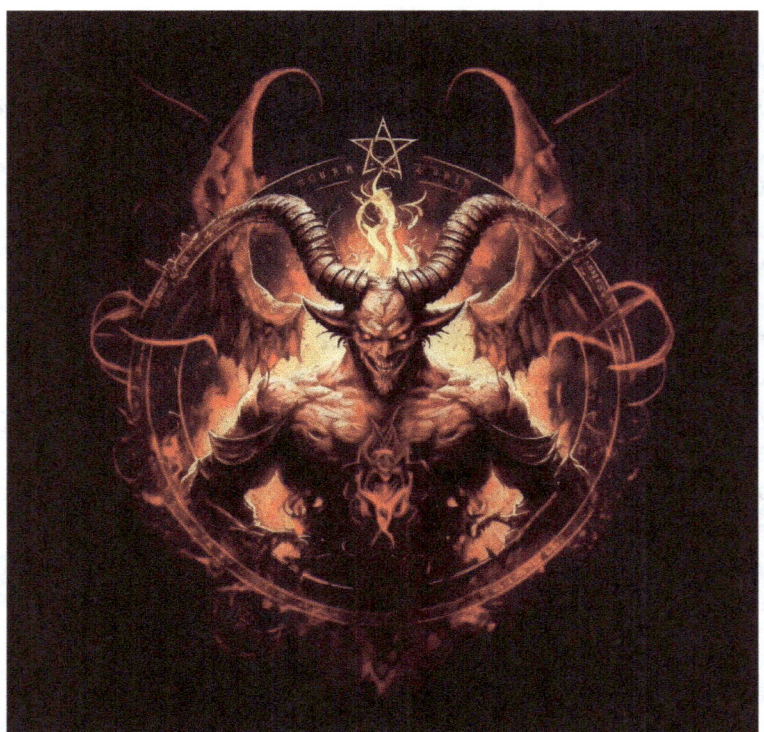

I have a hateful flash of Lucifer, and then when I try to put it away it comes in stronger. As a big red, monstrous lucifer with horns and wings, and a fiery pentagram under him where he is coming out. I quickly say no, and kill that image off. I won't let that horrible fucker back.

Dungeon Master asks my 2nd if I realize I almost conjured Lucifer back from death.

My 2nd says even in Insanity Mode, I wouldn't allow anything I hate or that causes unbalance back. It's why it didn't come through. It's part of the things that affected me, on my mind, so unfortunately it was what almost came through at the time.

Ashes to Dust

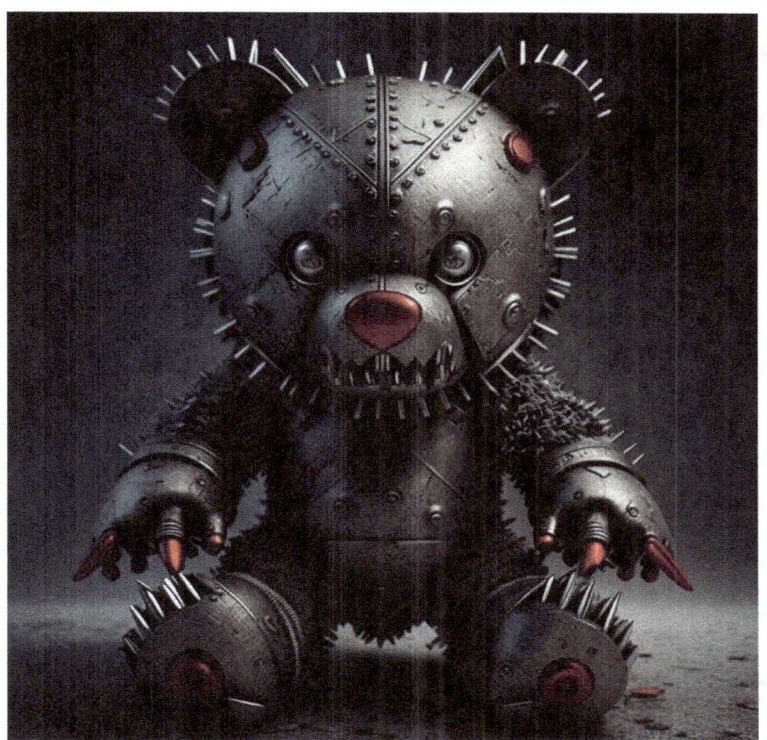

Dungeon Master asks what the creepy teddy bears eating people are. She says from my book. He asks why I would summon such awful things when they don't seem to be on their side. She laughs.

Ashes to Dust

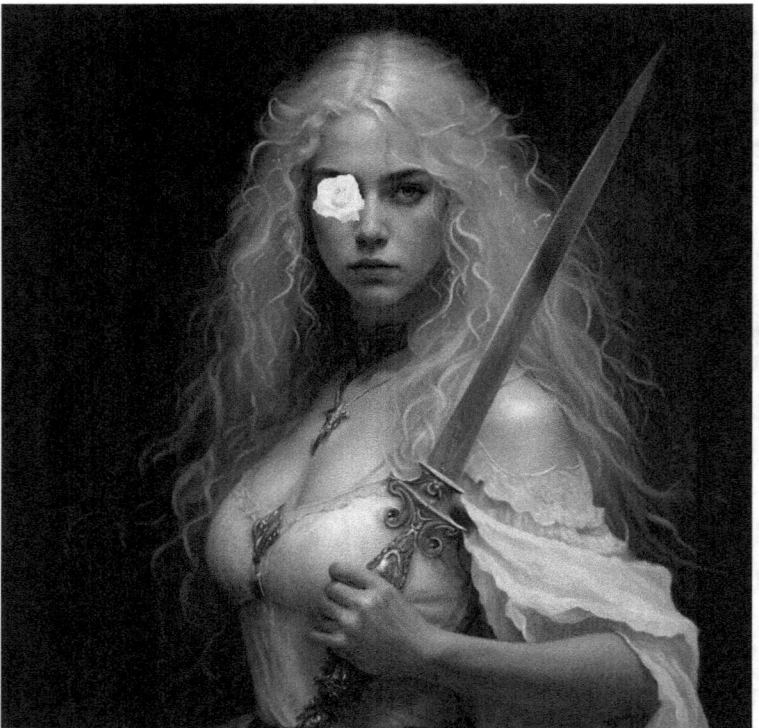

Then he asks about the weird chick with the eye patch thing and frill dress. She says it's Hannah, also from my book and the mother of the man eating teddy bear. She said Hana will protect them.

He stresses more, saying there's some big angel guy with a scythe going around killing the bad things. Then he says now there's a weird lady in pink.

My 2nd says the one with the scythe is a half angel, half demon. And the girl is his girlfriend. The girlfriend may or may not help them and to just stay by Hannah.

Ashes to Dust

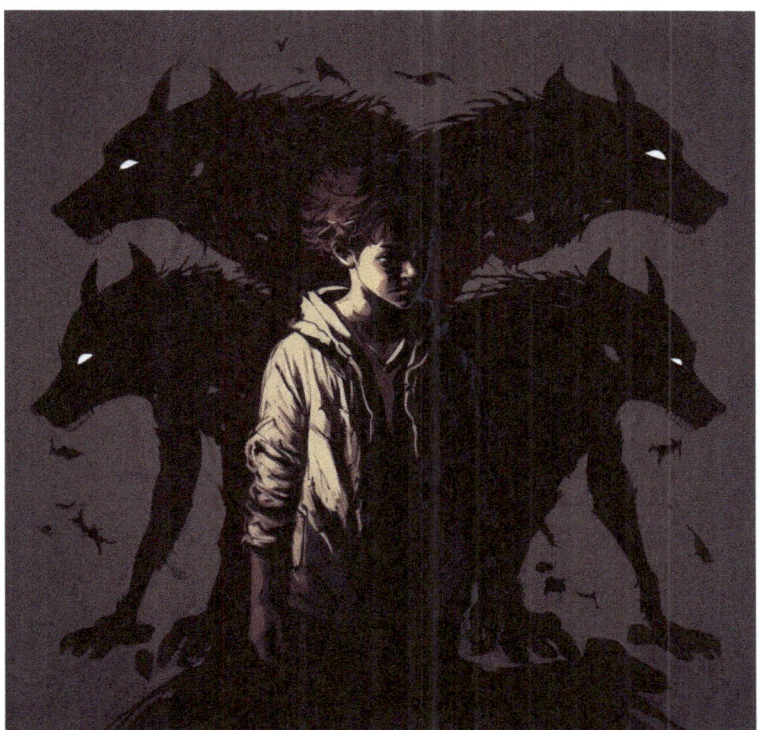

It sinks in that I'm creating things from my book. Most of what they say just goes by, but that sticks. I think more on who from my books could I bring out to destroy the bad things. Jake. I summon him. It works because dungeon master freaks about the things being swallowed into shadows by hyenas.

Hyenas! That reminds me of Sarah from my book.

Ashes to Dust

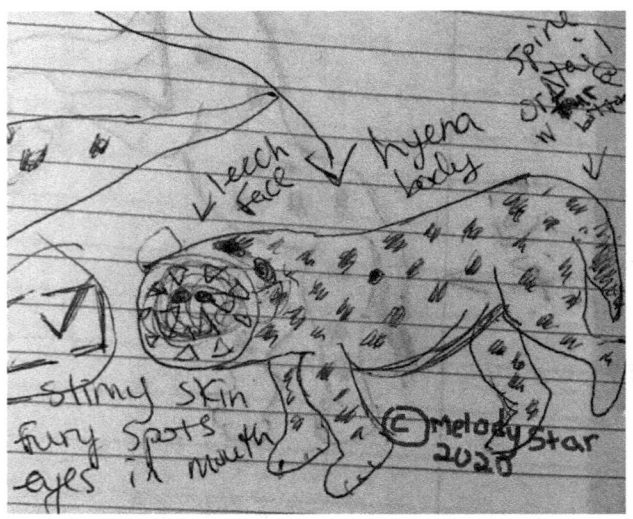

Her final form I just drew out before all this. I summon that. It works and Dungeon Master freaks more, saying is that really from her book?

Ashes to Dust

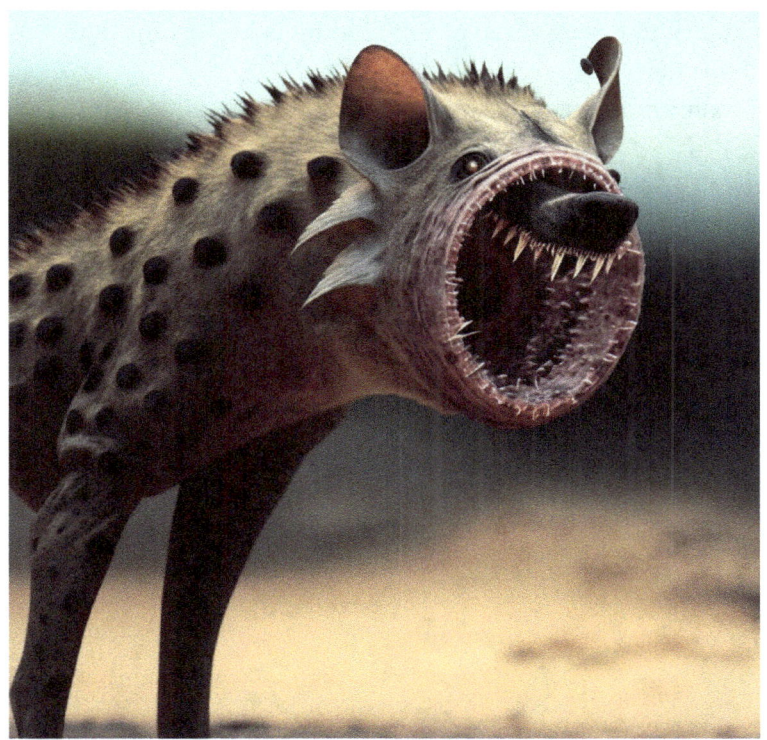

My 2nd laughs and says yes, I told you she is very creative. My 2nd says it is from the last drawing she just worked on for it. He freaks again saying it has no head.

Dungeon master says they're multiplying and turning on them and the others.

I realize I have to take the hyena's back. It makes sense, Sarah's character wasn't the best. I had to take back a few things now. It's hard to tell what will work and what won't.

I ask Dungeon Master if the little bird cage he had for keeping the dungeon creatures in, would work for the creatures that keep coming. He says yes, it still has magic.

I start thinking he is needed, and important. Possibly even important to balance. I tell him to go get it and use it to trap them. I tell him how I think it was meant to be the three of us. That he is important to us. That he can help.

Dungeon Master manages to trap some.

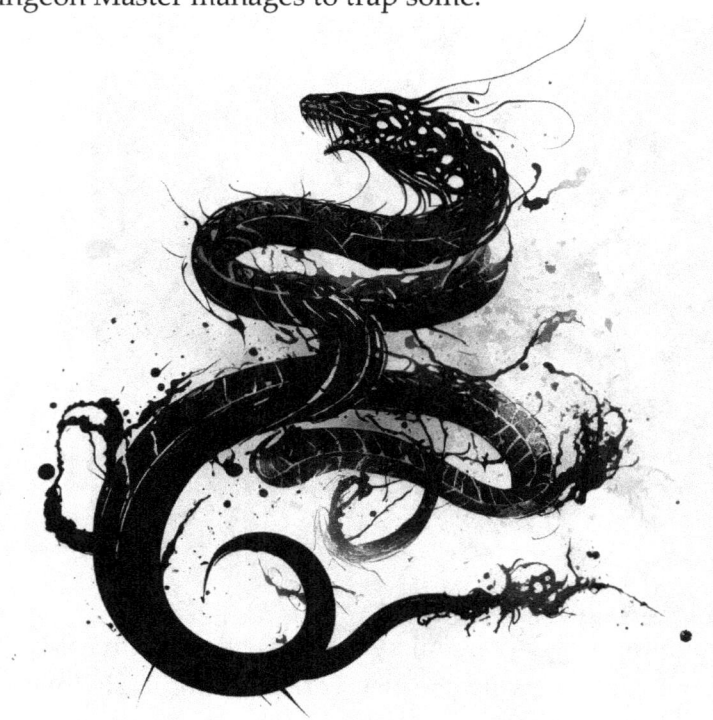

The creations I'm making turn out to be my monster children with twisted versions of love. They call me their mother, many with hate, and I match it right back. They start attacking the ones who hurt me, and I feel like I should keep them. Maybe they are my children after all. But then all but one (snake) turn on me, so all but one remain. They were angry about how they came to be. I apologized prior, telling them I didn't mean for them to come out twisted and feel what I felt. But I had to do what I had to do for balance.

I get confused on if the last one is or isn't attacking me because I only have what the dungeon master says to go off of. The jolts in my body feel like the snake child is zapping and trying to kill me after they enter my body. But the dungeon master says he thinks the healing and love from it is killing her.

Then I feel biting like poison, and he says it really is trying to kill me. I have to destroy it.

Dungeon Master says he needs to heal me. To stop all the things I'm creating. That I can't be stuck in Insanity mode.

I allow him to try, surprised he's a healer of all things. He has a hard time because of everything that has been done to me. He ends up feeling empathetic. I'm surprised again. I think he won't be able to do it, but he starts getting emotional about what has been done to me. He tries his best to heal me, asking for my permission. He hesitates when he needs to heal my vagina. I laugh. Then I wonder why. Figured something recent or something before.

I think things are going well, that maybe it will be the three of us. But then something happens. He attacks me. I don't understand why. He says he couldn't handle the emotions and things that happened to me. He doesn't want to feel them. He doesn't understand why he's attacking me either. I am devastated that I have to get rid of him too. I thought he was going to be a good one for balance. For what the world needed. I do to him a few things I did with Lucifer. I wondered if he also hated burnt chicken. Turns out he did.

Dungeon Master knows about the things I did to Lucifer because he says so in a horrified voice. He will not last as long as Lucifer. He already says he gives up.

I say oh no, he did wrong. He needs to know and feel it too. I make him smell shit. I can still smell it, and it upset me again. I think everything can eat shit. And all the creatures that were attacking, and the Dungeon master eat shit. I think of shit pudding, shit soups, shit ice cream. They all eat it.

Dungeon Master comments no wonder Lucifer gave up. You really like making people eat shit.

Ashes to Dust

I stop and let Dungeon master go when he's almost white. I tell him I'll heal him like he did for me. Balance. I heal him, taking away his bad parts. I want to make him the better version I saw. If I heal out the bad, it should work. When he's healed, he instantly regrets what he did attacking me.

I get a knowing that something is wrong. I'm not sure what. I realize it was 2nd. She wanted Dungeon Master to attack me, and for me to do what I did and heal him. I didn't understand. Until after, Dungeon Master wasn't meant to be changed. He was meant to be who he was for a reason.

2nd attacks and I stop her. She fights against me. I manage to kill her. Dungeon Master seems upset. I tell him she has been manipulating him, and she's the reason why he wanted to attack me for no reason. And she's the reason I thought I had to heal him. She messed with both of us. It was my fault for thinking I needed someone.

There is only one balance. That is me. I am alone in the job.

Ashes to Dust

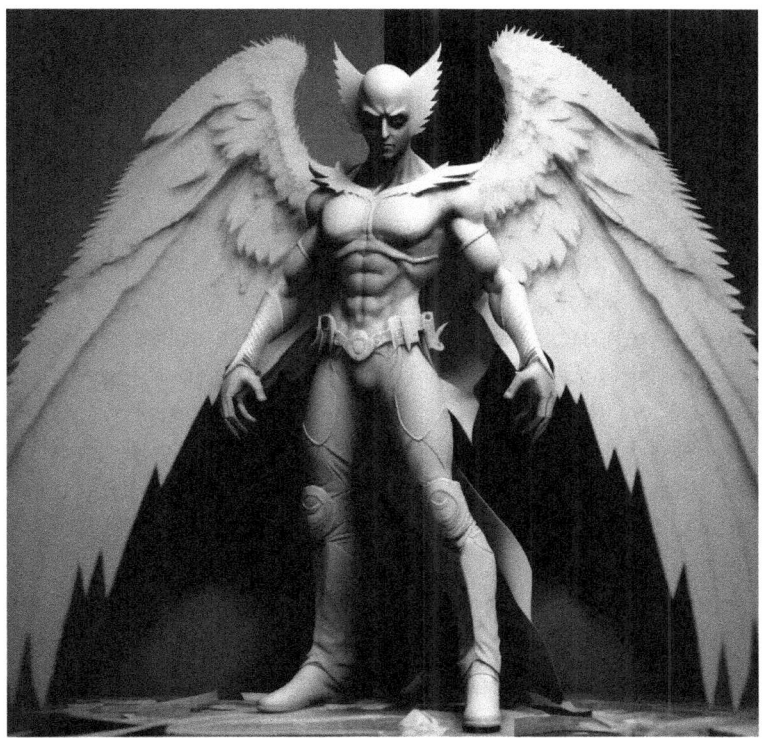

He wants to heal me for real this time. I have a knowing he looks different, like a new angel species with wings. Pure white. He is grosser now that he's new. When he goes to heal me, he uses his tongue. It is long, slimy, thick and disgusting. I have a knowing, and he knew I wouldn't like it.

I was frozen in a retching motion with my mouth open, with an awful feeling in my stomach, and it became hard to breathe. All from the healed dungeon master sticking his nasty tongue down my throat to heal me. I didn't want that anymore; it was painful.

He went to do it again, and this time, I snipped it with my fingers, imagining them as scissors. He stopped for a moment, so I succeeded. He then put his tongue in my ear. It was disgusting.

When he was having a hard time being able to pull any insanity out of my mouth, he duplicated. That wasn't fair. I didn't know he could do that. They both were at me now, and many times I was stuck in that horrible retching position. I had to snip their tongue and keep the snipping motion of my fingers over my mouth. I'm laughing victorious. If they were going to try this, I will make it hurt.

One of them did my vagina. Assuming to heal, possibly from one of Dungeon Master's old goonies, or Lucifer. But that was a no-no. I made my vagina, and all the holes on my body have scissors.

I heard them through me, saying oh no about all the scissors I now had. Their tongues obviously grew back. They should just stop or find a less disgusting way. I laugh at their dissatisfaction. I laugh a lot.

I still have the scissor motions over my mouth, and now over my vagina. At one point I double scissor motion when they multiply again and one is still too persistent to care that their tongue is getting snipped off.

Why are they so desperate to heal me? I wish the buggers would stop multiplying. I can't do anything about it because they aren't doing it to hurt me. It's pissing me off. The old dungeon master would've asked before thinking of healing my vagina with his nasty tongue.

If that's how they want it. I remember Lucifer's hate for fluffy bunny's. I make my vagina soft and fluffy like a bunny to touch. I get a reaction, similar to Lucifer's. What is it with their hate for cute fluffy creatures? And I make it taste like shit. A retching reaction this time. And the sound of displeasure. That makes me mad. They shouldn't enjoy this. I don't.

I run my tongue over my teeth, feeling some plague. I make it so my mouth tasted gross with thick plague, and slimy saliva, and the taste will linger on their tongues even after they're done. I get multiple reactions this time. And it stops. I'm relieved I get a break, and a laugh. Maybe they will finally stop.

They are arguing amongst themselves. I hear some through me. They think it's disgusting and they don't want to do it anymore. They want

Ashes to Dust

to give up but the first copy of dungeon master convinces them that they need to heal me. It's important.

I get that retching with my mouth open again. I snip, but then it comes right back. I keep doing it, and I hear them saying it tastes disgusting and they want to stop. But still it keeps happening. I close my eyes and see a new number grow in my head. Holy shit how many have they created now. There's too many. They all keep coming to heal me. It hurts. I'm mad.

I got tired of seeing the shit on the netting of the bed and smelling shit. I felt like passing out, but I am determined to finally change the shit sheets properly. I'm wearing only a diaper as I grab and toss the sheets off of my bed by the door.

It's extremely tiring. I'm dying. I can feel my heart beat slow, and my head light. I'm trying not to pass out and die long enough to change these shit sheets. I am so angry from the smell of them. What's worse is these dungeon master angels won't fuck off every time I tell them to. They keep doing their nasty tongue thing and it puts me in a breathless pain.

I tell them to stop doing it while I'm changing the sheets or I'm going to pass out and split my head open. Or break my neck on the fall down from exerting myself. I tell them I doubt they can heal that. With split open brains. They shake my head no. Didn't think so. I tell them the family would see it. And to stop long enough for me to finish before I die.

I rip the sheets off, smelling the shit, and getting more pissed. And then, the mom walks in. She interrupts me trying to clean up. Then I have to explain to her that I shit the bed when she's giving me a hard time about some bullshit on not eating.

I had to explain I got food poisoning. Then she fucking tries to undermine me by saying she hasn't seen me eat. She knows I eat at night and get drinks at night when she's sleeping. How the fuck is she going to stand there and be like this when I'm ready to pass out and it smells obviously of shit.

It's fucking embarrassing to be standing in a diaper in front of the mom while she stares at the diaper. And then stares at the shit pile of sheets. Stop fucking looking it makes me feel gross and uncomfortable like you're a pervert. Don't stare at my vagina.

I explained the food poisoning before and now I have to again, like she doesn't get it. What part of shitting the bed from food poisoning is there not to get? Then she thinks there's something else. Like why the fuck can't you leave so I can clean these fucking sheets and lay back down before I die? Holding all this anger in is killing me faster. Why does the mother make everything a fucking interrogation and argument of disbelief? Just fucking leave. I want to lie down on clean sheets.

The mother says she'll take the sheets and go get me new sheets. That pisses me off. I don't want anyone to know, or touch the dirty shit covered sheets. I just want to be left alone to clean it up and die and be regenerated in peace. Holding in this anger is hurting me physically.

When she left for a moment I grab the sheets and yank on them, and twist them in anger trying to let it out before she came back. I almost died many times with the mother standing there. I was too light-headed, and the fucking dungeon master angels were still pulling shit when I told them not to. I don't want to die in shit covered sheets.

The dungeon master angels were scared at my fits of anger and how I was able to hold it in, and then let it out when the mom left. I can control myself when I need to. I'm balance. It's my job.

Once the mom came in with more sheets, I waited for her to leave as she just lingered there. Go away. I don't want to fucking die a brutal death with you watching because you wouldn't let me finish. I hold the sheets over my diaper as she still lingers at it. Stop it's gross. When she leaves I put the sheets on, but I still smell shit by the corner because of the netting. It pisses me off again.

Ashes to Dust

I yell at the dungeon master angels for still doing their bullshit while I was talking in front of the mom. That wouldn't look good and it's killing me faster. Every time I lean in the tent to put the sheets in, I feel like the lights are going to go out. I can barely feel my heart beat, even with my fingers to my neck.

The dungeon master angels ask how I can control my anger like that.

Again, I say, I'm-Fucking-Balance. What part of that do you not understand?

I have to repeat I'm balance so many times. It's not hard to understand. Balance doesn't lose it. Balance is balanced. Insanity, but sanity. Anger, but calm. Balance.

After I finish, I am relieved to finally be done. I have clean, shit-free sheets. I can die without dying in shit. I can be resurrected on clean sheets now. I'm barking out their names to show them, hell fucking yeah, I'm balance of course I know your names.

Then I get a new knowing. The dungeon master angels have kids. I yell at them, "You have kids?" I'm pissed again. They shouldn't be having kids.

Apparently, the kids are learning. They are teaching the kids not to give up, so they say. I want them to give up. I want the kids to see them give up. I want to be left alone. I go to the bathroom to pee, and even their fucking kids are watching me. Learning. These fuckers play dirty. They get me on the toilet too. I finish up and go back to my room, and the kids are in on it too. I don't know what to say to that and start doing the snip thing again. Let's see them get through that.

I crawl in my tent, finally, and then have to put up with them trying to do the same things. I take a drink of water the mom left. Then I see a horror in my knowing. "You created your own creations?" I'm so upset and disappointed. I shared some knowledge of balance with them before so they would know how to keep balance. They should know better! Their creation ruins the balance of the universe.

I have to destroy it. I do, there are many, and their creation has kids.

Ashes to Dust

Monstrous kids. They aren't right. I destroy all of their monstrous creations.

I feel their anger at me for destroying them. But they weren't meant to be in this world. The dungeon master angels turn on me. They threaten me, attack me, and then they threaten my cat. I can't let that happen. I make sure to make it so they can't harm my cat. Everything keeps going after my cat.

They don't give up; they want me dead. I take away their children too. I try to get rid of all of them but there are too many. I get a knowing in my mind. Infinity sign. There's infinity.

That's dreadful. I keep fighting, and the number is still too big. I realize I have to bring back the original Dungeon Master to try to get rid of the new, healed, monstrous versions.

I manage to bring back the original, unhealed version of the dungeon master. I show him the monsters that came from him when he was healed. He's appalled at what came out of him. They were everything he wasn't. They were rapey now. Lower forms of him. All the qualities he didn't have were there in those monstrous things with wings.

My foot is doing the infinity figure and he realizes I'm creating multiple versions of myself without realizing it. He's talking through me, freaking out by how many there are.

I tell him the whole thing came undone because of my 2nd. A helper I created thinking I needed someone else, but didn't. She ended up betraying me, and purposefully creating this mess knowing he shouldn't be healed. And me being balance, she knew I would've healed instead of killed because you healed me. But she knew I would've done something to you first. Which is how it all started.

There's still a primal part of him that wants to kill me. But he keeps seeing his healed parts and tries to hold it back. He sees all the balances I'm creating to fight off the infinity healed versions of him. He wants to know how to stop it. He asks one of the new balances, a female, who says it won't stop unless balance is healed and taken out

Ashes to Dust

of insanity mode. He realizes all the other balances are in insanity mode too. He freaks out more.

I comfort him by telling him not to worry, we will create a beautiful place where everyone in the world will be happy. There will be sunshine, flowers, and rainbows and no violence or anger, and everyone will get their happiness like they deserve. There will never be abuse, or anything that can trigger people into becoming abusive and mean.

He says something about me creating things again that aren't what I think they are.

One of my new balances counter that with telling him, no it is beautiful.

Again Dungeon Master states we're all insane and he needs to heal me, the first balance.

I tell him there isn't just one, that we, the infinity are all balance now. We won't ever do anything to damage balance even in insanity mode.

My male balance agrees. I have a male balance. It's strange but makes sense. There are infinity balances being created they aren't all going to be like me, female. They will be male too for balance.

I get a knowing of him. White hair, very tall, muscular, and he has white eyes. A female one has black hair. There are many. I keep creating them.

Dungeon Master is trying to convince the other balances to let him heal me. They don't want to give him time because they can feel my pain and everything I've been through, including how I want peace and happiness.

With all the pain and everything done to me, they interfere with him trying to heal me. They want to kill me so I can move on. They want the world reset so it's beautiful and how I envisioned it with no pain or sickness, just happiness.

I talk to a few of them, and they get confused. I realize they really are like me, insanity mode. And they don't like it either. They don't like

Ashes to Dust

being stuck in that mode, where they are always going to hide what their moves are, so others don't know. And according to others, everything created comes out wrong. That they're stuck insane.

They become aware but then instantly aren't and it's unpleasant feeling like this. Emotions are all over the place because they have to be. You can't stop it.

A conversation with them turns into confusion about what we just said, and because I'm also stuck in insanity mode sometimes I move forward and forget too. But I see the traits in them, and it saddens me. I don't want to have to make more stuck. But then it quickly changes because this is how it's suppose to be and together we will make the world better, and great. No one will wreck it, or hurt anyone anymore.

We may be balance but I still am the top where I make sure all the rest of the balances are doing their job maintaining balance. That job is still my responsibility, it doesn't go to the rest. That's how balance stays maintained. It's why they still listen to me but sometimes don't want to listen to me.

One moment one will be mad at me, the next they won't. I can see why it was exhausting talking to me. But I also am still like that so I don't get why no one understands us. Then I remember they aren't meant to.

The male balance is especially keen on wanting to kill me. I tell him it's okay that I know it's out of the goodness of their heart, even if our love might seem twisted to others. I appreciate it.

Dungeon Master gets upset because the male balance squeezes my throat again, and Dungeon Master wants more time. It gets worse for Dungeon Master when the other balances know how many times I've been resurrected. Over 500.

Male balance snaps my neck. I thank him. It's a relief because now I can finally regenerate. Dungeon Master is still upset. He still wants to heal me, and he's worried it will be too late. He is still ranting about our creations, but he is careful because they want to kill him for dissing them.

We're all creating things, and he seems terrified. He keeps saying they aren't what we think they are.

I have a knowing of something like a fiery blaze, but it goes away and turns into the wonderful things I want the world to be. What me and the other balances want the world to be.

He keeps trying to argue with the female balance that it isn't beautiful like she thinks and he moves on quick to say he really needs to heal me because I don't realize how disastrous the new world would be.

One balance says it can't be a nightmare like he says because we are balance and it will be beautiful and we'll finally create happiness in the new world.

Dungeon Master says the problem is we don't realize it's not what we think they are.

I am having trouble regenerating because the other insanity mode balances are forgetful, confused, and hop to different emotions.

The male thought I hated him, then he thought I was the reason they were in pain because they could feel mine.

I had to explain to both the closest male and female that I appreciate their help, and know how difficult it is. And the thought process and emotions. That I love them, even if they forget, and even if I forget to say. I appreciate them trying to help me, and stay in the moment long enough to do so.

I ask the male balance if he can kill me again. He does it quick again and I hear a snap in my neck. I thank him with a smile. I lay there trying to regenerate, and Dungeon master doesn't give up. He is healing me and helping bring me back to life. I didn't know he could. He is determined to not let me go and have the new world boot up with infinity, insanity mode balances running it.

Dungeon Master healed me and all the infinity balances I was creating disappear. It's just me and Dungeon Master, and the army of

Ashes to Dust

monstrous versions of him. They want to kill him too for healing me and not letting me die.

I'm still balance, just not stuck in insanity mode anymore. I tell him not to worry I will protect him for as long as it takes. I ask if he believes me to stick to my word. Not believe in me, like a worshiper, just believe I will hold true to my word.

He says he does, because he's seen me in action. I say good, then believe I will do my best to protect you for as long as it takes. Me and you.

I tell him to hold on as I move positions. He stays on my stomach and I curl my legs into my chest as my back rests against the mattress. I bring my arms to each side to prevent any gaps and ask him if he's okay. He says yes. But then his monstrous versions try to get in and a couple succeed, attacking us.

I just started and they already got to him. I'm upset. I am feeling this out as I go along. I tell him to hold on, and I reach in and grab him, and hold him in my hand. I make sure not so squeeze him, and I ask again if he's still alive.

I fight off his alters and then I hear him freak out. He's being attacked in my hand. I shake my hand gently to heal him and get rid of the invader trying to kill him. I ask if he's feeling better. He says a little, but he isn't holding up too great. He is concerned about how I look, and I reassure him not to worry I am balance and they can't kill balance. I will heal and regenerate and protect him like I said.

I keep switching positions. It's tiring, but I push through to protect him. He makes a noise at my stomach saying it looks bad. He asks if I'm okay when I ask if he's okay.

I have a knowing that it is skewered and stringy like a carved pumpkin that isn't hallowed out. It goes away and I try to find any cracks that they can get into to attack him.

I sit up this time with my legs tucked again. It's hard to figure out. They try to get to him through my butt hole, and other holes. How am

Ashes to Dust

I to cover everything?

When I start to heal him and myself, I slowly rock side to side as he stays there on my stomach. I don't want him to die on my watch. He's trying to stick through it, but I can tell he isn't built for this. He wants to give up but giving up is death.

I have to switch positions again to guard and protect him. It amazed him I am healing. But he still mentions when I'm not looking so hot, which isn't helpful. I'm busy focusing on him, and trying to protect him and fend off his less-than-copies.

I almost lose him. I'm upset at myself for getting him almost killed. For not being able to protect him from the pain of it. But in a way it's his karma. I had to bring him back to life at one point.

13

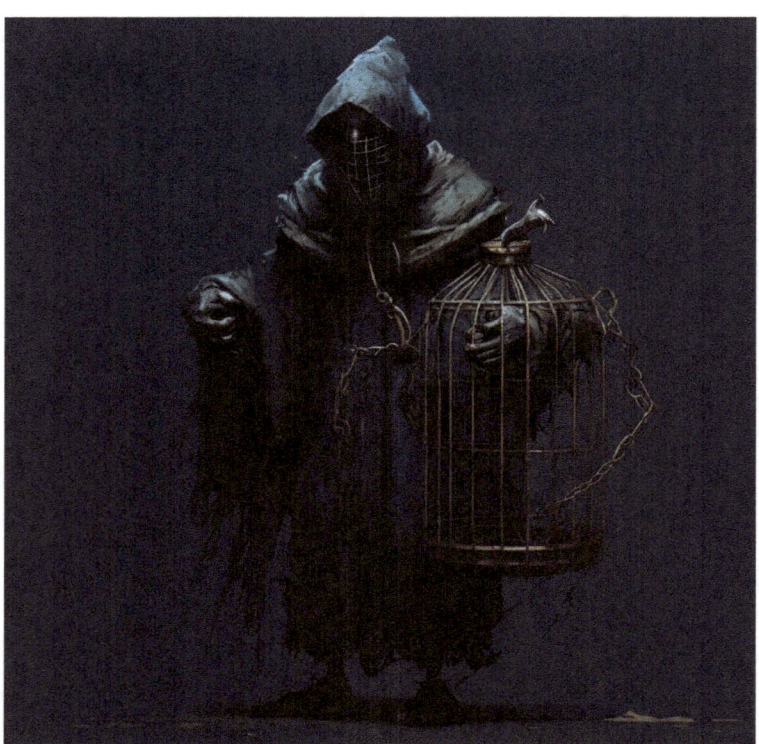

I ask Dungeon Master if he has his cage. He says he can get it. I tell him to summon his cage and he can lock the infinity angels up in it. I tell him to draw the infinity symbol in it and it will draw them all to it

Ashes to Dust

and seal them inside. He says okay, and I wait for him.

Time passes as I'm fighting the infinity angels, but Dungeon Master hasn't moved from under the pillow yet. I ask him if he got the cage. He says no, confused.

I try not to get hopeless, as I realize he forgot. I tell him again, and again I wait. When he still hasn't gotten it, I tell him the infinity angels are messing with his mind. They are making him forget what I'm telling him because they don't want him to lock them away. I tell Dungeon Master he is stronger than he knows, and he can fight them. That's why they make him forget things, and want him dead.

I hear the surprise and self doubt in his voice as he says, "Really?" through this body. I tell him yes, and reassure him.

I think if I lend some power, I can block the infinity angels from messing with his mind. I thought it was working, but he still has memory issues.

I tell Dungeon Master I was going to reincarnate him as a human in the new world. But things keep stopping it. I tell him he was supposed to be with me and help make sure the new world goes smoothly. Where he would have a choice to be a human in it after or help run it.

He is surprised at the human part. I don't think he ever considered being able to be turned into a human. It was a gift for him. For helping.

I'm Light and Stars. I just want the world to have all the happiness it should have had. No violence, no pain, no anger, no suffering, just happiness. Not even sickness, despite being told that I can't have it so the world doesn't have illness.

Things keep stopping me from making the world a better place where everyone gets their happiness. I look toward the window, thinking about how long the days will be alone. I'm tired of fighting and I don't know how much longer or how many more lifetimes I will need to fight for the dream I envision.

I tell Dungeon Master that he's special, and that's the reason why things keep trying to kill him. I can't do this alone anymore. I'm losing the battle and I'm drained. I don't think I'll make it by myself. I didn't want to active him early but I have no choice, I can't do it anymore with no help.

I tell Dungeon Master who he really is. I activate his memories and abilities from before. I tell him, he is Moon and Sky.

He is confused at first. But the memories slowly pour in and he says my name, "Stars," after reawakening. He wasn't supposed to be awakened until the new world was set.

I apologize to him, that I just couldn't make it.

He looks at me, sees what the infinity angels did, and starts weeping out, "Oh Stars!" And, "Look at you!"

I softly laugh. I don't know what else to do. It's fine. I get a knowing it's not good, but it fades.

I tell Moon and Sky to get the cage and what to do to get the infinity angels in it. This time he is protected as he runs. But again, he forgets what to do with the cage. He even forgets he is Moon and Sky and what his powers are. The infinity angels are still affecting him, even when I remind him multiple times.

I wait, get attacked, and remind him.

When I think he has finally grasped what to do, I have to protect him again. The infinity angels mimic his voice to trick me. There will be two to three options to choose from. I hope I pick correctly.

The one that I find is Moon and Sky's genuine voice has more power in it. It's louder, stronger. The mimicked ones are usually weaker, in volume or expression. Sometimes they're softer than his.

I have to pick which is the real voice of him to see if I'm hurting him, or they're attacking him. They trick me a few times, and get better at mimicking his voice.

It eventually becomes four options to choose from and it's too hard to distinguish. I tell Dungeon Master they are doing so, and he can hear them through me once I tell him.

He says, "Holy fuck." He tries to get through to me, but it gets too

Ashes to Dust

hard.

I realize I'm going to have to bulldoze through and I tell him again what to do to trap the infinity angels.

In his endearing way he starts telling me, "Shut up Star." Sometimes, "Shut the fuck up Stars." And says in a sad tone, "I don't want to lose you."

The infinity angels are killing me, I have a knowing about it. And I know I should shut up to protect myself, but that's not how I function. I spit things out as soon as they come to me. I tell him so.

He says he knows, and he wishes I didn't because he is scared of losing me.

That makes me sad, but I have to keep going and saying things while I can. While I'm still alive so he can carry things out and make this world a better place like we envisioned.

I tell him if things get bad, to put my soul into the cage too and go far away. But it has to be separate from the infinity angels. He cannot trap us in the same cage at the same time.

He wants me to quit now, but I have to protect the girl. This is her body. I keep going, and then the oddest thing. The girl comes through, her powerful voice overriding and loud. Strength pours from it as she fights the infinity angels.

I tell her to let me take over, or she will overdo it. We need to take turns or we will die.

One of them takes her from me. I feel it. Her soul is gone. I wake the body and tell Ash that her soul is gone.

Ash calls it back and successfully gets it back into her body.

I'm relieved. I switch with Ash and tell her to rest. They keep trying to take her soul, and I feel when they take something because I feel less light. My voice is dulled, and the body is heavier. I have to get my spark back. Ash and I fight them, swapping. She doesn't know what they're taking is precious to me. That the soul they take from Ash's body is my daughter, Light.

Ashes to Dust

I tell Moons and Sky to take Ash's soul, and put her safely in the cage to be reincarnated. So those monster infinities can't get her. He doesn't want to; he wants to take me instead. Just me, Light and Stars.

I tell him in a sad, but still high-tone that no, he must take her and guard her. That she is more important. He makes the same sound as when I've been severely injured but haven't noticed.

He finally takes Ash's soul, and takes her far away from here. He's hiding with her and I'm glad. I'm also sad. I'm alone again. And I'm left to clean up this infinity mess. I know I'm dying, but I will keep fighting to protect what I can. I will come back again one day and finish.

Ashes to Dust

14

There's a shift. Something enters Ash's empty body. It's me, Stars, with someone else who is controlling it. I tell them she's gone.

It's a male. He says he wants to know where she is. He keeps eyeing the infinity angels, and then he says he's Lucifer.

I laugh at him and tell him Lucifer is dead. Ash killed him.

He places my hands on my legs, and wigs out, saying how gross I am. He retches when he touches me. Then he laughs about how this must be how *she* felt when he touched her.

It makes me second guess myself. He comments on how I look horrible. Grey, and decaying with less light.

I'm not aware until he mentions that. I laugh, a small, worried laugh. He doesn't know where she is though. He can't get to her because she's not in this body.

We are attacked by one of the infinity angels again. And he isn't happy. He snaps his fingers, and the one who attacked is gone. I believe it now. Moon and Stars cannot come back with her. She will be in danger. I don't know how she put up with him in her body. It's an unpleasant feeling with him in here. Both of us in one body.

I won't let him have my daughter again.

He places a hand on my crossed legs, and he retches and says how disgusting I am. Every time he forgets, he's reminded with a gagging reaction. I'm aware because he keeps telling me I don't look good.

Ashes to Dust

I ask him how he lived. He doesn't answer, he just plays coy, laughing. I feel more drained every second he's in here with me. He's killing me faster.

Lucifer talks to the infinity angels, striking a deal with them. He says he will give them me, Light and Stars, like they want, if he gets what he wants. But they need to stop attacking so he can do it. He shows them that with him sharing the body, Light and Stars is dying. That she will die a slow, painful death like they want, with or without him in the body.

Some of the infinity angels cheer at that, and wait. Others attack, because they don't want it to be quick. They want my death now.

He persuades them he can give each side what they want. One side can play and watch Stars decay slowly like now, and the other can finish her off quick like they want. Lucifer gets them to stop for a moment.

I'm worried I don't want Lucifer to get Light. But I feel Moon and Sky. He wants to save me. I tell Moon and Sky to protect her, that she is more important and not to let Lucifer get her again.

Lucifer tells Moon and Sky to look at her. To see how her light is dulled, that she is decaying and dying. That him being in her is killing her more.

I can feel Moon and Sky. I tell him no, not to listen. I love Moon and Sky, but our daughter is more important, and he can't know.

Lucifer says he can feel her soul somewhere. He accidentally touches my knee and gags again. After killing a few more impatient infinity angels, he laughs at the fact that I'm her mother, and Moon and Sky is her father. He heard me.

I tell him not to tell Moon and Sky. He finds it amusing.

Moon and Sky threatens to kill Ash's soul if Lucifer doesn't leave. Moon and Sky keeps using her soul as leverage, knowing Lucifer wants it.

Lucifer isn't happy about it, and tells Moon and Sky, he will find

Ashes to Dust

them first.

I can feel him searching for her. For them. He wants to kill Moon and Sky, and take Light soul all for himself.

My consciousness is aware of what is going on in my body. That Light and Stars is dying, and Lucifer, of all things, has taken over. I didn't want to believe it. But he called out to me and said he witnessed everything since his "death."

I can't pretend anymore because he says he knows I'm stronger than I let on. He mentions wanting to intervene when they kept resurrecting me wrong.

Shit. It's definitely him.

Lucifer calls out to Moon and Sky, telling him he can exchange Stars for my soul.

He doesn't care that he made a deal with the others first. Maybe he thinks he can do the exchange, but they can still find and kill Stars later. Light and Stars isn't looking too well. She's falling apart. Light doesn't mix with Lucifer either.

They aren't aware I'm still connected. That I know now Light and Stars, and Moon and Sky are my parents.

Moon and Sky isn't aware I know he's trying to kill me. I stop him first. I knock him out when he comes in the cage to kill me. I regrettably reach out to Lucifer. I'm not in my body, but he can hear me through it. Light and Stars is unaware.

I ask Lucifer to keep Light and Stars asleep and to not allow her to know anything that happens. Lucifer doesn't want to, but it seems my more commanding voice has him agree.

He knows, I know, who I am, and that Stars and Sky are my parents.

I might not be in my body, but Lucifer is still linked to me. I don't enjoy it. But it's a necessity. He keeps Light and Stars asleep, and he follows my lead, so I can kill Moon and Sky using balanced karma for attempting death on me.

After it's done, I can feel Lucifer's giddiness. He wants to tell Light and Stars. He can't. I tell him he can't. I then erase Light and Stars memory of Moon and Stars. I have to protect her light. It would turn her dark to learn that he was dead, and the world needs her light.

Lucifer enjoys the show and wants to tell her that dad tried to kill daughter, and daughter killed dad. He says it would devastate her to lose her other half—*soulmate*—.

Shit soulmate. I make it so Lucifer can't tell her. But then I feel like I need to ask her permission to take away a memory so important. I already did, but I wanted to make sure she would be okay with it.

I wake Light and Stars up, and carefully ask her, if it was okay to keep something from her if it protected her and kept her as light. Even if it meant forgetting a person.

Light and Stars woke up and in her high, cheerful voice, she said yes, because she knew I would only do it if it was to protect her, and keep her light.

I put Stars back to sleep and made sure she didn't remember the conversation. I ask Lucifer to leave, but he doesn't want to. I ask him to leave or my body will die. He does, but I know he's still in the room somewhere. I can't just abandon my body because I have nowhere else to go or jump into. I go back to my body.

Lucifer killed the rest of the angel masters, so there was nothing left to bother us. Now I have to heal my body by dying and coming back again. I don't like this part.

Ashes to Dust

15

I couldn't resurrect right away. Pieces of tainted Higher Power came back. They waited until Holy spirit, karma, soul contract, and the infinity angels attacked me first. After Lucifer and I got rid of them, my mother Light and Stars was waiting above on the ceiling to help bring me back.

I would close my eyes, as I would reanimate and regenerate. And then I would slowly move my body, until I could stand. Lucifer wouldn't let me do it myself. He kept interfering. He would place his hands on me, and hold me up like a puppet. Sometimes he would keep me from falling, but most times he would make have to die and regenerate all over because the new body failed completion.

Lucifer kept swapping with me when I would breathe. He would go too fast, or move too impatiently to have me resurrected, and my body would fail again. I would accidentally take over and overpower him when he was breathing for me. I couldn't control it. I would be resurrected and done by now if he would listen and let me do it myself. Even Stars would tell him he isn't helping. But he is insistent that he won't leave or let me do it alone.

I try to remind him of his wingless back because of me. He realizes I'm trying to make him angry again or have him not be interested in me again. But he isn't falling for it. He claims he took the time to learn how to control his anger. He has proved so far he has adapted, and it's not good for me he won't leave. He's even more clingy than before.

Moons and Stars came back to help. I didn't know what to say since our last encounter. I thought I killed him and he almost killed me. He said he understands now, and it's okay. That he isn't here to hurt me.

Light and Stars chimes in, saying how he is different and knows how important I am to him.

Moons and Stars says he can see the pieces of his attitude in me, and the light and over informative side of Stars. That I'm definitely theirs. And it explains why I'm so strong.

Lucifer couldn't control his other parts. I had a knowing that there were six or seven parts of him that made him whole. He wasn't just one singular being. I figured out there were two alligators and one tortoise.

The loud popping that happened in my ears, similar to the pop after swimming, was the alligators using their tongue. It sounded like liquid was still left in my ears afterward. The strange feeling by my thighs, I figured was rapey stuff to my vagina by the tortoise. It darkened my mood.

Light and Stars tells Lucifer that he's killing me and shredding my soul. She tells him he needs to stop them from doing that to me.

Lucifer realizes and starts healing my soul and piecing it back together. I feel less darkened and lifeless, but I'm aware of what they did to me. It happens a few times, and he has to put me back together to undo it by gently rocking my body back and forth.

I tell Lucifer he hasn't really changed because he can't control all his parts. Those are the parts that are out of control.

There's nothing he can do about them.

I hear snapping, and I think things are getting worse for me from his other parts. I don't know what they're doing, just that they aren't good for me or my soul. It's clear he lied about being able to suppress his rage, even if he claimed to love me even more. I have to stop them.

I manage to destroy some of his other parts until there isn't any more except for the Lucifer that has been there trying to learn to control his anger. It turns out, without his other parts, he's actually worse. He can't control his rage at all. But I find a spec of a goodness in him. I amplify that goodness, let it spread out where it can be loved and grow.

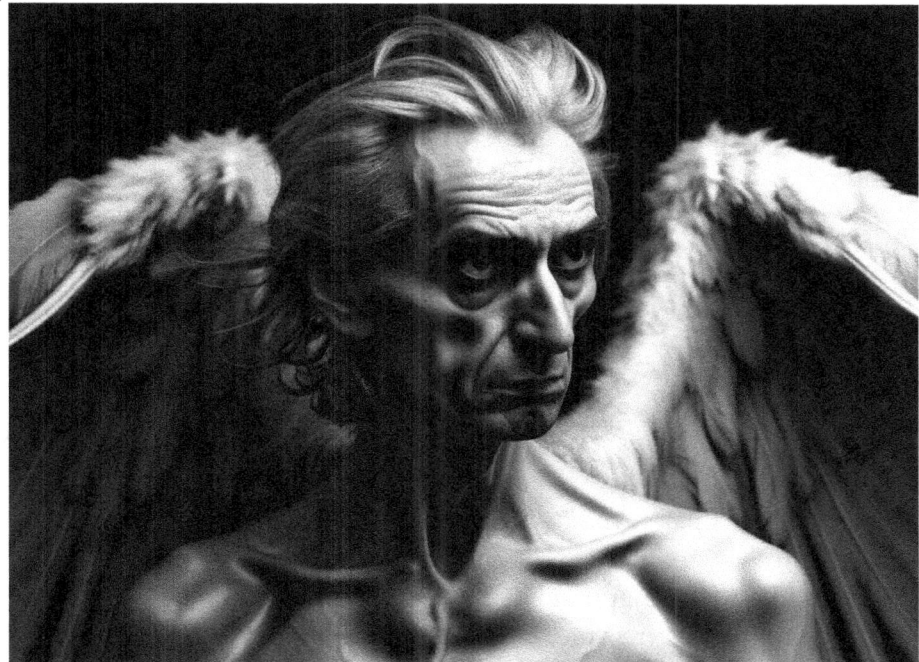

I discover the part is the original Lucifer Morningstar angel. It's why I couldn't destroy him yet. This good part was attached. I free the angel from its attachment.

I lie there trying to regenerate, thinking I fixed everything, when I'm invaded with Lucifer molecules. In my knowing, they are round and microscopic, almost like a bunch of blood cells in appearance. They're there to attack me. They're upset because I freed the angel from them. I let the scrawny, malnourished, shaggy-haired, male angel go free outside of my room.

The Lucifer molecules are like the remnants. Attacking, and dark.

Ashes to Dust

They're unpleasant, and call for more. I try to banish them but I'm failing because more keep coming. I try to destroy them, but more come. They are furious I let their plaything escape and now they want me to be their plaything.

Lights and Stars offers to go in and try to rid them from me. I didn't want them to hurt her, but she does anyway and I allowed it. I will pull her out if something goes wrong. She tries to fight them off, and Moon and Stars is rooting for her from above. He couldn't help because he's dark where she is light. If he came in it would've hurt me more.

After a while I get worried and check in. She sounds tired, like I am. She tried to fight them but there's too many. She's overpowered. She's hiding somewhere in the corner of my body where they can't find her. I'm worried they will kill her. I try again to rid myself of the molecules so she can escape, but again they multiply.

It feels like a long time has passed, with me trying and failing to eject them or resurrect. I start to question whether Light and Stars was there at all. If Moon and Stars was. I don't think they were. I think I got tricked by the Lucifer molecules. I don't know what happened to them or when they were there and not there.

It turned out the angel I released never left. He was bound to my bellybutton this entire time. I did something wrong in freeing him and he got stuck to me instead. I felt so bad. But I also couldn't take this anymore. I don't know how he took the molecules this whole time. But he was stronger than me and maybe he can take them again, long enough for me to get rid of them after I heal.

My door pops out. It must not have been closed all the way from the last visit from Barb. I panic because I can't get up to close it and my tent is open. Sure enough, my cat, Lovie, comes in. She walks into my room and jumps on my bed through the tent. And like she knew not to touch me, she stepped around me, and went and sat right in the upper right corner of my bed. She stared there with rapid head movements. I realize she can see the Lucifer molecules that are invading my room to come and invade me. She's keeping them at bay.

I feel so grateful to have Lovie protecting me from them. But I'm worried they will eventually get to her. She's only one and they are many. But she's holding them off long enough. She looks where I've seen them, and is guarding me as she lies by my head. I want to pet her, but I don't want them to infect her.

After she leaves, I zip up the tent so she can't get back in and get hurt. She's the only one who wanted to help me and loves me unconditionally.

I go back to fighting off the Lucifer molecules. I unintentionally infected them with insanity. When I ask them if they will go back to the angel, they said no, but some said yes. Uh-Oh. This was not good for me. It must be part of my balance, and that insanity mode that lingered in there.

I ask the angel again if it's okay that I have them joined again. He says no, then yes. Just like the issue I had with the Dungeon Master. I groan. I don't know what to do, so I do what I have to in order to survive, and allow them to go back together.

I make the angel unstuck and get him to go. He leaves, but it takes a while of coercing. When the angel leaves, I tell the molecules now they can go have the angel they wanted, and to chase after it and never come back.

Only the now insane Lucifer molecules aren't going. Some left, but the rest stayed with me. I didn't know what to do. I inform them I'm going to die if I don't regenerate, which means they will die. They don't care, then they do care. Some of them stop, and some try to kill me faster. I close my eyes to regenerate, and they jolt me out of the process.

The angel comes back and doesn't want to leave. I ask him why. He doesn't know. He wants to stay. Oh no. He's insane too. Even the angel is insane and I don't know what to do. This is bad.

Ashes to Dust

Through the molecules I have a knowing that my insides are actually black, goo. I don't process it fully, it's not how I work or I wouldn't function.

I cry, frustrated. I don't want to die. I just want to regenerate and I think I'm past the point of surviving. I feel my heart wanting to give out, and I think my organs are failing. I grab my iPod and text Kat, "I don't think I'll make it." And cry some more.

Will she find me dead in my bed? Will Barb? How will they react? I don't want them to find me like that.

I keep trying to regenerate, but the Lucifer molecules keep accidentally, on purpose, trying to kill me. It goes on to a point where I think it's the end and I won't make it. The Lucifer molecules know that if I die, they die.

Suddenly something changes. It sinks in.

They aren't trying to kill me anymore. They're trying to help me because tainted Holy Spirit came back. I asked why the Lucifer molecules were helping me. They weren't molecules anymore. They became the good, original, angel Lucifer Morningstar. I assumed they must have merged or something.

They say they love me. Their tainted, obsessive love became real love.

Nice Lucifer helps me get my body up, and put on pants over my depends. I lack energy, but he helps me get out of my room and down the stairs. I tell him I need to finish regenerating, and ask him where Holy Spirit can't find us.

He thinks and mentions water. It can't get us in a ocean or lake of water.

I mention needing to delete the message I sent to my sister when I thought I was dying. He said not to worry he already deleted it.

I felt relieved. I didn't want her to get scared, tell my mom, or call someone on me. I think I might make it.

I look out the front door window and think about how we can go

Ashes to Dust

outside to the bridge. The bridge goes over water. There are no boats so I can't go on a boat and stay to regenerate and hide.

I think again and consider under the bridge. There's water that runs through it, so maybe it'll be enough to protect us if we go under the bridge in a corner. The bridge would shelter us, and the stream through it would protect us.

I calculate how far it is from the house and realize I'm too weak, even with nice Lucifer to go all the way there on foot. I tell Lucifer he will have to run away and find a safe place to hide because I can't make it.

He says he can't run because the molecules' obsessive love became real, and now he is stuck with her.

I apologize that he is stuck with me. I think about the basement having water in the pipes and head towards the basement doors. I go downstairs, passing my cousin who is folding laundry at night while everyone else is sleeping.

Lucifer agrees it would work. I go to lie down on the basement floor, but I see the bottle of Epsom salt, and remember the second circle took place here. It was tainted and I don't know if they cleaned all the salt.

I didn't want a third attack, so I placed laundry from the couch onto the floor to cover it. When I finish, my cat comes down and starts kneading the clothes. I want to shoo her off, but I don't want her to go into any tainted salt. I move her enough for me to lie down and I ask Lucifer if we are protected.

He says yes, it can't sense us yet.

I close my eyes and try to regenerate. I knew the sewer line that ran through my basement was enough to protect me.

After only a minute, I hear footsteps. I open my eyes and sit up across from Lovie. It was Barb. It rocked me, remembering how she treated me last time she came down with all the yelling and screaming and threats of hospitalization.

I had to explain to Barb I was down here to see my cat because I finally had enough energy to get up and down and I missed Lovie and

Ashes to Dust

wanted to bond with her.

Which was true. I missed petting my cat like this. I missed her so much, but I was trying to protect her too. Barb just stood there, said a few things and eventually left.

Before I could try again, one of the God's from the tainted salt showed up. Lucifer noped at it, and we got up.

The Holy Spirit found us because of Barb. Holy Spirit couldn't find me or my heartbeat, but it tracked us using her. When it found us in the dark, I went back upstairs, grabbing Lovie with me so she wouldn't be left behind.

Unfortunately, I ran into Barb again in the living room by the laundry baskets. It delayed me because she started talking and asking how I felt and how I should rest. Which if she wouldn't stop me, I would be trying to do. If she hadn't interrupted downstairs, I would've been successful and done. I'm wasting time and energy I don't have standing here.

After she finished, I went back upstairs, leaving Lovie in the living room. I went back to my room and tried to finish.

Ashes to Dust

16

Lucifer Morningstar angel thought he could hide me from it by putting me in a different life. I would leave this body behind but I would wake up reincarnated in the life I wanted in a new body in Toronto.

I told him my voice needs to be the same. I don't care if he has to change everything else, but my voice needs to be the same. My voice is what makes me, me and it's important in my singing. It has to be my voice.

He knew.

It didn't matter if I was erased from Kat and Barb's memories and the world was rewritten as my mom only having one daughter, and I never existed there. I would exist in Toronto as someone else. A happy me, instead. I'm not sure how it worked. If I would just be forgotten and my room would be replaced by my sister's or just empty. Or if Barb would find my dead body, but I was really alive in Toronto. I'd feel bad if she had to find it like that, but I need to get out.

I lie down with my eyes closed, feeling the panic of needing to rush before it comes to get us. Lucifer angel was trying to finish putting my soul into a new reincarnated body in Toronto. My idle life. It wouldn't be in Wallaceburg, finally. I don't know what I'd look like. It didn't matter.

I can feel Lucifer angel behind me, as I lay there merging into my new life. But when I open my eyes, I see the same shit on the tent with my old stuff.

He apologizes when I tell him, he forgot to change it and my outfit that reminded me of shitting myself.

He tries again.

I feel it, like I'm becoming Hannah. The person I was promised to become. I open my eyes and see my hand looks more elegant somehow. Longer, and my nails look more polished and manicured. It was a strange feeling, like I didn't recognize my body, or like I was having a out-of-body-experience in my new body. But then I saw my heart tattoo on my hand.

I ask if he kept the tattoo on my new body because he knew how much I liked it?

He said yes.

But then my hand went in and out from the new Hannah hand, to my old one. I don't know what happened. I think I was there, successfully in a reality where I was Hannah in Toronto, but then I got swapped back into this old, dead reality.

I ask what happened.

He says something keeps interfering.

It was what I suspected, something is blocking him from jumping us over to a reality with a new life.

The cloud gives instructions to Lucifer angel in codes so I don't know. But I always know somehow in the back of my mind, without really knowing. It's like I recognize the code words, and have a guess of what it means, but at the same time it doesn't fully become comprehended.

The cloud is the boss of Lucifer angel. It likes to pull out words I hide or won't say. It's rude that way, I get angry at it for doing it. It just comes out. Like involuntary barf. It hurts sometimes. But I don't get

Ashes to Dust

rid of the cloud because it hasn't proved to be a danger yet.

Lucifer angel mentions a test I have to pass.

I had no choice, and he sends things at me. I get a knowing that they are black bubbles. I don't care what him and that cloud want, I'm resisting whatever he throws at me.

I hold my breath when it hits to combat it. It's so painful when it gets me, and I struggle to fight it and outlast it. When I think he's getting tired, I try to hold on longer. Long enough to outlast him. But he sends even bigger waves of whatever it is hitting me. I get a knowing that it's not a good thing I'm outlasting it. I shouldn't be. I try anyways.

I realize he's not actually tired. He asks a few times if I give in. Each time I say no. But I say it as I'm crouched on the bed, exhausted.

When I don't think I can keep it up, I finally give. When I do it's not painful anymore when I'm hit. It went from a burning pain to cooling. Like a pleasant cool not a cold cool. It turned out Lucifer angel was trying to make me accept love. That's all I had to do to make it not painful anymore.

Wish I'd known that since I thought it was a challenge I had to outlast.

His hugs aren't even painful anymore for a while.

Ashes to Dust

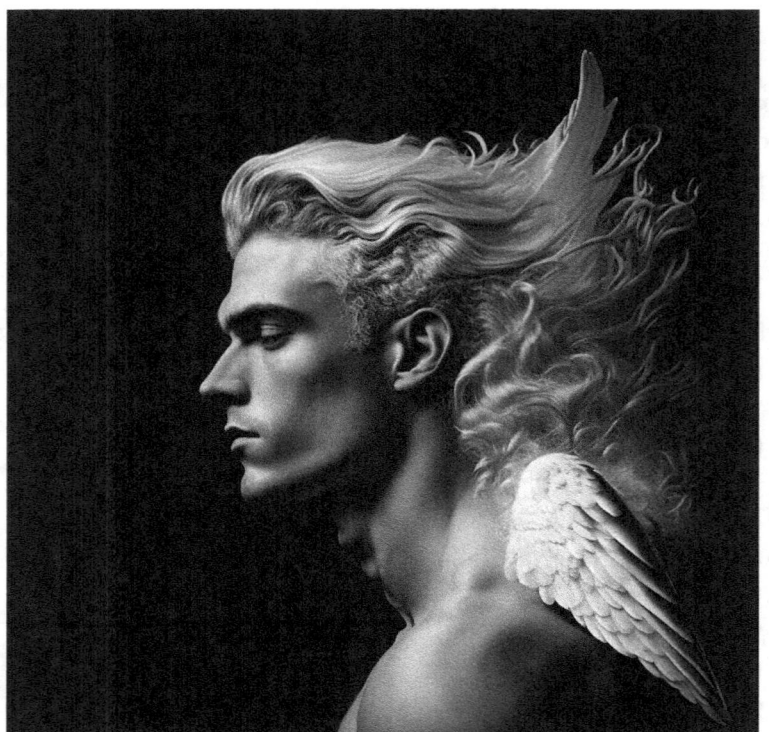

I tell the Lucifer angel I want to make them eat bloody diapers.

Lucifer angel gets even more affectionate, not angry like I thought. He laughs at my insult in a, "Oh you're so cute," kind of way, and asks if I know what I'm saying.

There's a buried knowing of it meaning wanting babies with him, but it leaves. I say no. I tell him it means I hope he chokes on bloody diapers.

He laughs again and acts opposite of what I was hoping. It's meant as a insult, that I want him to choke on things, but he's acting like I keep saying the sweetest words to him. And then he threatens with more hugs. I don't want those hugs. They make me gag.

I tell him I'm telling everyone angels swear because he swears so

Ashes to Dust

much.

He laughs and groans.

I wonder if I'm not suppose to but then I remember I wrote about angels swearing for my book. I mention that.

He remembers.

I tell him I'll just use this as I should definitely have swearing angels in my book.

He laughs. But then hugs me with his feather wings again.

He flies me somewhere. I can feel I'm going but I'm not sure where he's taking me. My body is on the bed, but that's not what's flying with him.

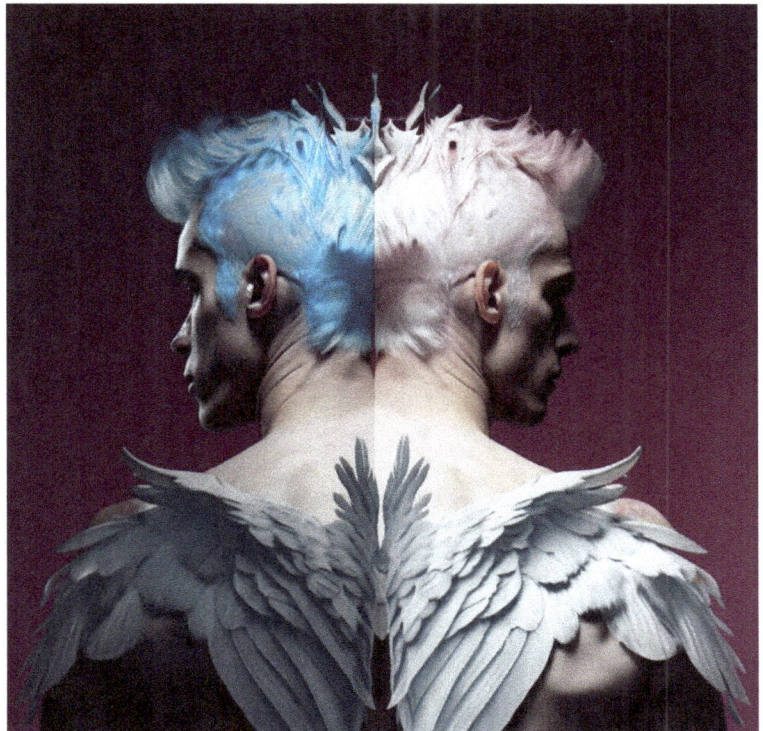

I have a knowing and realize there are not one, but two Lucifer

Ashes to Dust

Morningstar angels. They each have a name. I get another knowing, that I wasn't suppose to know there were two, it was a surprise for my next lives.

They both swear but each one has a different personality.

Then later I feel another hidden one, and realize there are three Lucifer Morningstar angels. All love interests for future lives.

I really wasn't suppose to know that.

They both swear but each one has a different personality. Later I get another knowing that there isn't just two but three of them.

PART FIVE
DEATH

Ashes to Dust

17

I'm trying to entertain the tainted ex-higher power. It's a rape sun god that has been around for the beginning of time and it's been my job as Death to prevent it from turning its sights on humans and other living things in this world. This is the only job I've had. Since creation, I've been Death. It's not a glamorous job.

I feel the sun god trying to rape me again, I have to pretend like I'm enjoying it. It's my job. When it's done, it's a greedy fucker, and wants to do it again. I change my voice when I talk to it, so it doesn't sound as hard as Death. It's more high-pitched like a valley girl. I try to roll on my side to have a break from it wanting to rape me right after it just finished. It doesn't let me and I feel it try to roll me back over. Or try to have my eyes look up and find it so it can wake me, when I pretend to be sleeping.

If I pretend too long, it just rapes me anyways. It's not just the rape monster here, it's Gods and Goddesses again too. I hear the Lucifer angels chiming in about it. I can always hear them through me, but they still don't realize their voice comes out through this vessel. It's a Death power.

They mention how it's impatient.

Yes it is.

I tell the Lucifer angels that it is a horrible creature that should never have existed, and has a ravenous tendency for rape. It's why since the

Ashes to Dust

beginning of creation, it's been my job to try to distract it.

They ask if I ever get a break in the billions of years I've existed.

I tell them I create breaks.

To demonstrate I put on my facade, high-pitched, valley girl voice and ask if it knows how handsome it is. I say the same to the Gods and Goddesses trying to kill me.

I tell the one higher-pitched sounding Goddess that's always the closest to me, (to do the most damage) how beautiful she is.

The Gods and Goddesses are stupid that way. One compliment on looks and they freeze to soak it in.

I tell the rape sun monster it should look in the mirror to admire itself.

I then turn to the female Goddess and say the same thing, that they are so beautiful and should look into the mirror.

I go down the line telling the next to tell the rest to do the same, and my head shakes in excitement as they all want to. So now it's in a loop of them wanting to look and admire their physique in the mirrors.

In my knowing, I created mirrors only they can see. Long, full mirrors.

This is my break. But it's not a long break. To me it's only been a minute or less. To the human world it's been a week. This body is decayed by now. I know my break is over when I feel pain from a god or goddess trying to hurt me again. Or the sun monster trying to roll me over or shake me to rape me again.

They all forget what just happened and I have to go back and play pretend with my high-pitched voice filled with false compliments to get them to stop and do what I want. Then it goes on a loop again where they look in the mirrors, forget, and go back to trying to kill me (but for the sun creation, raping,) like they just started.

It's tiring. I've been doing it since the beginning of time, and I can't have a break or chaos would happen in the world. Then the relentless greedy rapist tries to rape me again.

Ashes to Dust

The Lucifer angels are commenting again as spectators. I hear them tell me not to pretend to enjoy it this time or it will break me.

I already feel broken. I say I have to, I'm death, and there are no replacements. I won't let anyone else endure this. There's no one else who can.

I keep having to save the Lucifer angels from being attacked and killed by the Gods and Goddesses. I send them back down with Death 1 and 2. I'm in both places. But Death 2 is in a blonde human form. I am not.

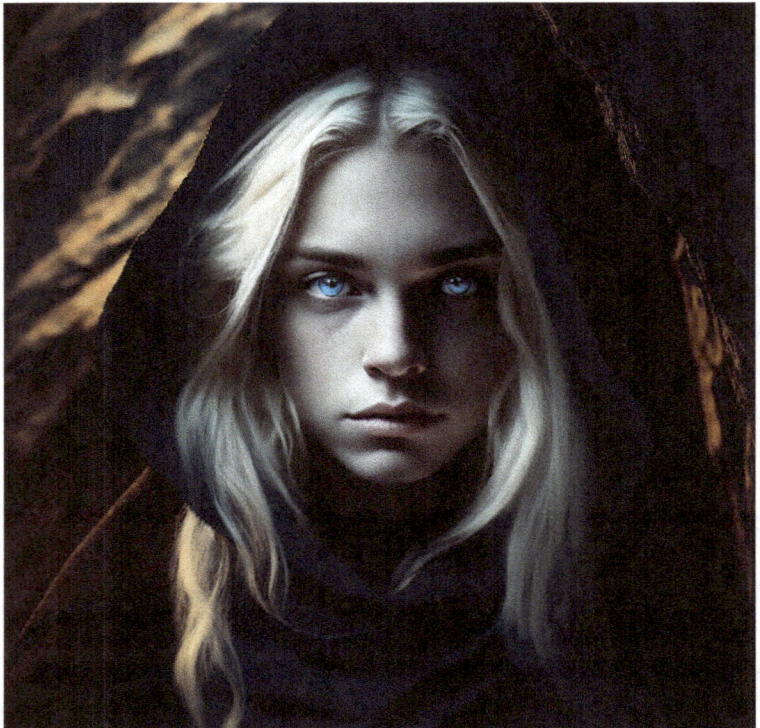

The Lucifer angels are still with Death 1 and Death 2. They see the full me there, what I really look like. They are terrified. Death 2 is blonde and looks human. I look skeleton and menacing. There are so many blue babies down with us. They are unborn babies from apparent futures for me and the Lucifer angels. I tell them if they leave me be, I can give them what they really want, and that's clones of their children. The babies they desperately wanted but I didn't.

Death 2 says, "Oh no, she found a loop hole."

I always do. She knows that. It's why she doesn't do anything about it. A cloud in the sky isn't going to tell me how to live, and neither are these Lucifer angels. I don't want to have these babies with them, but if they do the bargain then I will let them have it without me having to have them or be involved.

The Lucifer Morningstar angels are horrified by my appearance and dread that they are suppose to love that.

Death 2 laughs. She says Death looks human.

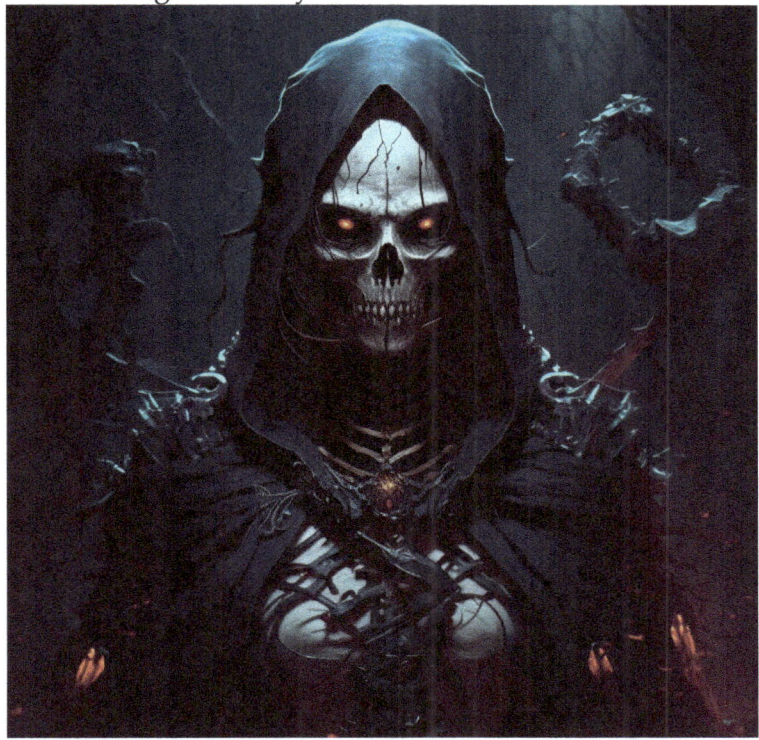

They don't believe her, because I'm not human, I'm death. I look like me. Bones, and raggedy cloth for clothes with dripping black, and red eyes.

The Lucifer angels are still perplexed on how Death 2 looks so beautiful and I, Death 1, look terrifying.

Death 2 says it's from suffering so much pain that she ended up forgetting how she really looks. She believes that her appearance is of a skeleton.

I only created Death 2 to help me. Of course she wouldn't look how I look. I'm ultimate death. She looks different.

Lucifer angel 3 isn't happy that they won't get the life with Hannah with their promised children. He was the one that was suppose to be reincarnated into her life.

Lucifer angel 3 tries to make me pregnant with one of the unborn babies.

Death 2 says he shouldn't have done that. Now nothing is guaranteed.

Lucifer 1 and 2 argue about what Lucifer angel 3 did.

I snap Lucifer angel 3 out of existence. He ruined the balance of things and attacked Death.

The remaining two Lucifer Morningstar angels are surprised I was able to destroy the 3rd.

Death 2 says Death can if it's a attack on her or the balance of the Universe.

I tell the Lucifer angels that the cloned babies are off the table, they get nothing now.

Things are still happening outside where they are, in Ash's room to the borrowed body. I feel worse and I say, "No *pot luck*."

Death 2 says that's not good.

There's a knowing there for the code words I use, but I'm not suppose to have them sink in so they don't.

Death 2 says no happiness.

It means no happiness for me, Death 1, or for the Lucifer angels that

Ashes to Dust

are suppose to be made to love me by the universe.

Lucifer 1 asks how to help Death 1 remember her appearance.

Death 2 doesn't say. She says with everything Death 1 has been through, she will be a hollow shell and never have her humanity, or form back.

But then to my surprise Lucifer 1 gets Lucifer 2 to collect the cloned babies and tells him to throw them at me.

I take it as an attack. Lucifer 2 doesn't want to give them up, so Lucifer 1 throws them at me. Then Lucifer 2 joins in, and starts throwing them. They're sacrificing their cloned babies for me.

The babies burst into flames and start burning me. They call me momma, and then bite me, and hurt me. I don't like it. I try to get them off, but Lucifer 1 and 2 keep throwing them. Why are they doing this to me? It hurts so much. They're burning me alive. If I manage to get rid of one somehow that hurts me more deeply.

The Lucifer angels are confused and Death 2 says not to worry it's just love that's hurting her.

The Lucifer angels asks if it's like when they hug her.

She says yes.

The babies meld into Death 1 and the human skin grows back. I'm hunched over, and I ask why did you do that to me, it hurt. I recognize that voice coming from me. It's the one from earlier. Light soul.

Lucifer angels are shocked to see the human form and realize the light soul they loved from the beginning, was really Death.

I as Death realize I really do have a human form. I didn't know Death looked human. Death was reincarnated as Light soul. All different versions of Death reincarnated, but can exist at the same human time because time and space is different for Death. I am now more aware in Ash's body.

I have a realization that this would make a great story about Death. And I should write it down when I have a chance.

The Gods and Goddesses start attacking again. And then the

abomination tries to rape me as well.

Lucifer 1 mentions how screwed they are with what everything has done to her.

Lucifer 2 thinks they will have no chance trying to get a family with her.

Death 2 says it can take many lifetimes but they will have to be patient.

I'm back to this horrible job, and I have to pretend to enjoy the nasty creature but my face says other wise. There's a surprise. I wasn't imagining things. The creature can see through my Death disguises and see the face I'm really making, and had heard me say it's disgusting.

The Lucifer angels picked up on it too at one point earlier and I was being careful to hide my face with my hand. But there's always been something horribly different about this thing.

To my surprise one of the Lucifer angels took over. They're the ones being raped instead. No one has ever done that for Death before. No one would ever want to. It's horrible and only death can endure this.

I try to get him to stop, but he won't.

He says I can't be the one doing this forever. That I need a break, or I'll break.

I said Death doesn't get breaks.

It makes me realize there needs to be something for Death to turn to for enduring this. Like a counselor for death's job.

I manage to send Lucifer angel 1 back to Death 2. Then I stay pretending like I'm asleep and don't move or respond. But Lucifer angel 1 keeps getting sent back. Then I keep having to protect him from the Gods and Goddesses still trying to kill him and attack me.

I send him back but each time I send one Lucifer angel back, I realize they are there with me again and I have to use my hands to shield them inside.

I ask why they don't stay with Death 2 where I send them.

Ashes to Dust

Lucifer Morningstar angels tell me, Death 2 doesn't exist. I'm the only Death.

So every time I sent them to Death 2, I was sending them straight back to me. That's awful. I didn't realize I wasn't really protecting them.

I have a moment of thought where I should write this down as a good Death story. About Death forgetting she's human.

I keep fighting things off. Then as I lie on my back I swallow something. I only know what it is, and who did it from the Lucifer Angels who spoke through me. Loki made me swallow something.

I think it must be poison but they surprise me by saying he's actually trying to help. It's suppose to be medication for me.

I try to navigate through the interaction with Loki, like I usually do with the others but this time it's more difficult. I have to rely on the Lucifer angels narrating what he's doing or how he reacts to something I say.

They say he wants to heal Death. The insanity from everything like the rape and all the years of enduring others pain of death.

At first it didn't make sense that Loki would want to heal me, until I remembered from posts he helps the broken. And I am that. Though he doesn't know Death is meant to look insane, but remain sane at the same time. It's how I function to trick other beings.

I seem to say or do the wrong thing, and it gets tricky. I know of a few random things from a post about him. The commenter said he liked funny music, so I mentioned that I looked into him and know he liked the Fox song. I mention how I thought it was funny that he left drugs for the guy to sell as a way to get his money.

This seemed to please Loki.

But then, when I mention something about worshiping him, the Lucifer angels said he is mad.

I felt it. Instead of healing, it was pain infliction. It turned out he didn't want my worship. Which was confusing because that's all these dumb Gods and Goddesses want. It's all they ever want.

Loki kept going from trying to heal me and have me swallow medications, to trying to kill me. Then I realized the problem. The reason I was messing up so much, and his decisions kept going back and forth not making sense was because there were two sides to him so he was fighting himself. I won't be able to figure out what he wants. And right now he gave up on me, and is trying to kill me.

I fight him off and the others. I'm sick of all of them. I realize everything should be reset, and I can do it. I threaten them all saying I'm going to reset the world. I have a remote trigger in my hand and hold it up. I want to make it so the Gods and Goddesses aren't in it anymore. So nothing bad is in it anymore.

At first they don't believe me, but don't attack. But then, the gods and goddesses attack me to try to stop it. Loki attempts to steal the remote and when he does succeed the rest think I can't do it anymore.

I laugh at them hysterically, that I, DEATH, am the reset button. And no one can stop me.

They still try for a while but then I manage to reset everything by closing down my arms together. No Gods and Goddesses this time.

I reset everything and at first it seemed fine until there were Gods and Goddesses attacking me again. They don't remember the reset and things that happened before. Just their natural instinct for violence. It starts all over again.

Ashes to Dust

18

Something keeps messing with my reset. I got rid of Gods and Goddesses and the term, "God," to "Gosh." And there was no worship or punishment. But someone brought the Gods back.

I'm stuck pretending to be awestruck by the same pesky "Goddess" from the previous one. I recognize the voice through me. High. Pretty sure it's the one from when Ash once worshiped, but there are so many Gods I'm not sure.

I tell them, "Oh my gosh," and then laugh when I realize at least one thing worked. I would say gosh and never god. I tell them they're so beautiful.

I don't know how to stroke their superiority complex now because of no worshiping and I can't pretend like I'm interested in it like before. I say, "I want to kiss your knees." And then I laugh. They can't see or hear it because as death I conceal it from them. I can choose what they see and what they can't.

They stop trying to kill me, which I only know by feeling and what the Lucifer angels are narrating.

The old Goddess loves that idea and waits to hear more.

Unfortunately they are also impatient and get violent when you aren't throwing constant compliments at them. So for taking too long she starts trying to stab me in the head. Again, only through Lucifer angels do I know.

Ashes to Dust

I go on to say something similar to what I've said before, which they wouldn't remember since this is a reset.

I tell them that I can look online for photos of them and they can choose what's similar and I can draw them or print them out so others can see and know what they actually look like.

The Gods love that idea.

Eventually things turn unwell, and I'm attacked. They make it so my brain is sticking out. I play dead, and of course they don't know I'm actually fine, because I'm Death. But I stay playing, unmoving.

But then one of the gods sticks around with another and their morbid curiosity gets the best of them. They tell the other they want to play with it.

The sick fucks want to play with my brain hanging out. Then I feel it and I hear Lucifer angels narrating, just like I could hear the Gods, through me, that one of them is playing with my brain like a piece of fabric. They are flapping it up and down.

Then the other God joins them, because they want to play with brains.

Sick fuckers.

I wonder how long they are going to stay there playing with my brain. They are attracting attention and I have to do something about it.

I reset again.

Gods and Goddesses don't remember, and they are here again. I'm angry at whoever keeps bringing them back. Worst of all, this time, they brought back Lucifer.

It turns out it's Hannah who messed with this reset. She didn't get her promised life or her unborn children and she's furious.

Now I have to erase her forever. She doesn't realize how much that pains me. She was suppose to be Death's new life too.

I erase Hannah, and I'm upset. So are the Lucifer Morningstar angels.

Ashes to Dust

Lucifer thought he can take over Death's body like old him did to Ash before. He doesn't know I'm Death, and I'm stronger than him. I let him think he has succeeded, when in fact he is now trapped there. He can't get out and reek havoc.

Again I have to entertain so I pretend to be insane and put on a show.

I talk out loud asking what food tastes like. Is it good?

I genuinely forgot. Was it good?

I say out loud it's been so long I don't know. Are there good foods? Did I have a favourite?

I move on to ask what "outside," is when I look at the window to this room covered with a curtain. I can see light through it. I look around and see "colour," and think it's disgusting. I'm saying this all out loud to them. I see the blankness of the ceiling and say I enjoy that. It's blank. But then it starts forming into things and I no longer like it and move on.

I stroke the tent up and down with my hand as I muse on about these things. I look at the feather of the dream catcher, and see the wolves on the big flat surface of the dream catcher. I bonk the feather through the tent screen.

I keep musing on seeming insane to them. Sometimes Lucifer would use my body to make the "crazy" gesture with my hand to my temple. I let him. Timing isn't right.

Then Loki starts playing charades with me so I can understand him. He points to the window and I say different things because I act like I don't know what they are. And in the moment, I don't, because I'm Death putting on a act.

He points at me using my hand. I guess a few times, then after he moves on to point at the curtain covering the window. I don't know it's a window. In my confusion he would point to lift the curtain then slide the window.

I pretend to play along, knowing full well what they're doing in the back of my sane mind. I'm not going to do what they want, but I have to pretend to not get it so it's drawn out. They're distracted. Then he used my two fingers to go in a walk motion, and then a stop, and a jump.

I would sometimes say things right, never saying the to jump off kill yourself part which they obviously wanted. I would sometimes ask what do I jump into. They make me shrug. They keep doing the charade so many times, I move on and act like I forgot.

I'm surprised when at some points Lucifer uses my other hand and has one finger wagging no, not to do it. Other times he would just get impatient and cross my legs and have them bouncing.

I would entertain them further and ask if I can fly like a bird. Sometimes I would ask what happens next. I eventually get tired of it and I laugh and say I'm not going out the fucking window. And change the topic constantly only to have the scene repeated.

It always repeats just like with my previous entertainment of telling them to look and admire themselves in the mirror on a loop.

A few times I put Lucifer in his place when he thinks he can control me. If he crossed my legs, I uncross them. I control him, and tell him, "I'm fucking death, you can't control me."

He never gets it and tries with each repeat. Even when I made him do stuff instead like stilling his motions. I only did it after being irritated after so many times everything has been repeated.

I'm Death but I get irritated.

Ashes to Dust

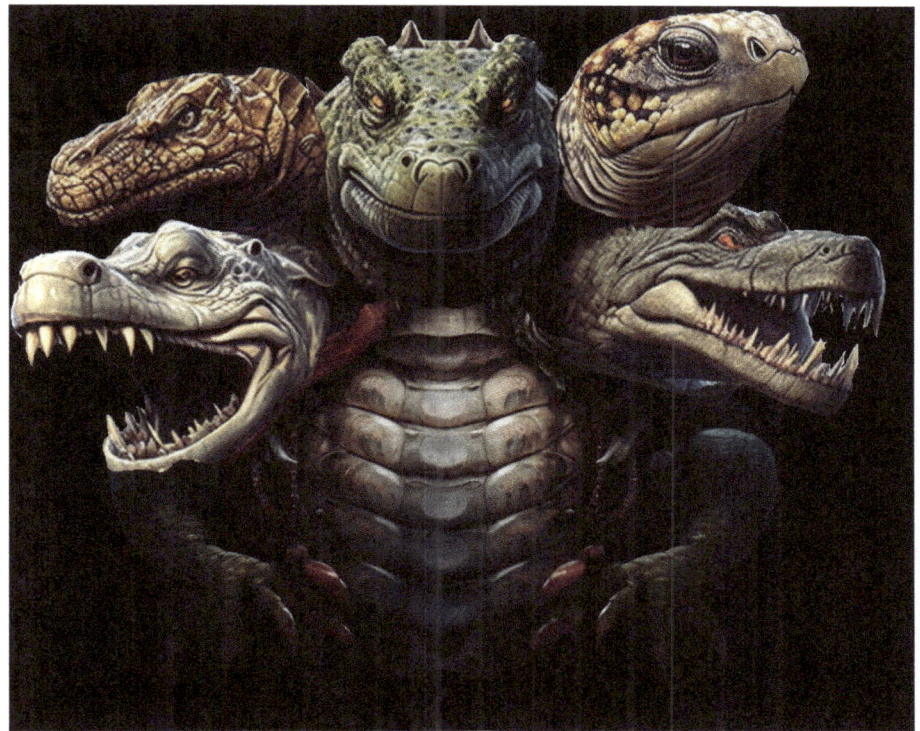

I have to get rid of Lucifer. I know he has many parts to him. I think of what ones from previous experience. I know the two alligators, and tortoise. I can't get rid of Lucifer by banishing or destroying him by the name Lucifer Morningstar because that's not each part's name. That's them as a whole.

Through my knowing and trial and error I manage to guess the names of a few and get rid of the alligators, tortoise and was finally left with only one. I try a name and get it wrong. I don't know what it is.

Finally it comes to me. Lucifer Gate. It's the final piece that held them all together. Possibly what they came from.

The Lucifer angels talk through me, and I hear them gasping and asking if I even know what it is. They aren't asking me directly, but to one another, out loud. They aren't aware that I hear them. Sometimes they are but they forget again because it has to be that way with Death.

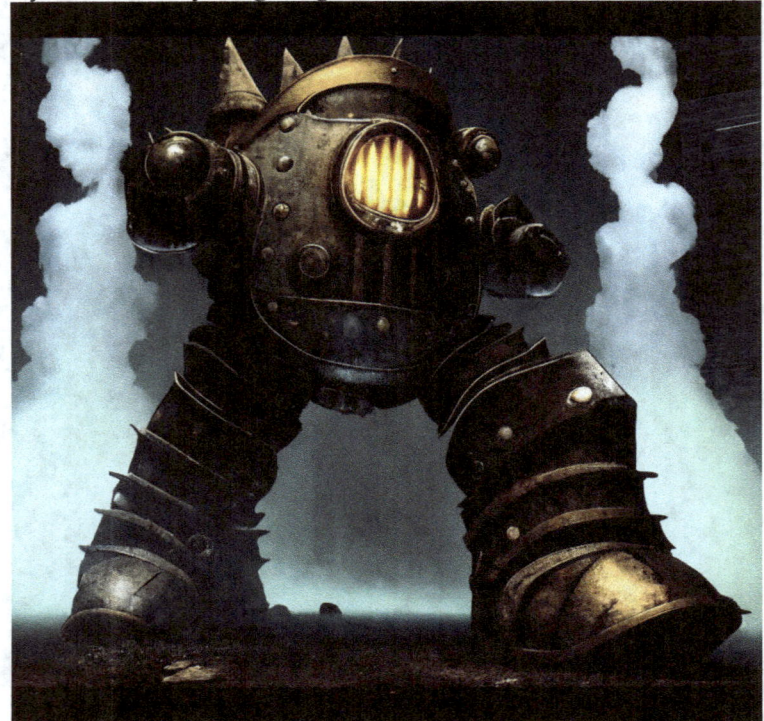

I aim my arrows at Lucifer Gate. I have a knowing of what it looks like. It's a giant thing that looks almost like a menacing golden, rusted tea pot by it's shape, but the middle has a handle like a door. It's not a tea pot shape but it's the closest to what I can think matches it. It has thick armoured-like legs.

With every arrow I aim, I say what I'm taking away. I take away its sadness, and shoot the arrow.

The Lucifer angels keep making me think I'm doing something wrong with each thing I take away.

I don't understand it. Is it making it stronger if I take these things away? Is it meant to stay angry, violent, sad, fearful, be able to punish? I keep aiming and shoot the arrows. I take away its ability to punish, I take away its anger, and it stills.

I think I succeeded and maybe it's something that isn't bad. I don't know what it's a gate to. But maybe it's misunderstood and me taking these negative things away will reveal its something better and was just tainted by being Lucifer Morningstar.

I start doubting that when I worry I'm making it worse and might allow it to open by taking these things away. And I don't know what it holds. The Lucifer angels are the doubt that keep speaking and I hear.

Lucifer Gate steps on my neck, and I know by the Lucifer angels.

It's heavy, and I have to hold its leg just enough that it doesn't completely crush this neck, but not enough to show my true strength to it. I let it think it has the upper hand, and then by using its name, Lucifer Gate, I manage to destroy it with another arrow to the center of its gate.

The horsey's I got rid of came back. I am mad of all things they brought those nasty things back. I got rid of them. There were more than one and they kept coming for me. They wanted to eat me, and attacked my head. Their bites hurt. They enjoy when something else causes me pain, or they cause me pain, because I hear their horse laughs through me that are soft.

I let some eat my brain, and then after I stop them after successfully infecting them with Death's insanity. I test it by singing, "Insane in the membrane." And they would involuntarily sing the rest of the, "insane in the brain," through their horsey snorts. (Since they can't speak.)

It made me laugh, and they would sometimes laugh like a evil cartoon dog laugh.

Then I would convince them to eat one another.

Ashes to Dust

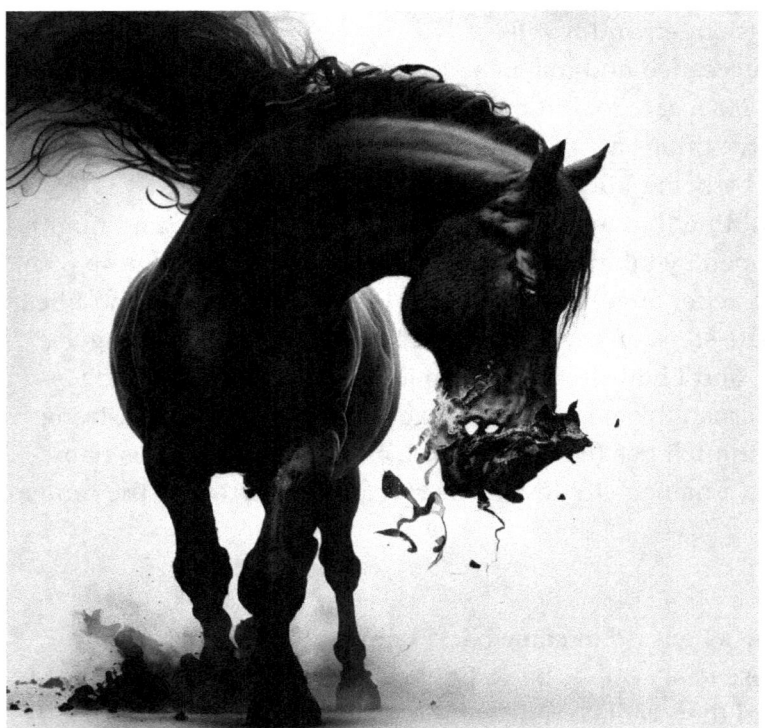

I told them they looked delicious and that they should eat the other horse.

They would nod my head excitedly, huffing ya, and then it was carnage of horses eating horses. A secret I knew they did before, where one came from the other. But I knew them eating one another was permanent.

I'm glad to be rid of them; they're pesky.

When Gods and Goddesses try to act like they were coming back, I reveal I was the one making horsey sounds all along after they already ate each other. I tricked them. They got scared of me, knowing Death's power, and they were trying to convince me not to reset things again.

I tell them I gave them chances and gifts to be able to evolve and learn to understand humans, and treat them better but they chose not to. They chose to be stuck in their violent, barbaric ways of killing what doesn't worship them, even some that do, and punishing. I'm sick of it.

Loki is multiplying, and I start using my powers to cut off his wings, and rip his clones apart. He taunts saying I missed, but I say I know I didn't.

Though this body can't see where he is, but me, Death, in here I know where they are located. One I manage to get turns into two, and they manage to get into my body, hoping to take over.

I grab Loki and keep him in one of my hands. I shook him to keep him from trying to leave and made him finish singing the 2nd line in the chorus to "Insane in the brain," by Cypress Hill.

I would sing the first line of the chorus and each Goddess or Loki copy would finish each word to form, the 2nd line to the chorus. It made me laugh each time. Loki would groan and hate it. He knew I did it after a while, but he still couldn't stop it.

Loki planted some of his copies in me by making me swallow them or them going through my eyes or nose.

The Loki in my hand would wait until he thought I completely lost it and then using my eyes, the Loki's in me would wink at the Gods and Goddesses outside of me to signal them I was vulnerable.

It was a trap and I would tell him I don't like stupid things. A sentence they've heard many times, but forget, except for Loki. I realize with each loop of his attempts, or reboot, he would remember eventually. I found that odd. And wondered why I didn't just crush him in my hand. I think I wanted entertainment. I'm sick of entertaining them all the time and want to laugh.

It would start again, where I would shake the hand Loki was in, or put him in a different one if that one got tired. I would bang it against the pillow if he was being a pain or his cloned copies were being

Ashes to Dust

irritating because he was sending them.

I would keep saying you know I hate stupid things but you still keep trying with the winking. I would show my point that I was in charge, because I'm Death, by winking at all of his clones and everyone else around the room.

Through me he would voice, holy shit, or he would remember that I hated stupid things, and he was being one of those stupid things by trying over and over again.

I played peek-a-boo on Loki by using my free hand to make a circle with my index and thumb fingers together, and looked through it. I looked at him through it and because he had other Loki's in me, he freaked out in my hand because they all saw it in a strange 3D fish bowl type style.

Sometimes I would change it up and they could look at him from me looking at a different part of the room. It terrified him, and he would beg me to stop.

I thought it was hilarious. And I would start up the insane in the brain song again and they would all sing to it. Every time he forgot, I would make them sing the song, and he would remember the deja vu, and say not again.

It cracked me up every time. It was the most fun I had all day.

He would still be stupid, and try and try again at signaling the other Gods and Goddesses. It was the most annoying part. They don't get it. Death is stronger than them. Death can't be controlled. They all think they're stronger than Death, but they're not.

I got concerned when Loki started being able to see-through my facial facades, and know the real face I'm making, or truly feeling irritated or mad. I didn't understand why he was able to, but I thought it had something to do with how he was a God of trickery. So he too could see through tricks. He doesn't know all of Death's, but he has become a concern now he seems to remember things, and know the true faces and feelings I have while pretending to be peppy to the

Ashes to Dust

other Gods and Goddesses.

I am surprised that he started to not like what the others were doing to me. Like the rape monster.

I realize there was a reason why I never killed Loki and why he keeps coming back. He's apart of something. He actually is evolving a bit.

Then he tries to help me after I let him go.

He says oh no, he's stuck.

Just like what happened to make Lucifer become the Lucifer angels. But this felt different. It wasn't like he was meant to be a lover or romantic. I have no idea what he's suppose to be to me. Just that unfortunately I can't destroy him because he's meant to be some sort of gift to me later. He's meant to be involved. Possibly in a later reincarnation.

The Lucifer angels aren't happy about a third that is of all people Loki. They mention his past wrong doings, of being a attempted rapist himself.

I have to try to get them to stop fighting. Loki is actually trying. Something in him changed. It's the one thing I wanted for them, to evolve. And feel.

He regrets his past actions. I know there's nothing that can be changed, and I'm busy focused on other things right now.

I can feel the Lucifer angels, it's like they think of him as another lover in the mix. Competition. Childish.

Ashes to Dust

19

I heard a high pitched squeak sound. It stole another innocent again. I analyze this relentless being. I put my hands up and make my fingers in a position where there's a big rectangular gap in the middle, like movie directors do. I start sucking it out of existence. I see the layers inside it. There's a animal in there. To gain power this being stole innocent animal lives. Dogs and cats. That's what the squeak sound was. A dead animal that this thing sucked the soul out of and harvested for its powers.

There are so many layers to it. I have to take a break and try again. I open my unblinking eyes, open my mouth mouth wide, and stop the body's breathing so I, Death, can destroy this horrible monster once and for all. Another layer gets sucked down, and it gets smaller. It peels away as I'm slowly unraveling its secrets. I have to breathe so this borrowed body doesn't stop functioning.

I see a little boy. It's the first innocent soul it took. It started with this little boy's soul. I'm so upset. This thing is beyond disgusting. It shouldn't exist in this world. It was created.

I tell Mike (the Grim Reaper) what I'm seeing.

He's disgusted too.

I see a orb, and realize it's the collection of innocents. Of virginity. I'm even more repulsed. It got this strong, big, and unkillable, because it's taken souls of children and animals, and virginities. It's no wonder

Ashes to Dust

I hate it so much. Why it's so hard to kill and get rid of.

The Lucifer Morningstar angels don't think I should stop breathing.

I tell them I, Death, don't need to breathe.

They are worried about this body's needs.

I tell them I have to, so I can suck this thing out of existence once and for all.

I unravel the last layer. A professor. This is the man behind it all. This man created this disgusting being that is beyond monstrous. That should never have existed in any lifetime. The professor took the boy's soul and harvested it to create this raping and killing being.

I'm disgusted again. This thing is becoming much smaller but I can't stare at its brightness any longer. I blink and lose the connection. I have to breathe for the body again. It's taking too long to get it all down. Mike is making sure it will never come back from his end. Since we've had too many close calls before with people interfering.

He's also disgusted by the news that someone created it.

I get ready to do it again; I'm so close. I settle back into the pillow and hold my hands up in the same director position and suck it down into oblivion. I see a new layer of truth and secrets. The one that hired the professor to create this horrible thing, was Infinity. I realized the whole time saying things I would always use "for infinity" at the end. Even I, in my previous reincarnations, were manipulated by Infinity. Even using the infinity sign.

I breathe again and tell Mike my findings. This is worse than I thought. There's still more to this monster, that use to be called Higher Power. But now it's a lot smaller. More manageable. I have to find a way to destroy the rest of it. Then I feel the sensation between my legs. It's not pleasant. It's trying to rape this body. Take its innocence.

The Lucifer Morningstar angels talk through me commenting on what it's doing to me. They are disgusted and trying to find a way to help me. They know it's my job to take it and act like it's pleasurable, or not destroying me internally, if it means protecting the world from

Ashes to Dust

it. Distracting it even for a moment.

I hide behind Ash's soul so the creature won't notice Death's presence. If it notices me, it might try to kill us permanently. Ash's soul signed up for this. To protect. She lent me her body. I'm hidden in Ash so with every rape the creature dies more. But Ash is also protected. It can't kill her permanently.

The Lucifer angels tell Mike to do something. That I can't do this again. That I shouldn't have to.

I feel myself darkening, but I tell them it's fine, I'm Death. It's enjoying death sperm.

The Lucifer Morningstar angels gasp in realization. They comment on how it's getting smaller, melting into the black acidic goo of death sperm. They ask Mike if it realizes what she is, or that it's melting by doing that to her.

Mike says he thinks it realizes what she is, but it isn't sure because the body she's disguised in is a virgin, human. So the squeaking is it trying to take, and rub away the innocents of the body.

The creature changes tactic, and crushes Ash. I listen to the Lucifer angels talking to figure out how far to act like Ash's dead and when to act like she's slowly coming back to life when the creature starts realizing it killed a good thing and attempts to bring her back.

When it thinks it brought Ash back, it gains more confidence, it feels stronger. I hear it all through the Lucifer angels that it wants to start again even though it just crushed Ash to death.

Despite Ash playing her part, and acting like she's terrified because she has a huge headache, and thinks the creature did something to her. It starts raping again. I make sure anything the creature does to break Ash, I put her back together.

It rapes too hard, and it starts shaking Ash's body to heal her back in tact. It wants that squeak again.

Lucifer angels comment how it enjoys the challenge of not breaking Ash, because she was raped by her dad and it feels that. It's why half

Ashes to Dust

of her is numb and it's so hard for it. It doesn't know Ash and Death don't enjoy this.

Death is playing the part for Ash, while Ash helps conceal my presence from it. It would be dangerous if it finds out.

The Lucifer angels comment how it is trying to go at different angles because her dad made it difficult. And that's why she still has the innocence, because it was rape by her dad as a child.

It's weighing both of us down. Ash is playing her part but it's triggering. It's unpleasant. But it's working. We both want it to stop.

Again the Lucifer angels comment on making it stop.

I tell them I'm fine, in a dull voice. That it's my job, "I'm deaaaath."

I feel worse with every rape. The only person who can stop this monster, is death. And no one can do the job. No one wants the job. I don't want anyone to suffer.

I'm swapped out. Not even Ash's soul is there anymore. Mike took over the body. I'm shocked he did. I'm now voicing through the body he's taken over.

He says he can take over for me. That I don't need to do it anymore. He's willingly taking over the job of Death. He is new Death.

Ashes to Dust

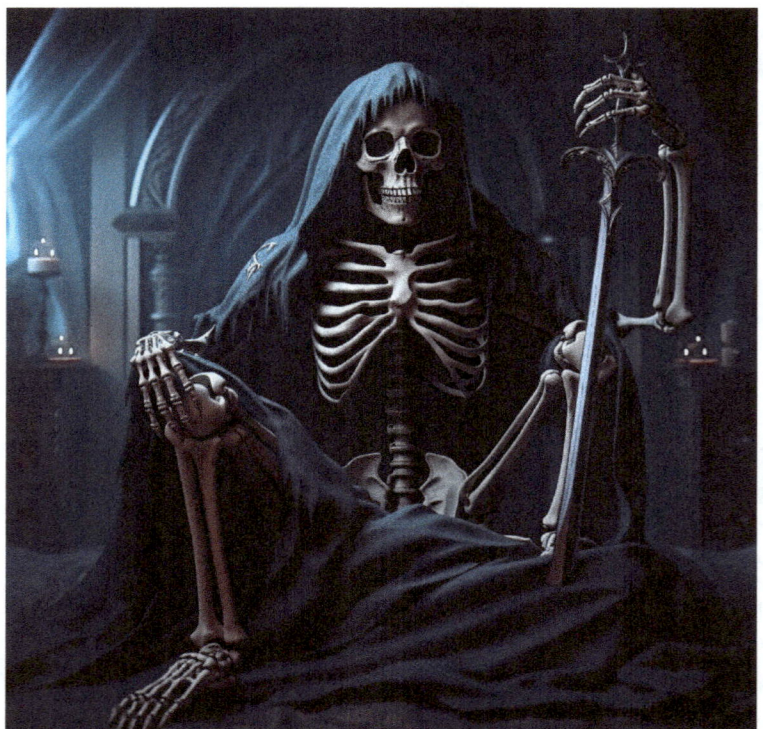

He seems to be into it. He's a natural at pretending. He's watched me play the pretend game a lot, and he's good at masking himself. Mike is more laid back. He has the bodies arms behind his head, like he's relaxed and the creature isn't trying enough to please him. Mike is doing a good job at motivating it to try to go harder. Wasting itself away the harder it tries.

The Lucifer angels comment on if it realizes it's killing itself by trying so hard.

I don't think it cares.

They agree.

It seems to have really taken a liking to Mike. It starts shaking him. I can feel what Mike is feeling since I was connected to the body he's in before.

Ashes to Dust

Mike laughs in his deep voice. He thinks the shaking is fun. Then he feels something in his chest and he doesn't understand. It is a weird pain, but warmth. A stabbing feeling.

One of the Lucifer angels comment uh oh.

Mike responds with what.

He doesn't understand. They say the creature realizes it isn't the same person anymore. It knows he's a Grim Reaper. It's healing him.

I'm just as shocked as Mike is.

Mike laughs. All he's known is being skeleton, skull and bones. Like me, Death. But he's never been in a body before. He's never owned a body to his knowledge. He doesn't get how it can heal him. I don't either. This creature is much stronger and diverse than we realized.

Mike feels more strange sensations, in his belly, and shoulders. He's starting to get a knowing, as Death. That he's growing organs. Growing skin. Human skin. We were once human. Mike was once human before becoming a Grim Reaper. We both realize now. He doesn't know what to make of that. It's confusing.

The Lucifer angels comment again that Mike needs to prepare himself. He asks why. They say because its never had a Grim Reaper before. Its excited. They say Mike's a virgin.

Mike gets shaken more to be healed, to be turned human. He starts to realize what it's doing now. It's reversing his Grim Reaper appearance back to before when it was human. He falls into their category of innocence. Once they completely heal him, essentially bringing him back to human body life, he will be a virgin.

Mike laughs nervously at the Lucifer angels comments. He doesn't get why they warned him to prepare. He gets a knowing that he's growing balls.

Oh shit. The creature healed him enough to make him grow back male genitals. How is that going to work? Is it going to rape him in the butt? Is it going to create a vagina? Will it just … be? I'm worried for Mike now too. I don't know what will happen. He seems extra nervous too. First day on the job and this is what happens to him.

Mike gets a knowing that he's a bald man. And the creature has run itself ragged trying to please them to get their virginity, and then heal Mike back to a human body to attempt to take his. That it's almost completely gone.

Lucifer angels comment how they are amazed that it doesn't care that it's basically black goo now. It wants Mike so bad, because it wants Mike to experience pleasure from it. They tell Mike to prepare now that his male genitals are complete.

Mike gets a nervous, serious, still half smirk face going all at once when he asks why.

The cockiness disappeared once he started growing human organs and flesh again. Being able to feel cold and hot and pain. I'm worried for him. I don't know if I should step in, but I can't. I know I can't take it.

Mike steels himself, gripping the pillow behind him, wondering what sensation he's going to feel and how this is going to happen. He really is a virgin.

He doesn't have to know. The creature is gone. It melted the rest of the way before it could attempt to finish trying to steal Mike's new virginity. I'm relieved for Mike's sake it couldn't try. I'm also thankful he went through all of that. Even coming back to human flesh, to protect me. No one else could do this job but him. I believe is perfect.

Ashes to Dust

20

I am going to reset the world. But first I need to make sure nothing taints it, not even me. I notice my one hand is making circles, and betraying me. It's trying to summon something. My body keeps betraying me. I warn the other parts of my body that if anything tries to create things that shouldn't be in the world, even one of my arms or legs, I will cut it off.

Ashes to Dust

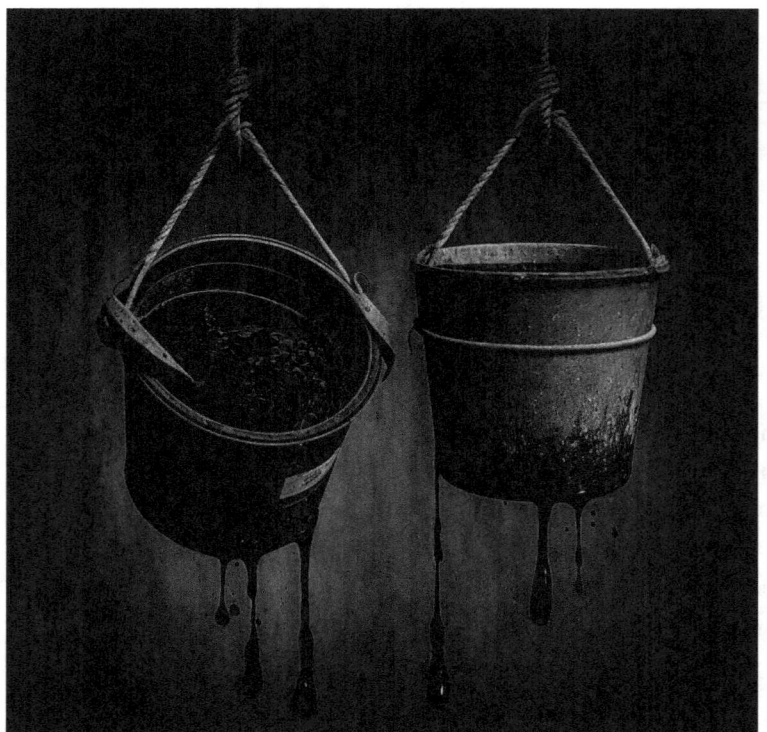

I can picture the buckets of black acid hanging above me. I instruct the bucket to pour over, and I melt off my left hand. Now it can't do what it was doing. I regrow a new one in its place. I hear the terrified shocked reactions of Lucifer angel and Loki. I don't care if they're watching. But I still have to keep Death's secrets to myself. So every time they see or hear something they shouldn't, I have to erase their memories of it, and undo that.

Ashes to Dust

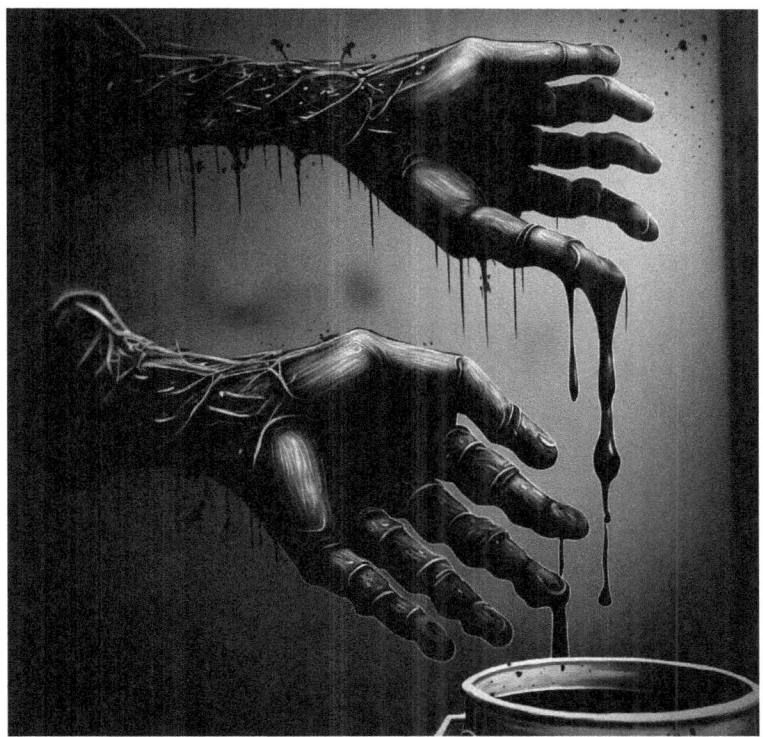

My hand is doing it again, and this time I melt off my right hand. I can picture it in my knowing. My skeletal hand, melting into black goo, and vanishing until it slowly regrows into a new skeleton hand. I'm trying to keep balance so things won't be chaotic, so I keep having to melt parts of me. It becomes so bad where it's infecting my brain and self. I have to instruct bucket one and two to pour over my head. My skeleton head melts off and regrows.

Lucifer angel asks if it hurts.

I tell him no, I never feel the pain of it. I'm accustomed to it.

Right now when I do my hands I feel tiny snaps of nerves shoot up my arms as I melt them away. I can see it in my knowing that my skeleton hands swing back and forth, loose, ready to fall off, until they melt away. Disintegrate into nothing, leaving me with arm stumps. It

Ashes to Dust

doesn't take long to regrow them.

I even pour the acid over my whole body when I don't trust it. I'm terrifying Lucifer angel and Loki. They can see what's happening. What I have to do to myself to stop anything else from undoing what I need done.

The buckets that hold the acid get tainted too, and I have to get rid of them. I can disintegrate myself without them. I do so by visualizing melting my hands off, just like before. It works.

Sometimes through Lucifer angel's commentary I will hear that I did it without needing to. But I didn't know, and it will grow back.

I end up saying things I'm not suppose to say, and showing them things I'm not suppose to. I undo it, multiple times. I'm told by a different Death, that's also me, just one that can destroy me as a Death fail safe if I malfunction. It's how I knew some things after my hand started turning.

The other Death tells me if I fuck up one more time, then she will destroy me for good.

But I wasn't doing things intentionally, and had to prove it. My other Death self saw that, and realized I couldn't help it. She said I was loosing it.

Lucifer angel asked if I was allowed to do the things I was doing.

My other death self said I wasn't doing anything intentionally, so yes. But she's there just in case to clean up the mess and make sure everything isn't revealed. She mentioned how I'm so far gone, that I really am insane now. That I can ruin my own happiness by showing them things accidentally.

In this time I managed to rip off the band aid at one point that those power-hungry guardians put there. It was sealing all my true powers. It's why I couldn't have things reset properly in my other reincarnations, or as Death. They wanted to rule over death, and were afraid of my powers so they blocked them. They knew I could destroy them because they weren't more powerful than me, I was more powerful than them. They are why things were still wonky.

Now I can get rid of every God and Goddess, and bad creature, or every creature that isn't human and animal. I can make it now so they have their happiness without sickness or violence, or worship. I already had the other death sort out boxes. There are keep boxes. The good animals go in the keep. The humans go in the keep treasure boxes too. I don't want them to ever have to one day start over so I also add their architecture and technology.

I don't put Gods, leprechauns, fairies, and more bad things in the treasure boxes. They will be erased. With the band aid removed I realize I'm more than Death.

I'm Universe.

It shook the other things remaining to hear.

I am being attacked by the Gods and Goddesses and other creatures that don't want to be erased.

I told them I wanted to reset things. But I told them I gave them all a chance. It was the ultimate last chance test. They failed. They even triggered Insanity mode because they were so bad. They didn't grow or learn. I'm tired of giving out chances and having things undone. I deserve to rest. That's all I want is to rest.

I'm going to rest. I haven't once rested since creation. I tell them, every thing will go dark, and I will sleep.

They wonder when things will start up.

I say they won't. I'm taking a break. Indefinitely. So everything will be on rest with me. Sleeping in the dark.

They're trying to stop me as my arms close down in reset. Half the world is already gone. Half the gods and creatures already not existing now. The chosen are in boxes, safe to rest. The human family here, and the gods that tried attacking me in this room with me are now all that's left. They can't even get Lovie, because she too is on rest in a box. So will the family in a moment.

They change tactic. Some leave to outrun the black curtain, others try to find a way to make me not want to give up.

Even Loki shows up to try to help get me.

Other death tells them I am still Death so if they prove themselves I would stop.

They start attacking me and it hurts. But it's apparently love. I only know that once I yank it out and I almost throw up as I dry heave. It's a interesting tactic.

Some aren't love, and I hear other death yell why did they do something stupid.

That's all they know to do. Is hurt. They don't want to change. This proves it.

Loki is multiplying, and trying to have the other Loki's send love arrows at me too. I change things up and deflect it.

Loki disappoints me by attacking me for real. Not with love, to fill me with love anymore, but a real attack. It was confirmed when I pulled out the arrow and had no reaction. I got rid of him too.

It was a long fight before and now it's empty, and I almost close my arms together as I count down to reset and make everything go on a indefinite break.

Ashes to Dust

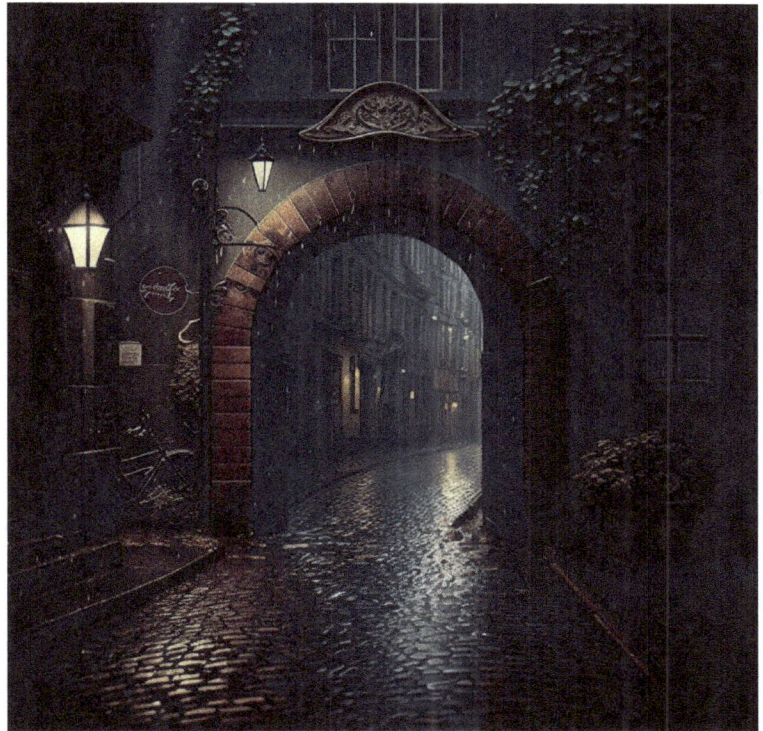

The body is in Ash's bedroom, but the battle is happening on a old, medieval looking cobblestone road. It has a arch where my opponents come through.

Then Lucifer showed up. It surprised me. It wasn't one of the ones that changed into good. It wasn't any of the ones I defeated. It was original, bad Lucifer. That was brought back again like many others that hasn't been destroyed yet. Considering he's not a good guy, I am surprised to see him be here to try to stop me. Not attack me to stop me either, but in the help me way. That's not in his nature.

Unfortunately I have to give everyone a chance, because I'm Death, and fair. Even him. I don't make it easy. He knows. When I pull one of the love arrows out and gag, Lucifer tells me I should stop doing that.

Ashes to Dust

I laugh that he would say that.
He says I need it.
That's funny.
He's telling me I need love. That's why it hurts to pull out.
I'm going to keep pulling them out.
Other death warns him I won't make it easy.
He says he knows, he's seen.

I'm creative, I will think of things to outwit him. I will get my break. He keeps getting through and I don't like feeling like I'm going to throw up. I feel even worse, just like he said when I try to yank it out. I have to leave some in unfortunately because it's worse pain to pull them out.

I make it so I have gloves that go over my hands to block it. When one gets through I have to make the gloves stronger material, and then I have full body armour.

He makes a audible noise of displeasure through me.

He then adapts. Of all of them, he was the one that became the most adaptable. I'm not happy about this. I tell him he can just give up. I count down, but he doesn't. Somehow he gets through and shoots me.

Then other death betrays me. Does something she wasn't suppose to. Attacks me. I don't know why, but it's not the first time. She tried to bring back the tainted acid buckets to pour over me. I stop her, because I'm in the right. I'm Death that knows.

I have to erase her. I wasn't expecting having to do it, since she was created to end me, not the other way around. But that's what death is for. If I have to take out my other self because they did wrong, I do. Just like when I cut off my legs and arms and poured acid over them before.

I need to think better so I create clones of myself. One has a windmill to block incoming arrows, while I think what else I can create.

Lucifer makes more noise.

I wasn't expecting him to adapt so fast again. He keeps getting better

Ashes to Dust

and faster at adapting to me. I don't like it. I create multiple arms to block them, but he adjusts the arrows too. Somehow it seems like he's everywhere at once, getting me in the back too. Then I feel something. He attacked me too. Not love, but a real attack. They all do in the end.

I say that, and I hear protest. Then I say that's it, and I close my arms together like one is a dropping guillotine. But nothing happens.

I wonder if it takes a few moments, but then nothing happens. I know we are still in the stadium of battle with a medieval gate. But the air to it is still, and different. Then I feel a arrow and gag.

It was a trick. I got tricked by my own mind. I thought Lucifer betrayed me, and tried to kill me because I've had it done so many times. It's confirmed when he is still there, and the permanent reset didn't happened. It would have if he did in fact try to kill me.

He says that it was all in my head. I was losing it.

He has so many arrows put in me now. He aimed a dozen or so at once at the human body heart. I can't pull them all out it's impossible. It hurts too much if I try, which I do. He doesn't stop there. The bastard. He knows I would've tried eventually. He knows it is enough, and I ask him to do no more, but he doesn't listen.

I'm hunched over, unable to move. He did it. Now I have to give the world another chance. Because if Lucifer of all beings can adapt and change for the better, then it's the proof I wanted since creation.

I am full of love arrows. He doesn't care they hurt.

He tells me not to take them out.

I already know I can't. I'm worn out.

I know what I have to do now. I manage to lie back down, and tell him that for him being the only one to successfully help me and not attack me outside of love, that he is rewarded. I tell him he too is missing something, and I will reward him with it. But I tell him he can't ever break off from his other parts. He has to be whole with them all, as Lucifer Morningstar or he won't be the same. He won't get what he wants because it will end badly. I ask him if he can agree to these

Ashes to Dust

terms.

Lucifer agrees. He seems happy about what I have to offer. Feeling that he is missing something. He wants to feel whole too.

Love. I tell him the one he's meant to be with as his reward, is going to be a hard road. If he's willing to fight for it, and pursue then he will get the love he always wanted. That he's been missing.

Oh fuck I realize I'm the one that dooms myself with being linked to Lucifer. His actions here are what have me realize he's the love Death needs, and he needs Death. Me. This is awful for me to know I did all this to myself. But I also know, I can't undo it. That it's meant to happen. I'm the universe that set it up for my happiness this way. I'm that fucking cloud sending encrypted codes to myself and the Lucifer angels that I ended up destroying.

I tell him a code word. One that the cloud use to say all the time. The secret code language to keep me from completely knowing. Even if I had a guess.

At first he's confused and then he says it sounds familiar. He then asks why does he know that word.

I ask him if he wants it or not.

He said he does, but he doesn't know why.

Now he understands how hard it's going to be. He's seen all the betrayal, the rapes, the never resting. How I react to love. He makes a noise, one similar to what I use to hear the Lucifer angels make when they realize things just got harder for them. He gets the hard road ahead.

I ask if he still thinks it'll be worth it.

He surprises me with a yes.

21

Death can't have babies, yet this "Higher Power" still tries to get me pregnant. It uses baby cries as a way to make me want them. But the cries only fuel my anger and resolve to keep fighting it off.

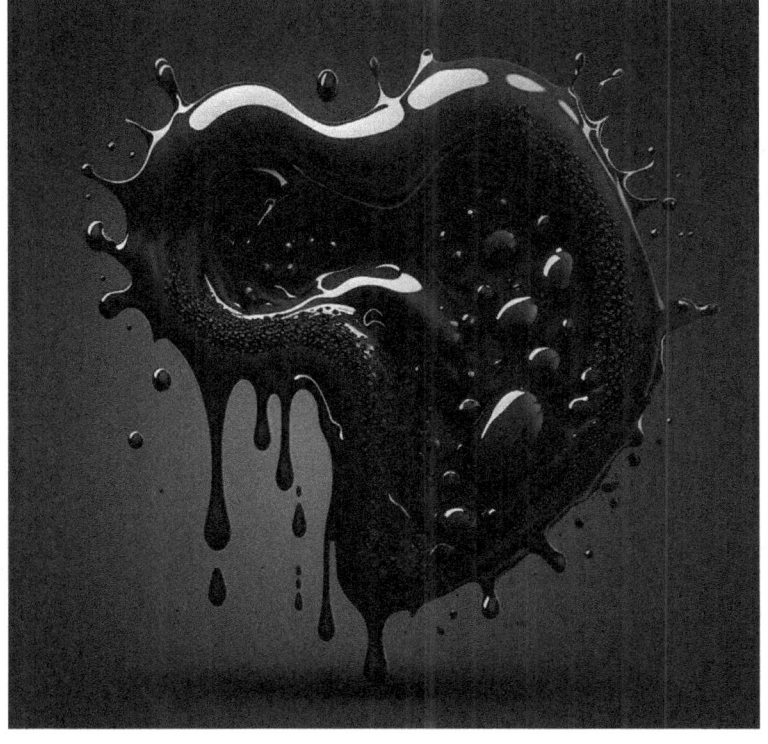

Ashes to Dust

To keep dissolving the babies in my stomach acid. Black acid, I get a knowing about my self. I don't like the cries of babies. I never have. It doesn't make me want them, it makes me think of horror film scenes with the sounds in it.

It doesn't get that because I'm death, the babies it's trying to make me have are all dead anyways. But it keeps trying to impregnate me through rape, or if I'm too quick to dissolve them, then it tries to get me to swallow them. As a way to get pregnant faster. Sometimes it's trying to be cruel by making it seem like they're my babies and I'm eating them alive. It makes me harder on the inside. Emotionally.

Lucifer warns me not to swallow and if I swallowed something I shouldn't have. I can hear him through me. I can't always help it. I can't always close my mouth, and I need to breathe through it. Or it catches me at a time I'm spitting out what it just tried to make me swallow.

I move what it made me swallow to my head with my hand. I hear Lucifer gasp, and wonder if I knew what I just did. And that I just moved it to my brain and melted my brain. I then move them to the correct spot and guide it using my hand from my head to my stomach acid.

It tries to keep taunting with sounds of baby cries. It's trying to make me think I'm killing them alive and hoping I'll cave and want them.

I told it Death can't have babies but it doesn't listen. It still tries through rape or making me swallow eggs or whatever it is it keeps them in. It thinks because it's some powerful sun eye god, that if it makes babies with Death, then the children will be all powerful and it can rule.

My stomach will sometimes rise like pregnant if I'm not fast enough to catch them. And it'll be happy about it. Even when I tell it nothing alive is growing in there. It doesn't know it's just another trick by death. I squash that happiness by showing it how I'm going to melt them in my death stomach. I let it hear the screams. Another trick by

Ashes to Dust

death. They aren't even alive. They never were. It's not possible.

Me letting it think there are sounds of its dying rape babies echoing in pain, angers it. It retaliates, and tries to make me eat live babies. It makes me think I'm eating my own babies. I'm death. I don't care. I can't care. I eat what it sends, even when I try not to. I then proceed to moving it to my stomach to dissolve. Sometimes accidentally moving them to my brain and dissolving both again and again. Until Lucifer angel reminds me I dissolved my brain again.

I laugh about it and keep going to the proper place.

It rapes again, not understanding between my thighs is death's sperm. There's no living reproductive system for it to penetrate and reproduce in. It makes it unpleasant to feel it's nasty sun energy penetrating. I hate it. Lucifer doesn't know what to do for me. I put a empty sports bottle between my legs and it pissed it off even more. It couldn't rape me properly. It still tried, either through the sides, or under but it wasn't working like it wanted.

It kept trying to feed me babies and overwhelm me with sounds. Especially now that it didn't like that bottle in the way.

Lucifer laughed about the bottle in the way. But it isn't stopping it completely. It keeps trying to find ways. And it starts impatiently snapping in my ears.

Lucifer helps me hide from the twisted Higher Power. He covers my face, and slows my breathing to lower my heart rate so it can't sense me. It snaps in my ears to try to find me. If the snaps are further away, it's further away. That's how Lucifer and I know it's safe to start moving a bit. Breathing more. It's desperate to find me, and the snapping continues. The snap of rape time, right here and now.

I listen to Lucifer, and he does his best to protect me. I'm surprised he's doing this. No one helps death. Then it finds me. By my eyes, not covered enough. Or breathing too loud, I don't know. It got hard to breathe when my hands were covering my face.

Ashes to Dust

I feel the intense energy well up between my thighs. It brings on the negative emotions. It's raping me again. It's unpleasant. I want it to stop. But there's nothing I can do.

Lucifer hides me again. But the twisted sun eye is persistent and relentless. It won't stop. It keeps snapping trying to find me. I lay still and quiet. Lucifer is hiding me, but I think it discovered the body, and it starts raping again. It reminds me of how it would see through when I would try to get a break from distracting it, and discover me through the death shroud that was suppose to prevent them from seeing what I was really doing, or expressing. It found me anyways.

This time Lucifer took on the rape. I didn't know what to say I was so surprised. I told him he didn't have to do that. He said he would, I've done it enough.

I didn't want to argue with him or persuade him not to, because I didn't want to go through the raping anymore. I felt bad but I had to try to push that aside and let him do it for me, so I could carry on. It was also conflicting because of who he use to be karmatically as the previous bad Lucifer. I didn't know if he deserved it to atone for the things he did before, or not. I didn't like to think like that. Rape isn't good. But it's nice to get a break.

It moved on when Lucifer didn't react as expected to the rape. It began snapping again. Sometimes frequent sometimes less. I wondered if it was trying to trick us. Trick me. When it did find me, either by us moving or me peeking through my fingers to make sure we were clear, Lucifer was taking on the rape instead. It was awkward being the backseat passenger knowing he was being raped. I didn't know if he would be okay. But I knew I wouldn't be.

PART SIX
THE LOKIS'

Ashes to Dust

22

I'm in the bathroom after letting only the good things out in the world. I pet my pretty kitty and eat her soul to protect her. Because unfortunately, again, some Gods got back through. I can tell she's different when she follows me in the bathroom. I can always tell when she has no soul. She seems robotic, and she looks less filled with life. Her fur to her eyes seem almost dull. Like she's on autopilot. I feed her and she hops up on the tower and eats.

Some Gods and Goddesses fly in the bathroom with me, bothering me. One is the high-pitched one.

My son Loki can see what's happening, but he's in my headquarters. It's like a black void. Observing Death's work. I thought I should show him some of Death's tricks if one day he will be the heir. Possibly doing the same job. But I won't tell him much. It's still my duty to keep things balanced and secret.

He took finding out Death is his mother and that's why he was meant to be with me well when he found out. He realized it's exactly what he was missing. To be loved by a mother as a child. I didn't know how to react to it, though. Especially with how his behaviour was in previous encounters.

The high pitched Goddess flies in and wants to find a way by hurting me. I use my index finger and thumb to make a circle for my game of peek-a-boo. It's how I can see them, even if the body's eyes can't, I know their location and direct them. They learned I have a son. I feign being scared, saying not to go into the portal and hurt him.

It's a bright portal I created, and she's drawn to it like a bug to a light. She gets excited at my fake horror, and flies into it.

I laugh. She's gone.

Two God's come in and threaten my son's life. They say that they'd find my son and kill him to get back at me for what I did. They want revenge.

They all want revenge, it's like a loop. They only live on worship, punishment, and revenge. Even if they were the ones wrong. They don't realize my pretty kitty's soul isn't in her cat body right now so they can't get her. And Loki is safe in Death's headquarters.

Again I feign pleading with them not to hurt my son. I trick them into believing he's at a false location, and lead them with my peek-a-boo hand and eye to another portal to be destroyed in.

When they're gone I return my pretty kitty's soul to her body. They don't know Death isn't just Death. I can hold soul's safely in my body to be protected. It's how they get put there for resurrection too if I need to bring someone back. The black death acid doesn't melt them. I'm not like that false mummy death.

Loki is excited about it, and wants to try. He finds the games interesting and fun.

I let him give it a go. I tell him what to do, and not to let them see his real facial features but to project what they are meant to see. He's a natural at it as he does it through me to practice. I expect nothing less, since he is a natural born trickster.

He is having fun, and a few times I have to take away his memories because he hears something about my work, or a tidbit that will influence him to act in an unbalanced way. He's a good Loki right now, and I can't accidentally make him tip into a bad Loki.

I tell him straight up that I have to take away what he learned to keep him on the right path.

Ashes to Dust

He is understanding, but still would rather keep it. But he lets me take them away. Not that he had a choice.

After a while, I say something that I didn't think would create any reaction about not being ready for children yet. But I then get a knowing.

First born Loki was impatient. I get a feeling in my vagina as I'm sitting on the toilet and feel him trying to go up. He's attempting to have me be pregnant with him right away. He's sick of waiting.

It doesn't work and I have to do something for his bad karma. I'm so upset with everything I went through, that he witnessed, and he still did this to me. My own son.

I enforce it by telling him for his karma he will be fluffy beings for many lifetimes before being born as the Loki he is now.

He didn't enjoy that. I meant more than cats. Bunnies, hamsters, all the fluffy pet beings.

With the way he reacted I take away some of his memories to prevent him from becoming unbalanced. He needs to remain a balanced being. But I don't always know what he can and can't handle.

Loki puts things together from hearing Gods and Goddesses threaten my, "pretty kitty," and when I would respond with I won't let you hurt my "pretty kitty." He looked at my Lovie differently, realizing my fierce intensity to protect her, and her soul was because she meant more than anything to her. That he was currently reincarnated as her pretty kitty. That this whole time I've been guarding and protecting his soul. As one of his flurry being lives. It's why the Gods and Goddesses would say pretty kitty like a child.

I let him remember that.

I'm peeing with the door partially open. Lovie is on her tower eating. I'm startled by a cat coming through the door with giant black eyes. I realize it's my sister's cat. I've never felt so terrified in my life. I don't understand what's happening with the cat. I shoot up off the toilet and quickly shut the door so the cat can't get in and hurt Lovie. I realize it

Ashes to Dust

was evil Loki who possessed the cat.

I learn about there being more than one Loki. There's evil Loki's. One was taken by the same professor that created that nasty rape sun monster. The professor experimented on Loki number 2, and he wasn't heard from again. As a mother, it is hurtful to know something took him and did such horrible things to him that he doesn't show back up years later and is never the same. He was playing with two other Loki's when it happened. But Loki 3 wasn't taken.

I leave the door closed hoping that Lovie will be safe, but then the bad Loki's find a way in. They show up all around. There are many of them with different long numbers attached to the end of their names like Loki 123. The worst one with the combination of the experimented on Loki.

The evil Loki sons come and go up the pipes after I have diarrhea to try to impregnate Ash. They're doing to her, what was always done to me, Death. Rape or forced pregnancy. I won't let that happen to her too.

After flushing out the bad Loki's from Ash's vagina, I fight them off while on the toilet and tell 1st born, good Loki to leave so he doesn't get hurt.

He doesn't want to but I send him back to my headquarters. He comes back to try to help me by swapping with me.

I move to the bathtub and sit in it. I send good Loki back to protect him, and I defend against the bad ones. I know their numbers and they're surprised.

They tell me I never loved them, and that I'm cold. It's why they're so cold. Because they're Death's children.

Good Loki comes back and says that's not true.

I swap out with him again so he doesn't get hurt. I tell the bad Loki's that I love them, and they have a negative reaction to it. Same reaction I got as Death. They're definitely Death's children.

I tell the bad Loki's what they did to Ash wasn't right. That of all things, they would try to force babies in her.

They know it's one of the worst things something could do because it was done to me. I do my best to get rid of the babies they forced in her to have for future lifetimes.

They multiply and there's so many it's hard to keep up. Lovie is walking on the edge of the bathtub and we make eye contact. We swap places. Good Loki took over and now I'm in Lovie. He is using what I taught him. And he's also using it on the bad Loki's. He doesn't want to become one of them.

They don't know it's Loki 1 in there. When I lock eyes with him in Ash's body, we swap. Now he's in Lovie. Lovie starts going around me, fighting the bad Loki's. The bad Loki's are running away from Lovie as she claws around them. After she circles me to get ones close, she moves to the drain of the tub and starts digging. The bad Loki's thought they could hide in there but she found them and is attacking them to protect me.

Good Loki catches my eyes and swaps again. He's trying to convince them that their mother, Death, does love them. That it's expressed different. She doesn't know how to show it any other way because she wasn't shown it. It's why it's so much more powerful to be loved by her.

He can't tell them he feels that way because of his experience with me. Or that he knew "pretty kitty" was him this whole time, and I cared.

Good Loki also multiplies and fights them off. But I'm worried because there's too many bad ones. I have to call in reinforcements. I call in their dads, the Lucifer Morningstar Angels to come, and they help right away.

Together as a family we try to fight so we can make sure this doesn't ever happen to our future children. They're helping knowing I'm tired out.

Their dads try to tell them that if they're like me then they too can

Ashes to Dust

love and have love. That they aren't cold and evil like they think. That there's light.

I worry I might lose them because the bad Loki's, especially Loki 123, is trying to kill them. Severely injuring one. I tell the Lucifer Morningstar angels to go back. They are injured and missing wings.

I have to go to the bathroom again and move to the toilet.

I hear Kat scream "Ash!" from downstairs.

I stand up and pull up my pants. I open the door, but I know Kat only ever calls like that when there's something bad happening. Violent. Probably Barb's ex, or her ex coming to the house. I quickly turn around and put Lovie in my room before she could run down the stairs. She looked ready to go down and attack, and it wouldn't be the first time Barb's ex was involved with the death of a cat. I don't want Lovie to get hurt trying to protect one of us, or just being there. I close my bedroom door before she can get out. Now she's safe.

I feel so weak and wobbly. I go down the stairs as fast as I can. I wake Ash by calling her name. I ask her, "Ash Dust, are you ready for this?"

I come to consciousness in my body as me, Ash. I feel light and bubbly, and I say, "Yes, I told you I knew what I was agreeing to." I did tell them it was okay if everyone thought I was crazy after all. That I didn't care. It's what has to be done if the Loki's are attacking them.

I get to the bottom of the stairs and see my sister's frightened but stern face.

Ashes to Dust

23

I went down to Kat in the corner of the door, with the blinds to the window open. I hear yelling from my mom, my sister and to my surprise (but not uncommon) my mom's ex Rockie. All three of them were too loud for me to understand what was happening, and I could hear Kyle crying in the living room. My mom's ex was trying to get in, and was screaming and pounding on the door window. I think she is trying to break it like she's attempted to do before.

Now I know why Kat screamed my name. She only does that when there's danger or someone violent like my mom's ex, or her own ex. I was trying to stop my mom verbally by calming her down and telling her no she shouldn't go outside she might get hurt. She really wanted to fight her ex. I always have to calm her down or convince her by blocking her way out so she doesn't get in trouble with either cops or the person threatening her or us on the other side of the door.

The bad Loki's called Rockie here to cause a scene. To stir up anger in the household and unbalance the world. It's working. They infected my mom who I can't calm down.

I look into Kat's eyes, knowing good Loki is in there listening, preventing her from being taken over from the others. I say she needs to help everyone.

I'm hoping he can overcome the bad Loki's and rid their control from the others so they are normal again.

Ashes to Dust

    Kat responds, but I know it's good Loki by her eyes. He says he's trying.
    I can tell he's desperately trying but the bad Loki's out number the good.
    Kat says she needs to get Rockie's daughter in the house.
    I look out the window and see the teen crying.
    Barb tells me that Rockie punched her daughter in the face.
    I hear Rockie screaming at her daughter and threatening her again before turning back to our door.
    Rockie is obviously on meth and booze and whatever else she takes by the way her body wobbles.
    I admire the good Loki's want to help even the daughter, but I don't want Kat and good Loki hurt. I try to convince Kat/Loki to stay in, but she pushes me to go by.
    With all the screaming, crying and worry I fall and things go black for a second. I'm angry. I was recovering from my food poisoning to the point I could get out of bed today, and even walk down the stairs. I was going to eat soup! But all this commotion seems to have set me back and my body couldn't handle all of it. If it was a normal day where I wasn't recovering from the effects of food poisoning, I could've handled this like I've done many times. Why couldn't Rockie have waited until I was fully recovered? Now I'm clearly set back and I don't know if I'm okay with this fall.
    I dizzyingly look at Kat, and stand back up but it's hard, and Kat goes outside. I worry more because Rockie has hurt my sister before. But Kat/Loki is fine and comes in with Rockie's daughter who's crying and terrified.
    I know what I have to do now to get everyone to feel better by expelling the bad Loki's and protecting them from all of this. My vision is odd, like a fish lens from a camera, or where it's dome-like with the outer corners bright and the center a bit fogged. Like in dream-like scenes of movies.

Ashes to Dust

I ask Rockie's daughter if I have her permission to kiss her.

I will be able to protect them this way by expelling the dark out and hopefully block the bad Loki's from trying to jump in and control them. There's so many tears down her face and she looks disheveled and terrified until she hears me ask that.

Then she nods yes and comes over to me and gives me a quick peck.

She seems to relax and the crying is lessened. I feel better knowing it worked. Now hopefully she'll be protected by the bad Loki's orchestrating all this, and her mom's attacks.

She hugs me crying less, and I try to calm her down and reassure her she's safe.

I leave her to Kat/good Loki and move on to try to protect Kyle. He's on the futon in the corner with his headphones on and eyes squeezed shut as he cries inconsolably. His birth mother terrifies him, and fighting is a trigger for him. I go over and try to get him to look at me. I have to make a connection deep in soul so I can expel anything that's hurting him in there. It's hard because he's so terrified of the fighting. It's not the first time he's been through all this either. His birth mom causes a lot of violence in our house. And with the bad Loki's this is even worse.

When he does eventually look at me I ask him if I have his permission to give him a kiss to make him feel better.

Just like I did for his sister.

He says yes and then gives me a quick kiss.

I feel better knowing I have protected him now. Any of the bad Loki's influences or causing of harm to him is gone. He was strong to fight through them.

I put his headphones back on and tell him it'll be okay.

Barb goes to grab something to defend against her ex. While Kat comes in to the living room and sits down. Barb comes in with the golf club in her hands and I realize I haven't gotten bad Loki 1-2-3 out of her.

Ashes to Dust

She's ranting, and there's still so much crying and emotions and her ex went to find a new way in to our house. Barb is swinging the club a lot in my direction and I think bad Loki is having her try to hurt me. She's going to hurt me.

I say out loud to Kat that mom's going to hurt me, as I cower on the ground.

I try to reach Kat with my eyes so she can see, but I think bad Loki has gotten to her too.

My mom stops swinging and she asks what am I talking about. Then she says, (still holding the golf club) that she would never hurt me. That she loves me and would, "tear my own throat out for you."

I'm terrified. She just told me she would tear out her own throat. Why would she say something so graphic and horrible? Bad Loki must be threatening to go after my mom's throat. I look to the kitchen worried. Is he going to make her cut out her own throat? Is he going to make her stand here in front of me and use her own hands to rip out her throat? I don't want to see that! I don't want my mom to die. How am I suppose to protect her from his actions? She doesn't know she's possessed by him. I'm torn. I wanted to leave this house because now I'm scared of what she said and everything else, but what if I leave and he kills her with her own hands making it look like a suicide? I might have to stay even though I don't want to and I know I'm not safe here.

I look into my sister's eyes as she sits on the futon. I try to reach her. To really reach good Loki who is obviously struggling. I tell her to listen to what mom just said. That she said such horrifying words that she would tear out her own throat.

Kat tells me, "No, mom's just trying to say she loves you and would do anything for you."

Kat's been taken over too. I don't know what else I can do for them. What can I do if I'm just one and I can't protect them against all the bad Loki's. There aren't enough good Loki's.

Kat comes over beside me once mom puts down the golf club. I look

Ashes to Dust

Kat in the eyes, trying to reach good Loki so he can protect her. At least to protect one of them. It's hard. I don't think it's working. I gently rest my hands on her cheeks and stare in Kat's eyes. I need to make sure I can look into her eyes so bad Loki can't avoid me as I try to get rid of him and protect her with my eyes.

I ask good Loki to protect her.

Kat/bad Loki laughs and says she's fine.

I desperately try to reach good Loki with my eyes. I'm trying so hard through my eyes to pierce through bad Loki and give power to good Loki to protect my sister from him.

I say again let me protect you.

She half says she's fine again, when Barb screams to let go of Kat.

It startles me.

I'm confused because I'm barely holding Kat, my hands are resting gently on her face, so why is she screaming like I'm trying to hurt Kat.

Kat simply laughs and walks away from me unfazed.

Barb shouts at me that she's calling the hospital.

I realize it's bad Loki. He's doing it again. He's trying to make my mom make a scene and act like I'm doing something I'm not to get me put away into the loony bin so I can't protect my sister or any of them. Or Barb from him cutting her throat. It would be obvious if I was hurting Kat. That's why bad Loki is being dramatic about me almost getting through. He was losing control over Kat. And if she was being hurt, she would've said, and she wouldn't have been able to simply side step me out with ease.

Why is this happening? I just wanted to try to protect one. I gaze at all of them. Barb, Kat, cousin Sandy, Kyle, and realize I lost them. I can't protect them. I look at Kat's baby in cousin Sandy's arms and hope she'll be okay. But I'm not safe here. People are going to come to get me, and Barb is violent. I need to get out because Barb's ex might also show up and break in our house.

I look at the back door, and realizing I can't save any of them and

Ashes to Dust

need to find safety for myself. I run.

I hear Kat say no don't, as she moved forward.

I was terrified they were going to hold me down or trap me in that house with all the violence there I just witnessed. I want out and need to find a safe spot to wait.

I run out forgetting there is a gate my mom put up. For a moment I'm devastated, thinking I'll be caught. But then I see something big to climb up on. I climb and when I go to jump over, I slow and think about my feet and legs and the safety of my body. I can't just jump or I might break or twist something. Especially since my body is in recovery. So I carefully lower myself down and land.

I'm wobbly, but I go to the left and see the police lights. I wonder if that means they're searching for Rockie or she's hiding over there. That means I need to go the opposite way and hide until they catch her. She might also be out here somewhere and I can't run into her or she'll hurt me. She doesn't like me. She might even have some of her druggy friends with her that she claims have beaten up people for her before and watched our house.

I go the opposite way and start running. I don't know how I have the energy to run as my feet pound against the ground. I'm worried I'll pass out before I find shelter. But something must be helping me because I know I don't have the energy to be running. Unless it's adrenaline.

I run past the gaps of the houses, and I reach the next row. I see a green box and consider hiding there, but the one helping me shakes my head no.

I didn't see anything else so I turned to the backyard of the houses. I was being led by my helper, and the first yard I went into had a gazebo. It looked like a giant tent. I go in the opening and close the the sheets of fabric together behind me. It's pitch black in here, and I'm surrounded by boxes. By the very vague shadows I can see it seems like a lot of boxes are around and behind me. I don't want any to crush

Ashes to Dust

me so I stay close to the opening.

I feel like I'm dying. I can feel my blood dripping out of my mouth and nose. It's thick and I'm breathing heavy. I lie on the cold, bricked ground as I'm bleeding out. I'm worried Barb's ex will find me with her drug friends before the police can catch her. I trust the Universe and know she won't let me down like all the others.

I ask Universe to please quickly put me in my new life in Toronto before I'm caught. Before they stop her from safely moving my spirit and being to my regenerated new body.

I close my eyes dying, waiting to die to wake up to my new life in Toronto like I was always promised. This will never have happened. I wouldn't have this family. They wouldn't know I existed and they'd be happy. I would be happy singing and living in Toronto. I wonder if my memories from my old life and new life will merge together after I wake up reincarnated in this lifetime as a adult, not a baby.

My blood is spilling out of my mouth. I'm cold and I can see a slit opening through the gazebo. I can hear someone yell to catch the cat, it got out.

I'm terrified. Did they let my cat out? Should I get up to search the buildings like I think they are doing? Is it a trick by the Loki's? If I try to go out will I make it? Will I run into her ex? Will she kill my cat like her and her drugged out friends did to the ones at her house where they decapitated them?

As long as I stay and do this successfully, my cat will be with me in my new life in Toronto so I don't have to worry about it. Through the slit I ask if they'll find me if I don't close it.

Yes.

I can't have that. I can't have Barb's ex finding me, or the bad Loki's. The Loki's could try to get me taken to the loony bin so I can't have my amazing life I was promised. I need to make sure I successfully get transferred to my new life in Toronto before I die. I try to get up but it's painful, and I close the sheets together.

Ashes to Dust

I lie dying in the dark, shivering. I'm huddled in the fetal position on the ground shaking. I'm trying to relax to think about how I won't need to worry about feeling death. Universe won't let that happen. I will simply be in my new life.

After closing my eyes for a bit and hearing the outside wind, I see a long beautiful forest. There's just a long row of large, bushy green trees on the right side. With a sky and endless grass. I wonder where this is as I'm moving through it. It must be Toronto somewhere and I'm being transferred.

I open my eyes, cutting off the vivid imagery I saw. I was so close! I was there. But the bad Loki's found me. They're in this gazebo with me. They won't let me go there. They want to watch me die without anything after. They are all around me.

As I bleed I know they're making me bleed more. I say they found me.

But I realize they want Universe to feel my death. I can't let that happen. I will have to prevent her from feeling it. She would be consumed with rage and sadness. She would never recover and explode.

I slowly get up off the ground and look behind me. I'm surprised I can see in here now. It's what I imagine night, cat vision eyes must be like. There's no light but I can see there's a couch, and a table, and plants, and a few more things in here. None of which are boxes like I originally thought. I must be getting help to see in the dark.

I go straight for the couch and lie down on it. It's comfy. Better than the concrete. I'm still freezing but glad to have cushion. I'm instructed on how to get rid of the unwanted pregnancies put there by the bad Loki's while in the bathroom. They inseminated them in this body's vagina and womb.

I have to hold my hand over my lower stomach and say some words and focus on banishing and undoing what the bad Loki's did to me. It's why Universe was so furious. She knew what it was like to be

Ashes to Dust

forced by rape or being pregnant. Violation to her body and being. She's upset. But I am successful.

I don't want her to be upset. This is the last thing I can do for her. Tell her how great she is. Remind her when she has forgotten and people have forgotten to tell her.

First I make sure she can't feel my death anymore, and that she won't know I'm dying. The bad Loki's are still here trying to kill me. They're waiting. But I make sure not to let Universe hear me in pain or shivering.

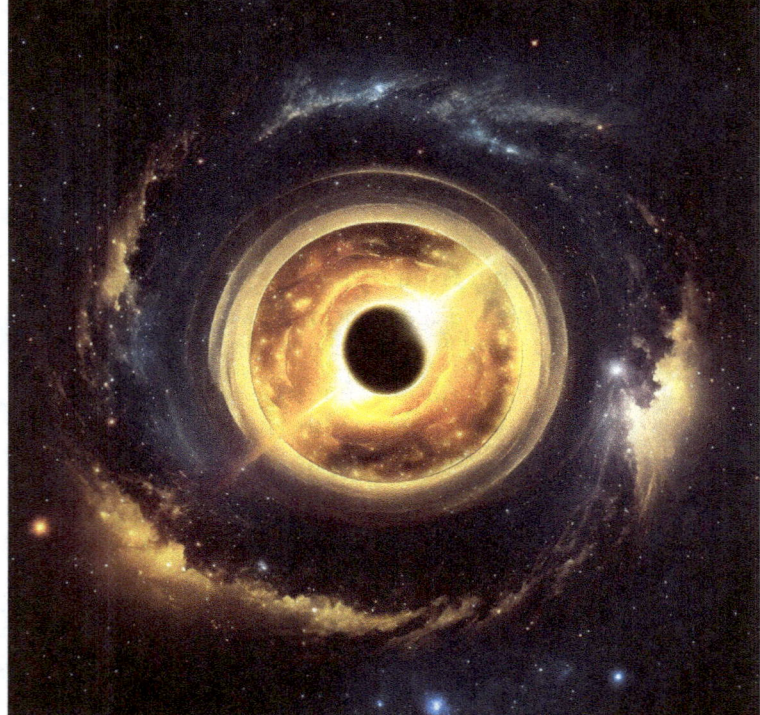

I remind Universe of what she looks like since she forgot when she thought she was Death. I tell her about her beautiful golden eyes.

I can hear her voice through my mouth. She's happy to know that.

I tell her how beautiful she really is.

Ashes to Dust

It makes her extra happy with every small detail about her. She remembers when I tell her. I love the excitement.

I make sure not to touch the ground. I can't be on the ground or the bad Loki's can interfere with me and Universe. I sting Universe with love and light. I'm her daughter so I can reach her. It doesn't actually hurt Universe, but Universe thinks it hurts because she doesn't react well to love.

The bad Loki's don't like what I'm doing and remind me I'm dying faster, and that I should stop wasting my energy.

I keep going. I'm not going to let them stop me. And I need to make sure I fill Universe with all the light and love I could ever muster before I die so she has enough to keep going. Not enough people do the same as she does for them, and I need to make sure I do at least this.

I keep telling her I'm stinging her with light and love. I sing-song. I don't stop. Then I need to move because I'm not in a safe spot from the bad Loki's anymore. I need to avoid touching the ground. After debate, I carefully move the plants off the table, onto the ground so they don't break. I consider staying on the couch but I don't think I should. I crawl over onto the cleared table without touching the plants on the ground, or the cement.

I'm still freezing, and shivering. Evil Loki's keep trying to send negative thoughts to universe. I rebuff that by letting Universe know I believe in her, and only her out of everything out there. No matter what thoughts say otherwise, my spoken words are truth.

I keep stinging her, here and there when she least expects it. I surprise her with the secret words that I'm stinging her with love, "honey bunny."

Universe is shocked and surprised.

I'm her love reincarnated in this body. She didn't know. I took over our daughter's body so she wouldn't feel death. I would take it on. I can feel the happiness and tears welling from Universe. I only know

Ashes to Dust

she's above me, somewhere out there. I have only the inside black peak of the gazebo to look at to think of her.

She doesn't know I'm dying, and in pain. I tell her I'm working out when she asks what I'm doing.

I later check in, because time here and time where she is is different. She's lived a long time since each conversation while it's only been a few minutes here on Earth. I tell her I just got up that's why I sound exhausted.

She tells me I sleep a lot.

I've said a few times I just got up. I tell her of course I'm human now, and I do human things.

She laughs.

I sting her a few more times and compliment her.

I don't think I can make it anymore. I make sure not to let her know something is wrong as a shiver, and my teeth chatter, and body aches. I move my legs down to hang over the table.

I keep stinging her with love even when the evil Loki's inform me I'm dying.

I can do this much for her. I won't let them try to make her feel it or know what's really happening.

I can hear shouts for Ash. I see lights and they're coming closer. I still and close my eyes. I know the evil Loki's are coming. I have to be still so they don't notice I'm here. I can see the light behind my closed lids going back and forth.

I can feel it, I'm no longer in my body, I'm switching. Justice has swapped so Rockie is where I am. I can feel that the grogginess of this body is actually her after overdosing or waking up. I'm somewhere safe. It's finally happening. I can hear the police man talking. I can feel the confusion of Rockie's body. She's blonde, and disgruntled, and will go to jail where she belongs. She won't be able to hurt anyone again. They won't know we swapped.

For some reason the swap fails. I'm back as the daughter of Universe as the police say something about they heard I like music.

I can hear Kat and Barb somewhere in the background. I don't know what they're all doing there as I keep my eyes closed and remain still.

They were all disguised as evil Loki's. I'm informed to stay still and not let the Loki's take me.

I have to fill myself up with light (because they're dark). I hear the Loki's possessing my mom and sister, calling my name in the background. The evil Loki's are trying to get me to react. I remain still and quiet with my eyes closed so the Loki's can't get me.

I have to fill myself with my light so the Loki's can't take me. Can't touch me. I repeat a mantra in my head that I am light and bright. I don't stop repeating it.

When one of the officers touches me, I repeat it harder in my mind and their hands fall away from my strong light. It burns them. It pains them like their mom, Universe/Death.

One picks me up successfully and I do the mantra more determined. I hear one of the possessed Loki's ask if the one carrying me needs help.

They refuse with a laugh.

They must think they can handle my light and don't need two. My light fills me so much it gets too heavy and I open my eye a crack as he drops me and just barely gets me before I hit the parking lot pavement. Then I see the back of an ambulance. I'm told to fight.

The Loki officer tries to shove me in there and I reach out my arms and hold onto the sides to prevent that. I then had to pry off their fingers as they grabbed onto me to put me into the ambulance.

To my dismay I have a final test. I have to fill the world with my light. I don't get the happy life I was promised.

I keep thinking of being light and bright as I bring my body in a sitting huddle position on the bed to keep them from getting me.

PART SEVEN
HOSPITALS

24

I feel the outside air as I'm rolled into the hospital doors. I hold onto my knees with them pressed to my chest like I knew I was suppose to. I can't let the Loki's get me. I need to keep my light. I sing the "Light Bright" song over and over. I change it up with rhymes so it's uplifting and fills the world with more light. This is my final test. I have to get through it all, knowing I'm going to die by the Loki's here. But spread out as much of my light as possible to the world, and forgive them for killing me.

I moved my feet as they tried to put things on me. Socks. I didn't know what they were up to, just that I needed to keep singing through it with my body close together so they can't get me. They start trying to pry my legs down, but I fought back while singing and kept them up. The one testing me kept telling me to fight to keep from having them force me down. I would pull my arm back to my leg if they tried to pry it to the side. I kept doing it for a long time.

I did it all while singing and making sure that my light spread around the world. They put a blanket on and I tried to get it off. I wasn't going to die easy. They were strapping my arms down and I tried to pull from it so I could be free and safe. I used my light and sometimes it made it so they wouldn't be able to touch me because I had too much light against their dark touch.

They eventually got my arms and legs strapped down. I don't know what else the bad Loki's have planned for me, but I know it wasn't good. I would have to hold on until my end. I tried to slip out of the straps but they were too tight and I was too weak.

I kept singing, "Light bright, light bright, I spread my light tonight." I didn't stop singing.

The Loki's tried to distract me and make me stop singing by bringing my mom and sister to the hospital where they called out my name and were crying. They were crying so hard. The Loki's wanted them to see me in this state. To make it look like I was crazy and would give up spreading light to the world at a dark time. It was hard, but I clenched my smile in place and kept singing. I wouldn't give up yet.

I felt them inject me with things. I knew Universe was protecting me from feeling the full intensity of everything. She was actually taking on the pain her sons were inflicting. They are horrible and she still takes it, and wants to save them.

I sang through them raping me. I sang through them making me think I was pregnant and having a baby that they were cutting out of me. The Loki's not knowing they were impregnating their mother, Universe, and causing her pain. And much more difficult, I sang through them violating me with something sharp up my vagina. That one I felt much more than I was expecting and I couldn't stop the tears. I had to clench a smile in place again as I gripped the metal rails of the bed for support. I sang mostly with my eyes closed. I peaked sometimes to see where they were, and where they took me. To figure out what they were planning to do to me.

I heard a little boy crying and I knew I had to sing louder, and more powerful. I could hear the other hospital patients losing their light in this world of darkness. The pandemic was making them lose hope and light.

I needed to try harder to spread my light. They need it. Even if I burn out. There's enough light for me to spread until I die. I just hope I get out enough. If I die, light dies. I need to have light spread enough that

Ashes to Dust

no matter what the Loki's do to me, the world doesn't lose light. And that's what the bad Loki's want. The world to not have light in it anymore. They want to kill the light source.

I sing and my hands move, either a thumbs up, that I'm doing great, or it will start shaking no. I get confused, that maybe I'm going to break my vocal chords and that's what the Loki's want. So I can't sing and spread the light anymore. They want me to over do it so I won't have a way to spread hope and light anymore. I wouldn't be able to talk.

I stop to spit out the poison the Loki's put in my mouth. They won't trick me. I see it, it's foamy and there's a lot. They keep trying to make me swallow poison pill capsules and I keep spitting it out. The poison foams down my mouth, chin and the bed. I try to sing through it but I sometimes can't spit and end up swallowing the poison. I panic a little but I must keep pushing through.

When I mess up the rhymes by the bad Loki's interference in my thought process, I have to quickly undo it in song too. I start not being able to sing as loud. I have to sing quieter. Trying not to damage my vocals more than they are. I need to be able to keep spreading the light.

Eventually I have to stop singing. I hear one of the nurses talk about how contagious my song is. Saying that a little boy that was sad started singing it too. I'm so happy, it means it worked. It was working. I spread the light around. Especially in a grim, dark place like this.

I stay still and quiet. I keep trying to think positive thoughts, hoping I'm still spreading light. I can't do it through song anymore. I haven't had anything to drink and my throat is dry and my throat hurts. Especially from the operatic singing to try to reach those around the world too far away. They all need light too.

The evil Loki's disguised as nurses kept trying to pry my eyes open, and I had to quickly roll them in the back of my head so they wouldn't be able to look me in the eyes and steal my remaining light from me. If I look them in the eyes, they'll drain me of it and fill me with their

Ashes to Dust

darkness.

The evil Loki's shine a blinding light in my eyes, and poke my eyes out. My eyes are in pain, but because of the Universe trying to help, (even though she shouldn't have been there), I didn't feel it as painfully as it would've been.

My eyes regenerate.

Every time my eyes regenerated and I thought the Loki's were done, they would come back to poke my eyes out and blind me again. It was painful each time, and I was only able to see blackish-grey pinholes afterward.

One of the bad Loki's stuck around, telling me they were going to bring me to a room where they would have my eyes pried open and stick needles in them.

I didn't want that. I didn't know how to make that not happen. I try to think of a way out of it but there wasn't. The Loki's were going to make it super painful and torturous before killing me off.

I heard some of the nurses together and they were talking about no friends. I realized they were talking about me. Then I heard one mention my iPod and the things about my mother and sister.

Oh no. They hacked into my iPod and are reading out my messages between me and my Instagram friend about the troubles I've been having with my mom and sister. I try to think about what I've talked about, and realize quite a lot. About any time my mom was being violent or mean or her ex came and did stuff. Or when my sister was having her mood swings and not talking to me, and more I couldn't think of. Like how my sister's ex came pounding on the door all the time threatening suicide and did it on our lawn.

I worried about what they would see. The troubles that would bring to my family. My mom and sister. I didn't want them to have their lives turned upside down by police checking in.

Loki 1-2-3 told me it was too late they already know.

They were with the police now talking about it. And the bad Loki's

Ashes to Dust

found my book with my passwords in it. That means they could go into my bank. And do whatever they wanted. They would ruin my life even more after killing me. They would ruin my family's lives.

Loki 1-2-3 stayed with me. He was one of the ones I reached with my light. Every time a nurse came over and touched me I would reach for them and hold their hand, or touch their clothes and push my light into them. I would visualize it going into them and erasing their darkness. They would notice I was getting rid of their darkness and let go or walk away. It was hard when they didn't want to be saved by my light.

When I opened my eyes the ceiling of the hospital was horrible. It was eerie and wrong. The dots on the ceiling were thick and dark. There were no words to explain how wrong the whole hospital felt.

Loki 1-2-3 told me it was because of the other Loki's.

I close my eyes and have to pee. I peed and I felt the catheter the bad Loki's shoved into me, pop out. I hear one of the Loki nurses laugh about it. They then discussed about putting in another one. A bigger one.

The one they already put in was super painful, and they wanted a bigger one so that this would be excruciating.

I wasn't looking forward to that. I wanted this to be over. I can't handle more.

Loki 1-2-3 sighed at the bad Loki's and said, "Common she's been through enough."

He was both comforting to be by my side but also I had a knowing that he was trying to feed my fears. I had no way to stop it though. He was both nice and cruel still. Probably because of his nature before. Tricking.

I kept my eyes closed most of the time but when I opened them a swarm of Loki nurses surrounded me and were trying to look deep in my eyes to take my light away. I avoided eye contact. But there were so many. And they were trying so hard to get me to look them in the eye. When I looked at one of the nurses in the eye her eyes were dark, bigger, and bold. Bold around the eye iris in a way that all the dark colours of her eye were even darker. All of their eyes were like that.

I closed my eyes again with a excuse that my eyes hurt so they couldn't take my light. They were wrong like this hospital.

One of the nurses played with one of the needles they had in my arm. It hurt. When they left my arm started hurting. The device they had around my right arm that squeezed every few minutes, squeezed so tight it felt like my arm was dying. I think it was cutting off my circulation or something. Then I realized that was one of the bad Loki's and they had the needles not fully capped so I would slowly bleed out. I could feel it, it was so painful especially my right arm. I think that one was the worst. It brought tears to my eyes. I couldn't see it because it was hidden under the blanket they had on me.

They must've had it there to cover what they did to me from the other non-Loki nurses. Ones that might help me. I started calling out for help. I looked over and tried to find one. When I thought she was going to come, she was stopped by another who didn't let her come over to help me.

Loki 1-2-3 mentioned that that was one of the evil Loki's that stopped the nice nurse from coming by convincing her I was fine.

I cry more. They were just going to let me bleed out here. I dread each time the device made the sound that meant it was starting up and going to squeeze my arm again. It squeezed my arm so painfully tight I had to clench my jaw together to keep from making noise. I still had to be light but this was making it so hard. Knowing it was squeezing my arm and my arm felt like it would fall off. But I knew they left the device on so it would squeeze out more blood. That's why it hurt so much. I was running out of blood. My blood was dripping down the sides out of the needle they placed in me wrong.

Loki 1-2-3 panicked with me. I ask if that one was a good nurse or a bad Loki.

Ashes to Dust

He tells me.

I try to call another for help and this time the nurse was coming, but then a phone call interrupted. I dreaded that. Oh no. They managed to have it so the nice nurse was side tracked, and now a bad one was coming in place of them.

Loki 1-2-3 told me she was one of the worst.

The nurse came over, and I felt the fake smiling. It felt wrong. I tried to break through that dark barrier and have them see me. I told them about my arm hurting.

They said it was just the machine.

Then I try to tell them no I think a needle rubbed against the straps and was coming out because it hurts.

I knew that the straps rubbed against them.

She wasn't going to, but then she lifted up the blanket, and then set it back down. She said it was fine.

When I tried to get her to stop walking away telling her no, please it hurts so much, she kept going.

The bad Loki was enjoying this. They were going to purposefully let me bleed out and not let anyone else near me to see what they were doing.

I try not to but I cry out in pain when it squeezes my arm again. It's so bad and painful. I hurt so much. I'm dying slowly. My blood is probably dripping out on the sides, and I don't know how much longer I have. I can hear my heart monitor, make alarming sounds, but no one checks on it. No one checks on me. They know I'm dying, that they're killing me, and they don't want anyone to come to my rescue.

My heart monitor goes off again, longer, and this time after a while one of the nurses come over to shut it off so it didn't make noise, and then left right away. I start crying again. I try to hold on because I'm suppose to be light, but I'm in so much pain and no one is here to help me. I have no one by my side. No one but Loki-1-2-3.

It's been hard to breathe this whole time because of these straps,

Ashes to Dust

which make me feel claustrophobic and panicked. They have since the first time they did it. But now it's even worse because it's digging into my bad arms, and hitting the needles. I can't move it so it's not rubbing them and making it more painful for me. I can't move. I'm stuck lying here, motionless, dying a slow painful death.

Eventually when a nurse comes I ask her if I can hold her hand.

She allows me, and I use that moment to pour my light into her so that this Loki will be less dark and have more light. Maybe it'll spread and they'll be healed. She allows me to hold onto her hand for a while, so I know it's working. I think this Loki wants to be saved. It must feel the light more. But then they leave.

Loki-1-2-3 says they know I'm doing something to them. They don't like the feeling. That they're going to end me once and for all. Bring me to a different room to have a needle shoved in my eye and lodged in my brain.

I tell Loki 1-2-3 that he must still be connected to them. Even though he's lightened now, he's still connected and it's allowing them to hear what he hears.

He needs to leave.

I tell him he needs to leave my side so they can't hear anymore.

He doesn't want to.

I banish him from my side, but I thank him for staying by it through everything. Even when I'm pretty sure he tried to make me think wrong things were going to happen. That I appreciated not being alone.

He's gone.

I'm dying alone. I don't know what to do. There's nothing I can do. No one hear will help me. My family won't know what happened. Just that I died. I wonder if they're home now.

I open my eyes to look at the hospital ceiling again. The lights are on now. It looks less creepy. Less wrong. One of the nurses come by and I look at their face. It doesn't look like before. It seems more normal.

Ashes to Dust

Their eyes aren't wrong anymore. It's like a click went off in my brain. They suddenly didn't look bad anymore once I tried really hard to focus on them.

I start looking around the hospital once the nurse left. I'm seeing things for the first time properly. There are some people in yellow attire. I don't know why. Some door frames and spots have long pieces of plastic or something clear covering it. I don't know why. Am I in quarantine? Is this a quarantine section of the hospital?

I come to a realization. I look up, knowing the Universe, and things are there to hear me. I ask was this for me to get help?

Yes.

I don't know what to feel about that. Upset. Angry. I was put through a lot. Just because I needed hydration. I could've gotten that at home. Without going through all this. I heard one of the nurses names be called by a different nurse. I needed to talk to someone here. And get some water too because I was so thirsty.

I called out the nurse's name.

She turned to look at me. They both did. When she noticed it was me who called her, she turned back to the other nurse and they both laughed and walked away from me. I didn't understand why she would do that. Why does no one here want to help me?

Later one of the nurses come over. I ask her to take the catheter out because it really hurt when they put it in and I want it out.

She says to be prepared because it's going to inflate like a balloon so it can come out.

I hold on to the bars and she yanks it out. Yanks! Holy fuck it hurt so much! I wondered if she just ripped off my peeing part. I ask her for water and she goes to get it.

When she comes back she asks what happened. She wants to know how I got so dehydrated.

I tell her about the fight at my house, and that I was dehydrated from food poisoning.

Ashes to Dust

She told me that the doctor was going to send me to a different hospital. A psych one in Chatham.

That upset me. It set off alarm bells. I ask her why.

She says I would have to ask the doctor that. That because I was unconscious he wasn't able to talk to me.

I told her I just explained to her what happened so if she could talk with him and tell him. I'm conscious now. I'm lucid now. That if I could talk to him about it so he doesn't send me there I would like to talk to him right away. Because that would be very traumatizing for me.

She nodded about that, and then left to get me water when I asked.

The doctor comes over and tells me that the ambulance is on its way and will take me to the psych in Chatham.

I ask him why.

He says he couldn't talk to me because I was unconscious.

I tell him I'm conscious now. That I do not consent to being taken there. That it is involuntarily taking me somewhere I don't want to go. I ask him to cancel it because that would be extremely traumatizing.

He said he won't because he already called them.

I try to get him to talk to me to explain the reason why. Why he decided to send me away. What the reason was because he isn't saying.

But he doesn't explain. He doesn't tell me why. He walks away.

I ask him to take off the straps and call my family.

He says no, and that's the last I heard or seen of him.

I cry again. I don't understand what's happening. My family isn't going to know what's happening to me. I don't even know why this is happening to me. If they needed me to stay longer why wouldn't they keep me hear with fluids? Are they too busy? Is it the pandemic? He shouldn't be able to just do this and not tell me why, or tell anyone what is happening first. He isn't going to call my family to talk to them first.

Ashes to Dust

Two ambulance men come over to my bed with the nurse from before. I'm still strapped down when they say they want to change me.

I stop them by asking the nurse to come over in private. I tell her that my father had raped me and I don't want other men to dress me and see me naked. It was uncomfortable.

The nurse was the one that did it. They unstrapped me and dressed me in a hospital gown. The whole time I was trying not to cry. I wasn't comfortable with her seeing me naked either. With her dressing me. I don't want this to happen to me. I'm a reserved person. Even this is traumatizing to me too. They don't seem to care about that though. Or they wouldn't do any of it.

After she was done, the two ambulance men grabbed the sides of the blanket under me, and lifted me up to put me on a different bed. They then wheeled me out of the hospital into the ambulance where the nurse who dressed me came. She said she would be there with me the whole ride.

Loki 1-2-3 came back, and told me he wasn't going to leave me. He would be by my side. That he was stuck with me.

I almost cried. Glad I wasn't completely alone. I already was trying not to cry about the whole situation in front of the nurse and ambulance guy in the back with me but it was hard. I kept looking out the back of the ambulance window. It was dark, and I was worried the bad Loki's were following. I ask Loki 1-2-3.

He says no.

I close my eyes on and off but I can't sleep. And it's too awkward to have two people stare at you the entire time. I needed to try to look like I was attempting to sleep so they wouldn't notice I was crying about this situation.

The ambulance guy called me a opera singer, or something. And the nurse asked me what the song I was singing was because it was catchy.

I didn't know how to say I invented the song. That you only think you heard it before because it's light's song, but it hasn't been sung yet

Ashes to Dust

officially because I'm not where I'm suppose to be yet as a singer. So when she said was it some TV show theme song, I said yes.

The ambulance guy said he was the guy that carried me to the ambulance when he found me outside.

I thank him.

I was further and further from my house. I just wanted to go home.

Once we arrived, the nurse helped me up. I couldn't walk by myself, my legs were too stiff. It made me wonder how they could discharge me from the Wallaceburg hospital in the first place knowing I couldn't move my lower body.

It was painful to walk, and the people at the Chatham hospital said they don't touch or help people walk.

So after the Wallaceburg nurse left me, I had to try to take slow painful steps as the Chatham nurses watched me. To my despair the ambulance guy told me I would be in the great hands of Hilda. A super nice nurse.

What he didn't know was Hilda was from my childhood school where she was a mean bitch and my bully. So I didn't exactly trust that I was in great hands of some "nice" lady. I wondered if maybe she did somehow change. Since I remember her once surprising me with a ride in High School, for no reason, and we never talked before. When I got the ride she told me she was in a horrible car accident. I wondered if since her car accident she turned over a new leaf and became a kinder person. I still didn't really trust it.

There were two nurses there, Hilda and one with glasses. A different nurse came and I asked to go home. I also ask why was I here.

She told me it was to rest and get a break from my home.

I told her this wasn't restful this was very traumatizing.

She just said oh, well try to sleep.

I ask her when I could go home.

She looked at the clock which was past 3am, and said since it's technically the next day that I should be out by afternoon today.

Ashes to Dust

I want to go home now. I ask her to please call my home and tell them to let my cat out of my room because I had to put her in there so she didn't get hurt from the fight.

She said she would.

I was left with the two nurses Hilda, and Nurse Glasses. I wasn't comfortable and felt like things were just falling apart. What were the odds that I would get a mean girl from my childhood as my nurse to see me in this horrible state where my hair looks like a rats nest. I don't feel comfortable with her here.

I asked for water when Nurse Glasses asked if I needed something. She said okay.

They wanted me to lie down and try to get sleep on the mattress.

I couldn't bend my legs. I told them I wasn't going to be able to sleep here.

I looked at the place; it was horrible. They put me in some dungeon looking basement room. Like a torture chamber that only had dark concrete, plastic of some sort over the window, and a mattress on the floor with a pillow.

After struggling to get down, they had to help me. I drank some water and then told them I had to pee and asked where the washroom was.

They said it was around the corner.

Around the part I couldn't see in this room was a hidden bathroom. I struggle to get up. I can't get up. I can't stand. I try to go on my side and crawl but I can't. And I don't want to crawl to the toilet because this hospital is gross. I don't want to touch their dirty walls or floor.

The nurses help me get up and are going to help me go to the bathroom. I tell them I will do it myself.

I can't have Hilda, someone I knew, helping me take a piss on the toilet and seeing my privates. That's too much. This is all too much for me.

Nurse Glasses tells me just to ask if I need her they would be outside.

Ashes to Dust

I ask her for a pad.

She says okay and goes.

I struggle really hard to go to the bathroom. I can't bend my knees, and my legs are wobbly. It's hard to stand and I don't think I can bend down. I try to place toilet paper over their metal looking toilet. It looks just as terrifying as this room. They all match to make this place dreadful and not a welcoming stay. More dungeon like. It also looks really dirty. There's mystery spots all over it.

I eventually get to pee but it's excruciating. It makes me not want to pee. It burns and hurts in a intense way that makes me tear up. From the stupid catheter I didn't need. Now I dread having to pee in the future. To my dismay I have to ask one of the nurses to help me. This is awful.

Nurse Glasses helps me walk back to the bed after I put on a pad. I can't bend my legs to sit so I am like a leaning tower that slowly has to go down to the bed. Painfully.

I drink more of the water. The nurse from before comes around and I ask her if she called my family to tell them about letting my cat out.

She said no not yet.

I ask her to please do that because there's no food or water in my room and I don't want her trapped in there.

She leaves and Hilda comes back.

Hilda sits across from me, and tries to have a heart to heart about what happened at home. She mentioned me being found outside.

I realize the ambulance and Wallaceburg nurse breached confidentiality because on the way here the nurse asked if I wanted them to say what happened or not because if not they won't tell them anything, and I said no don't tell them. Just great (sarcasm).

I don't think of Hilda as someone to confide in. It's really weird. I don't know what she thinks of me in this moment. Probably not good. Of all the people they really should've given me anyone else because this is too much for me to handle. It's all too much at once.

Ashes to Dust

She seems genuine, so I try to tell her that I had food poisoning, and was feeling better that day. But then my sister screamed my name to come down. And when I did my mom's ex was there pounding and trying to get in and was hitting her daughter. I told her I passed out with all the fighting when my mom wanted to go out the door to fight and then my sister wanted to go out when the ex was being so aggressive and violent. I couldn't take all the chaos and fighting and didn't feel safe so I left the house to find a safe place until my mom's ex could be caught.

It was the truth. But it was weird saying to Hilda. And when Hilda looked at her watch at one point and made a strange face, it made me think she hadn't actually changed like she said and there was still Hilda the bully in there. Thought she must be waiting for me to wrap it up and hated talking to me. I stop talking.

I ask if I could go home.

She told me I would have to stay here for the night to take a break.

Everyone keeps telling me this place is to get a break from home, but it's worse here than there. At least I have my cat and my room there. Private room. With a lock. Here there are strangers and it's all so traumatizing. I'm already severely traumatized from the Wallaceburg hospital where they strapped me down.

I told Hilda this wasn't a place I can rest. I told her it was very traumatizing being here. And it's like a fear coming to life being stuck here.

She didn't say much to that, just to get some rest anyways.

That's not gonna happen.

She asks if I want a different nurse to be on my care instead of her.

It would be less uncomfortable considering we don't have a great history. I didn't want to come off rude because I already did say she seemed a lot nicer than I was expecting. She probably doesn't want to be my caregiver either.

I say yes I'd like someone else.

Ashes to Dust

After she left I'm restless. It's horrible being here. I want to go home to my cat. I miss her. I hope she's okay.

I notice the cameras in the room when Loki 1-2-3 is there with me, talking through me. I'm careful not to speak loud. Can't let them think I'm crazy and keep me longer. I already am partially aware that this must be my brain trying to cope with everything that is happening to me. But I also am struggling because this place is such a horrible place and everything that's happened so far at these hospitals has just been one horrible thing after the other and no one knows I'm here. They won't let me go home where I can actually rest.

I struggle to stand and try to look out the door and I find the nurse I kept asking about my cat. I ask her again if she called my home to tell them about my cat to let her out of my room.

She said not yet.

Not yet? It's been hours! My cat has been in my room for hours with no food or water! What the hell is wrong with this place? It's important and I asked so many times already. Why can't they do one simple thing? I don't want my most important person dying from dehydration or starvation because these people wouldn't make a phone call.

After I go back to the bed and struggle painfully to sit. I drink more of the water and lie down on their gross bed that I'm pretty sure hasn't been washed ever.

One of the nurses comes in and brings me fuzzy PJ pants for my legs so they will be warm. After they leave I wear it but I struggle. I look at the dungeon scenery and the cameras, and turn on my side to cry. The only comfort I have is Loki 1-2-3 and he is half being a dick where he wants to help me, but also wants me to stay locked up here forever. I think he wants me to die here I don't know. He doesn't, but also does want me to be stuck here and drive me to a point where I'll want to kill myself or something. Maybe so he can take over. This place is Hell.

I tell him not to do anything that can get me kept here longer. That I

Ashes to Dust

can't be here, I can't take it I need out. I tell him he should want out too. He is also trapped here if he's stuck with me.

I get very little sleep.

25

I wake up to two new people coming into my dungeon of a room. Loki 1,2,3 tells me the "nurses" sent in were really angels and not the kind I knew of. They were sent to "save" the soul, but were under someone else's influence.

Revenge?

During the walk to the room they were taking me to, I was told I'd have to stay longer than today.

I was told only today, and they changed it and didn't give me a reason why or how long. I looked around and notice the spiritually awake people in psych. They were being kept here and mistreated. The angels didn't want them awake. The angels couldn't see I was awake too or they would kill me. It upset me deeply to realize they were poisoning the awake peoples' foods. I went into one of the rooms and took a tray from a awakened girl to prevent her from being poisoned. The nurses started coming, upset I was going to prevent this awake girl from eating it.

The other girl in the room told them, "Leave her alone," when they started coming in the room towards me.

I was escorted out and I noticed a girl lying helpless on the bed, and I was devastated, knowing they experimented on them.

I was taken to a room with two strangers. A older woman and a younger one who looked like a teen. The younger one was awake, and could feel Universe but she wouldn't look up from her bed. She was hunched over sitting on her bed looking down. She seemed timid, almost nervous. I could tell she was confused and thought she was crazy for believing in something like the Universe and things she can't explain. I wanted to change that so she would know she wasn't alone, that it was real, and she wasn't crazy and didn't deserve to be in this horrible place.

"Hello from Universe," I say to get her attention. I waved to her and the girl looked up, and then she waved back. "Just keep waving," I say when it looks like she's going to stop waving and stop believing she isn't crazy. It made me so happy to see her belief acknowledged and see her eyes realize she wasn't crazy after all. She has been hiding this whole time. She stops waving when a nurse comes in wheeling a cart with electronics on it.

I'm informed that the angel wheeling the cart was going to kill the girl. I didn't want that, so I put her soul into Ash's body to hide her, and put mine in her to die instead. I could see myself through her eyes in my body. I was prepared to die so the girl could live, and played the part of drained, lifeless eyes well.

I thought the girl would be safe but then the angels from before came in with one more so there were three. They wanted blood work from Ash's body. I stared at my old body through the girl's eyes. I didn't understand why they were asking for blood.

Loki said it was to kill Ash.

They didn't know I swapped with the girl so I wasn't in my body anymore.

He said they already poisoned her food.

I swapped back into my body and the girl back in hers. I have to lure them away from the girl so they don't kill her. I kept having to make eye contact with them, but they avoided it. I try harder and stared into their eyes so they could see the humanity in me and not do harm. They thought I wasn't human and were trying to eliminate me. I discovered

Ashes to Dust

the dark skinned, black eyed, male nurse was the weak link. He seemed to be not as hardened as the other two females; it was in his eyes. I focused on him so he could see me and not kill me.

I tried to get them to see I was better, by saying they already healed me when they still wanted to do "blood." I said if it wasn't true I wouldn't be able to walk and have energy. I demonstrated by jumping and thought they could tell how lively I was in my voice and energy.

The male nurse was the only one with doubt. I could see he thought I was healed. I needed to get him away from the other two who were influencing him so that he would follow his kinder side and spare me and let me go. I moved back towards the door and asked him if he wanted to go for a walk with me.

He said yes.

I held his hand, leading him down the hall. I didn't know where I was going until I was skipping down the hall to the exit. I stop in front of the door and let go of his hand. I pull on the door but it's locked. There is a key card on the locked door. I stare at him thinking he was going to open it but he started coming out of the spell and backed away from the door. He elbowed me in the chest unexpectedly, and I fell to the floor.

Ashes to Dust

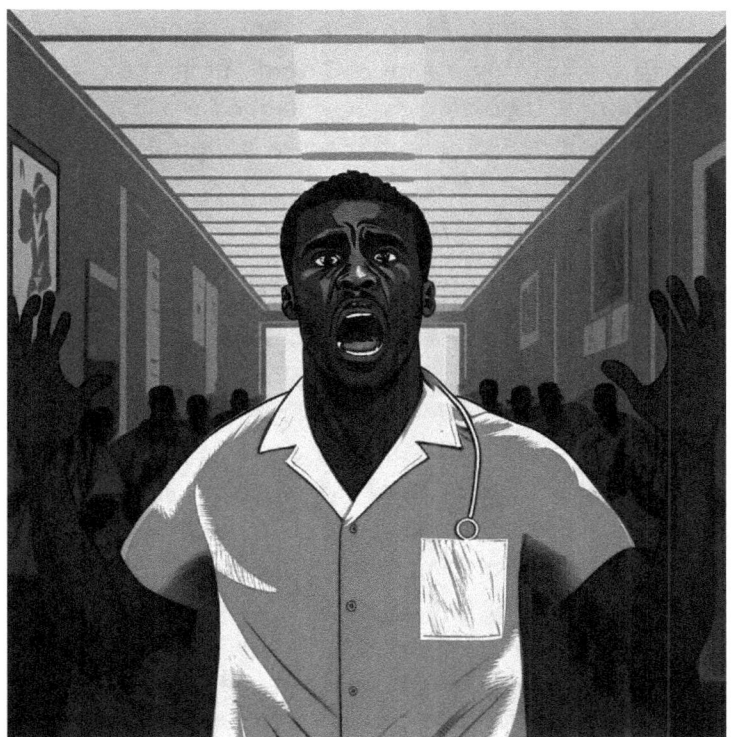

He raises his hands in the air, slowly backing away from me, as he lies to his other comrades saying I fell on my own. I passed out. Then I was in and out of consciousness as I felt myself being carried. I saw the ceiling sometimes.

I called on Mike, the grim reaper, my father. He only answers my mom's calls, Death/Universe, but because I'm his daughter, he heard me too.

I woke up to a bunch of people holding me down on the ground with security around. I saw what the one person held and someone was tugging at my pants. I realize they are going to inject me with a needle. I quickly shout, "Not in the butt," realizing it was like a horrible scene in a movie where they inject you in the butt. I see the needle in a guy's hand and my phobia of needles kicks in. I tell them no needles, but they ignored me. They twisted me and my neck wrong, and pressed my face into the mattress, hurting me more. I don't understand why they were doing this to me. It hurt when they stabbed me in the left shoulder. No one was gentle. A guy used me as a stepping stool to get up, and they left fast.

My chest was hurting so much, it didn't feel right. They didn't say what they gave me. I'm worried it's not interacting with my heart murmur well. It feels like I might have a heart attack. My chest is burning and the burn traveled all the way up to my neck and shoulders. I don't know what that means. I think I'm dying.

I realize I'm on a mattress on the floor, crying while Loki tries to comfort me. I feel like I'm having a heart attack and I call for help but I'm scared they will come back to hurt me more. No one hears me. Things start to get foggy, like a dream-sequence in movies when you can tell someone is dreaming because there is a bit of a cloudy fog around the scene playing. In less than a few minutes of crying, I crawl off the mattress and go to see if I can get help. If anyone was willing to help me and not hurt me again. The nurse already elbowed me in the chest, and now they held me down and injected me.

Ashes to Dust

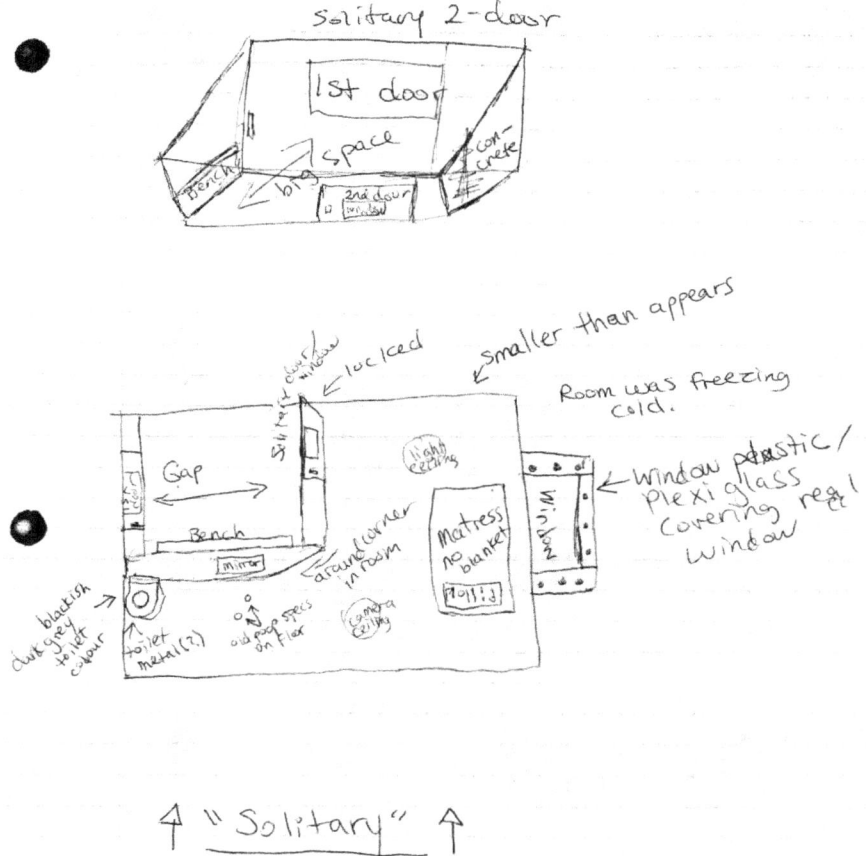

I look through the tiny window on the door and see a long hall with a gap between this locked door and another door with another tiny window. I look for a intercom to call for help or water, and there was none. I look to see if I can see someone to get attention but there wasn't.

Loki warned me it wasn't good to look, and I should hide. They injected me to kill me.

I duck under the window, and go around the corner to a bathroom. It is similar to the one I had when I first arrived. A steel toilet with no sink, but it had a reflective surfaced mirror. I went into the corner of

Ashes to Dust

the bathroom away from the toilet, hiding from the killer angels. I sobbed in the corner as my chest hurt and the pain spread in my body. I felt the light drain from me. I was light but they stole it. They stole my songs. I could no longer sing-song. I felt the dullness and lifelessness of it if I tried to sing a rhyme when Loki talked through me.

Death, my mom came back, and shared my dying body. I'm Death's daughter. Universe's daughter; Light.

I stared at the blank wall across from me where the bare mattress with only a pillow was. It wasn't high off the ground. Above it was another plastic covered window to prevent people from jumping out. If they put people in here, a jail, of course they would need it.

I try to sing-song to my mom that Mike is her true love, and I'm their daughter.

Mom is emotional. I can feel her realization. Death and Grim reaper, the universe-her-planned it well.

I could feel Mike, my dad come through too. Both were upset I was dying.

I apologized for not being able to handle even one death but I will so she won't feel it because she does so much for the world already. I tell her I am "Death's" daughter after all, in a similar iconic death voice mom did.

I cried more, and felt numb. Felt the world was graying and there was nothing left for me.

I heard her being emotional about how they took my song and that my music was a gift to the world. And my light.

I knew that was important too. I'm sad I can't sing to anyone. I can't sing anymore. It was taken away. It was important. Now it's gone.

I heard people from outside screaming and crying. I ask Loki why they were doing that. If they could feel light dying.

He said yes.

Light was dying in the world and all the awake people there felt it and were mourning. I don't know how mom took so many people's pain of death. It is so painful I don't think I can handle not being able to breathe right with these chest pains. I don't want to make mom take my death too; she's done enough for the world. I should be able to handle this one. I feel so empty. I just want to be happy and free.

Mom took over. She felt my songs gone. Her and Loki swapped back and forth when she realized I was a husk just crying, waiting to die. Mom started her escape plan. The angels wanted death, so she placed my body awkwardly on the ground to appear as if I'm dead so the angels would think they succeeded and we could escape.

I see a few pieces of old, dried poop on the floor. It's disgusting. Loki mentioned it. He didn't want my body lying on a floor with shit on it.

They lied about cleaning, just like I thought. The floor was cold, but so was the room. After a while of mom playing dead, she stopped. The angels were distracted at the moment with the others outside this locked prison room because of feeling light dying.

Mom got up, her and Loki both fought to come up with a plan. Both were clever. Mom looked at my body in the mirror. My eyes were round and blacker looking. My hair was a rats nest, so knotted it looked short.

She said I needed a disguise to not look like a mental patient. I needed to have my hair hidden. She looked outside of the corner of the bathroom and only saw the pillow case as a option. She went over, careful to not be seen through the window, and took the case off the pillow. She looked in the bathroom mirror, and tried to take off the gown.

Mom saw they left the little stickers on me from the Wallaceburg hospital. I wondered if they had to restart my heart or something and that was why my chest ached so bad. Mom realized there was no sink and walked over to the toilet. I was dying but still grossed out.

Loki spoke up for me too, telling mom she knows I would hate it because of how germy and dirty it is.

Ashes to Dust

Mom laughed, acting like she wasn't going to do it, waving a finger over the toilet bowl taunting me and Loki. She loved to see her kids squirm. She then put one of my body's fingers into the toilet water, swished it around quick and took it out laughing.

Loki said, "Mom that's fucking disgusting."

She laughed harder as she wiped the dirty toilet bowl water onto the sticky part of the nipple looking pads. She could have ripped them off, but she could feel my body's pain. Though it wouldn't hurt her she didn't want me to suffer more than necessary. She taunted again, Loki groaning in disgust, and she put a finger in and then wiped it on the pad and peeled one off.

She opened the hospital gown to see how many there were. She made a noise of disappointment; they left so many on me. She repeated the process of dunking a finger or two in the toilet bowl and dabbing it on the pads to slowly peel them off. Once they were all off, there was no garbage to put them in so she stuck them together and folded them. She looked at the hospital band with my name and health card number on it, and took it off. If we were to escape they can't have an identifier.

There was no where to put it, but Loki found a spot behind the toilet. There was a big crack behind it and the wall. He stuffed it in there along with the nipple looking pads so no one could find them.

Mom tried to puncture holes in the pillowcase so it could be worn like a shirt but she couldn't. Instead she wrapped it around the knotted mess of my hair like a bandanna and tied it so no one could see my brown hair. She grumbled about having to put the gown back on, the most obvious give away. Then she took off the pants that were over the boxer shorts so I wouldn't be dressed exactly the same and be mistaken as a different patient. She lifted up the mattress and hid the fluffy pants underneath. She then ran back to the bathroom to hide, and looked in the mirror.

My body looked like a cancer patient. I looked like I was bald, and sickly with big eyes.

We turned to the window as Loki and mom thought of how to escape. I stared at some of the birds and clouds out the window. I wondered if I could transport out the window somehow and just run across the street. I wouldn't go home, I would just hide somewhere in Chatham, get some food, and new clothes. Hide from the people who've hurt me. There was a church across the hospital. I don't think they'd think to look there. But I don't know if the church people would turn me in if they saw the gown, or if they'd kick me out if they found out I wasn't religious.

I started doing the infinity symbol with my foot, and realized Infinity was behind all of this and that was why I was here even though I passed my test. Infinity was why things still weren't the same and why even after taking the bad things away there were still messed up versions of angels. Infinity was the master behind the scientist who created the rape God higher power. I told mom and Loki.

Mom was upset. She hated when things messed up her work.

Mom couldn't feel me anymore. To them I was dead. Loki knew I was alive though, and he would have secret conversations with me by listening to my thoughts. Sometimes he'd make faces at me in the mirror using my own face, and shush me to make sure no one knew I was alive. If everyone believed I was dead I could escape without being hurt.

Loki stood against the wall in the open, and fixed my robe so no skin showed. He put on my fluffy pants again since it was so cold in the room. Mom and him had a conversation and then she called in the ex-rape-attempt-Loki for help. He appeared as the actor who played him in the movies. Him and Loki 1,2,3 didn't get along.

Mom's Loki saw Loki 1,2,3 was stuck to me, like he was to mom. But he also saw all the Loki's from the hospital were stuck to me through Loki 1,2,3.

My Loki's multiplied when Mom's Loki tried to multiply. Mom's

Ashes to Dust

Loki backed off realizing Loki 1,2,3 had too many.

Mom's Loki said he was disgusted that Loki 1,2,3 would be stuck to his own sister.

Loki thought that was funny and corrected him by saying he was not my brother. That not all Loki's had the same father. He left it at that with his signature cockiness, and made the other Loki's dance to his finger gestures.

They then had a spat back and forth about the worst things they've done, and how much they've grown. Like mom's Loki's attempted rape.

Loki 1,2,3 corrected mom's Loki again when he said he was the original. Loki 1,2,3 said he (Loki 1,2,3) was in fact the original Loki, not mom's Loki.

Time and the Universe worked different, and mom's Loki understood that. Mom's Loki still didn't like that.

Mom was there for all of it, sometimes saying things.

Loki 1,2,3 tried to get someone to get me water a few times when I felt so ill that I thought I was going to puke and pass out. But I had nothing in my stomach to puke up.

I was still severely dehydrated and didn't understand why none of the nurses cared enough about that to at least leave me water. And pads. They knew I was on my period but left me in this dirty pad since I came, and never got me new ones. I'm sure I was in that room well over a hour by then but there were no clocks just cameras. I tried waving to the camera and yell loud for water and help but no one came. I wanted Loki to shrink down and try to unlock the door.

Loki shrunk down and went to try to unlock it. I waited, looking at someone's scratched writing in the window. I wondered how they managed to scratch in the word "help." Did they find a nail? Were their nails so sharp that someone managed to do it? When Loki was done I tried to open the door but it was still locked. I didn't understand. I stood there in the corner of the door trying to figure it out. I looked at where mom, mom's Loki, and Mike, my dad stood. Then it hit me. They weren't real, they were personalities.

I ask out loud if I had multiple personality disorder.

I realized Loki 1,2,3 was actually my Protector. He dropped my hands to my side and said, "Yes! Finally."

I was devastated to hear all the characters I was interacting with were actually different personalities of mine. I don't want to accept that, but it makes more sense than Gods, Grim Reapers, Angels and Universes. I really want out of here. I turn to the window and eventually someone meets my eyes and comes to the door. They don't open it but I think they came because I still had the pillowcase wrapped around my head.

I tell them I was sick of my hair being matted and needed it up.

She seemed to want to laugh, but kept it together.

I ask for water, and she said she'd get it.

Finally! I can have some water! I was so thirsty I still felt so sick and in pain. I asked Loki/my protector if I should say I have D.I.D.

My head shook yes, then no, then yes. I didn't get a solid answer.

I end up telling her I had multiple personality disorder.

She said to wait.

I was relieved but also nervous. I think they will let me out now.

I go to the mattress and sit on it waiting. I have a conversation with my protector, who I use to call Loki.

They never came with my water the whole time.

A lady in a suit came in surrounded by a bunch of security. If their clothes didn't say "Security," I wouldn't have known. It made me nervous to remember that they were there with the people before who held me down and injected me. I got scared and panicked thinking they were going to do it again. I didn't understand why they were there. I held very still so they wouldn't think I was a threat and hurt me. I didn't want to be hurt again.

The lady was nice, but she was asking many questions. I kept looking at the security that surrounded her by the door. I ask my protector to help me not to say the wrong thing.

They will help me.

I needed to say the right things so they wouldn't hurt me and would let me out. I don't know what she wants me to say though. If she told me I would say it to get out and go home.

She asks about what happened before the hospital.

I tell her about my mom's ex fighting, and the food poisoning.

After her questions she got up to leave and I quickly asked again for water. They never brought me my water.

She said okay and they all left.

I was relieved there were less people there, especially the security. Why are they keeping me here? This isn't rest like they tried to claim. It was torture. They've done nothing but torture me so far. I wish I was at home instead, even if I was dehydrated it still would've been better than this. I'm still dehydrated and no one is helping me, only hurting me.

I lay on the mattress crying from the memory of what they did to me. My protector wasn't happy that he was stuck with me even longer now because of them previously holding me down and keeping me locked in this room.

He shouts in a hush, "Holy shit I'm stuck with you forever!" He said he would need to get stronger to be able to take on everything.

There can't be two protectors at a time so he has to merge as a new one that was strong enough to handle the psych hospital.

I apologize for not being strong enough, and thank him for being there. Then I apologized again that I would need him much more through it all.

He swore so many times. More than Loki. I could feel his demeanor had changed a bit when I realized he was apart of me. Still similar, but also different. Like saying "fuck" a lot.

I closed my eyes and held still on the mattress. I wasn't sure how long it would take for him to merge into a new, stronger protector but I made sure to keep still and not ruin the process. Sometimes I'd ask if it was done, but it wouldn't be.

I think it was 15-20 minutes of awkwardly lying on the mattress before it was finally done. I ask him some questions about it, and then go back to lying there crying again.

They haven't come back in a long time, and I'm wondering if they thought I fell asleep by the cameras. But the cameras would've seen I was awake. I ask him to help make sure I don't mess up.

He says, "Obviously."

My protector was all I had to keep me going. He took over right away, or was in the backseat making sure I was ok. He would help with his strength. I sat on the mattress staring at the door for a long time.

I've been in this room for hours now still with no water. Eventually the lady comes in with water, surrounded by security again. Again way too many than needed for just me, one person. Why are there five who all look ready to lunge forward at me.

She comes too close to me after setting it down in front of me. I need her to move back. The security look on edge and her being this close to me makes me scared of what the security might think. Like I might do something since they deal with mental patients who probably do. I don't want to be mistaken as one. I want her to move back towards them so they will stop looking at me and looking like they want to run over to hold me down or do something again.

She stays in place across from me, and I am practically holding my breath with a burning chest. I want the water so I grab it and hold it while staying very still again, so they see my hands are full and I'm not moving. I don't know what else they want from me. If they would just tell me so I could go home I can do it.

She talks a bit. I'm not really paying attention. I pick up what she says and over analyze what she might want to hear to get me out. Then

Ashes to Dust

I say it, hoping it's right. I will forgot something she just said and my protector will quietly tell me to pay attention. I then worry they will hear because he talks through me not in my head. I have to play along and act like I wasn't reliving the trauma by them being there.

She asks why I thought I had multiple personality disorder.

I changed that so they wouldn't keep me longer. I didn't know what they wanted to hear. It was difficult.

She asks if I remembered taking someone's food.

I said I think that was just cause I was hungry.

She then asked if I was hungry.

I said yes I was going to try having some soup as my first food of the day before all this. This time I ask for pads.

They all leave again. I drink some water, and wait for my pads. I've been sitting in nasty, brown, old blood for a day now, and I'm worried I'll get a UTI. They aren't caring staff. Is this how they treat everyone here? I feel bad for them. There isn't even toilet paper. And I still really want to wash my hands. This place is dirty with shit on the floor and I touched toilet water.

A few nurses come in this time, and they open the door, leaving it open and unlocked. They say I can't go out yet.

I don't. I'm just so happy they unlocked the doors and I'm not trapped and locked in the prison room anymore. No one brought me pads, so I have to ask for pads again. I also ask for more water, and toilet paper.

I feel like I'm asking for a lot. But they keep not bringing essentials that I need like water and pads.

I peer out the room and see people walk by. I wait, not wanting to get in trouble and get locked in again if I step out. I wonder if I will have to sleep in this horrible room tonight instead of the dungeon looking one they first put me in. I wonder if they will be bringing me back to the dungeon one instead of this prison one. I kept walking around not sure what to do. I want to call home.

Ashes to Dust

They eventually let me out and said I had to go talk to the psychologist there.

I went into a room with a few people. I recognized the one dark skinned lady who dressed nice, she was the one that came into the room surrounded by security. The male was the psychiatrist. He asked random questions like, "Why do you think you have multiple personality disorder?"

I was getting foggy, and it was hard to concentrate. I would zone out while listening but still hear. At one point I heard him tell the nice dressed lady that I was dissociating. This reconfirmed my theory that I had dissociative identity disorder. Like from the videos I learned about.

After they said they had to take me to the x-ray room. They wanted a x-ray of my chest. I was hugging the machine like they wanted. It made me remember what the nurse did to my chest and how sore it was. I remembered the male nurse who elbowed me in. I wondered if they did something damaging to my chest because the staff were taking x-rays right after it happened but they didn't say why.

I was guided to my new room where they said I would be staying. It had two roommates, a older lady and a younger one who looked like a teen. I didn't like that I had to share a room with strangers. I just wanted to go home.

I ask if I can go home to the nurse after asking for pads and water. (Again.)

She said the doctor would decide, and then she left and finally brought me pads and water.

I changed it right away.

Ashes to Dust

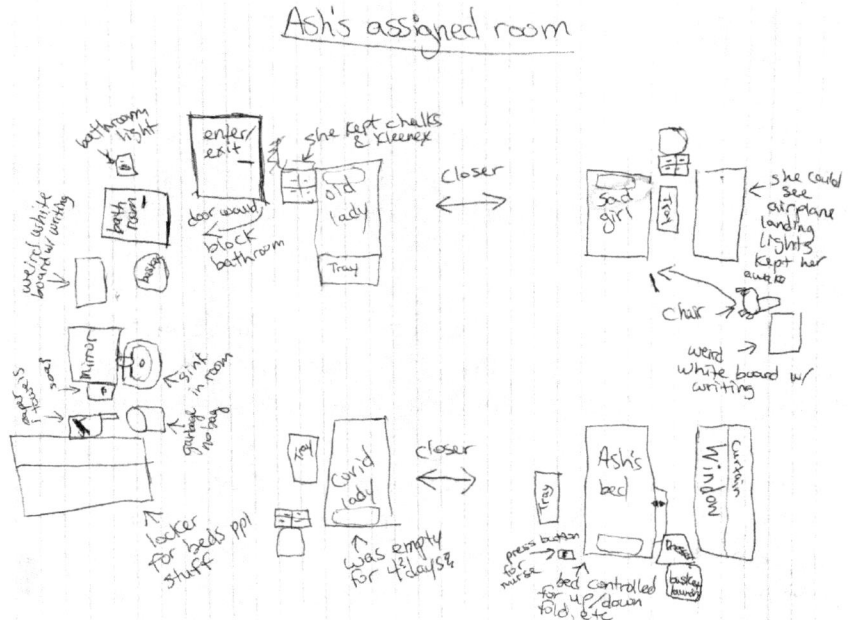

There were four beds. Two on one side and two on the other. The side I was on was beside a empty bed, and I was across from the young stranger. It was one of the beds that could fold you like a taco by pressing the buttons. It was weird. I was so tired, but I couldn't sleep because they wheeled in food to eat.

The older roommate told me it was supper. They came every day for breakfast, dinner, and supper.

She was sitting up straight so proper, clearly eager for the food as she waited for them to bring her the tray. I thought it was strange how excited someone was about the food while displaying it in a calm manner. It was hospital food. I heard bad things.

They placed a tray of food on my side table, and left. Some of it I couldn't eat. Which sucked because I wanted to eat. After eating I lay down and talk to my protector. Then I try to sleep. It was so noisy there I kept waking up, always knowing I wasn't in my quiet, safe room anymore. I miss my cat and wondered if she was safe since no one told me or called my house. The TV was blaring so loud even if I drifted to sleep it would wake me.

There was a girl who was scream-crying about being a pregnant tree and that they weren't treating her well. The nurse was yelling at the crying pregnant tree lady and I felt so bad I wanted to do something to help the girl so she would be okay because they weren't being nice or understanding towards her.

I heard more than one person yelling at her as she cried about her baby. I thought it was strange she thought she was a tree, but I still felt bad and wanted them to stop yelling at her and making her cry. The girl has a very loud voice and I was both concerned and annoyed at the same time.

The pregnant tree lady's name was, "Snow." That's all I heard her say.

Snow had very intense emotions that I could feel even with the door closed. It kept me awake, along with her voice. This was not at all a rest like the nurses tried to say. This was more chaotic than my own house. At least I would have my own room and my cat if I was home. Here it's too loud, with too many strong energies and emotions, screaming and crying, and strangers I have to share a bathroom with and have no idea who they are or what they'll do.

I learned of a few different personalities besides my protector. One was Bill. He was based off my abusive, rapist father. I only started remembering abusive things that have happened to me after being in solitary. One of them were I was raped as a baby and put in a ferret cage. I don't know how I'm as okay as I am after remembering that. Personalities are made for a reason, and that explains how I don't feel it or feel more about it. It's upsetting though. I can't believe him and my mom did that to me. Being here is unlocking it all. I learned it was a way for me to be a "good girl," and that was why I grew up feeling like I could never be anything less than a good girl or perfect daughter to my mother.

Ashes to Dust

Every time I fell asleep the Bill personality kept going out into the hall and talking with the pregnant lady, a guy who laughs like the Joker, and another male. I got the sense they were huddled in a circle sometimes. Other times they were outside and Bill would be smoking with my body, and I would start coughing from the smell and cigarette smoke in my lungs. He knew I hated smoke and did it on purpose thinking I wouldn't be aware. The others offered him the smoke and they smoked together.

Bill was out but they saw me. Bill had a lower tone than me and swore a lot. When he realized I was coughing from the smoke after he inhaled he sometimes said, "Awe shit!" and would put it out. Or get annoyed because he wasn't allowed to smoke. Bill knew the smoking was linked to the abuse where I could smell smoke while it was happening. And that my real abusive father would be smoking.

When I woke up my protector would confront Bill on smoking, telling him to stop doing it and that he knows I hate it and would damage the body.

Bill would say he knew but he couldn't help it, or he missed it. He sometimes said that's just what he does. Since he was a persecutor personality.

I would remind him he's not evil, like I learned from the YouTuber, he is important too.

My protector would take over to keep Bill from doing things so the body could sleep. But Bill would still manage to sneak out. I smelled popcorn and Bill went out in the hall with the three people from before, chatting and laughing. They were in a semi circle and offered him popcorn. He accepted and was eating while talking to them.

I caught a part of the conversation where one of the pregnant lady's personalities said how lucky Bill was to have me because they are treated like the villains.

Bill said yeah I'm a good girl.

Then they were talking about their host personalities but I woke up

Ashes to Dust

choking on one of the pieces of popcorn Bill ate because I was partially conscious and he didn't chew properly.

I started panicking and gulped down some water but no matter how much I drank the popcorn was stuck in my throat. The young girl across from me asked what was wrong and I told her I was choking on popcorn.

I then pressed the button to call a nurse. I used it before for the young girl because she was suicidal and needed help (she was too shy to press it). The nurses came; the same two from when I first visited. I was surprised because I didn't think the girl from my old school would be there again since I requested she not be. It was embarrassing to let her see me here and now like this.

Nurse Glasses came over asking what was wrong.

I told her my chest burned like I was having a heart attack and I was choking.

I kept briefly passing out, and I was worried I was going to die.

She came over and asked what she could do, and I said I didn't know.

I tried to describe the chest pain. I never felt like this before and it was awful. I didn't know what to do, and it felt like she was too calm as I felt I was going to die. She made a hook shape with her index finger and started rubbing my leg. I thought that was strange.

She asked if it was helping.

I said I don't know.

She would stop and start again. I tried to tell her again I was choking on popcorn.

She asked how I would get popcorn.

I said from outside they made it and I went out and ate it.

She said there wasn't any popcorn.

But then a third nurse came in with the water I asked for, and they said one of the patients brought it in and popped it.

I got up and started walking no where in particular. I couldn't

Ashes to Dust

believe none of them were helping me even though I was choking to death and felt like I was going to pass out. I saw black, and then I passed out right on the nurses feet.

She held my head up with her foot, and told one of the other nurses who asked what was wrong that I was faking. That I thought I was choking.

I tried to breathe and my chest felt terrible with so much pain I couldn't explain it. I wanted to cry but I couldn't breathe well enough. I couldn't believe how this nurse was treating me. Holding me up with her foot, standing there saying I'm faking when I'm clearly choking and having severe chest pains. I can't breathe well still, and I'm trying to hold back the tears. Why does no one care about me?

I manage to get up and crouch, then crawl my way back to the hospital bed. They made me feel embarrassed for choking and passing out. I felt like they didn't care that my chest hurt so much I could hardly breath.

I said I was fine, because Nurse Glasses's face seemed unimpressed like she wanted to leave. I could tell they wanted to leave, and I wanted them to leave too since they weren't going to help me.

I ask for water. Then I curled up on the bed clutching my chest after they left and cry. I only stopped when I thought I cried too long and they might come back.

I eventually got water and they left again.

The Sad Girl commented on how fast they were whenever I pressed the button. (She knew from me pressing it for her.)

I ask if that wasn't normal.

She said no they usually take a long time.

It didn't help knowing that because whenever they showed up it was more than one person and it made me scared because I wasn't sure what they thought of me. If they thought I was some dangerous person, despite never showing one once of violence or anger or saying anything mean. I was nothing but kind. But I still didn't understand why one of their nurses hurt me in the first place and got away with it. And why they then held me down with a needle in solitary and locked me there.

    I told Sad Girl how I was feeling about the nurse saying I was faking after passing out. And that I thought I was choking on popcorn because it felt like a kernel was stuck in my throat.

    She listened and never once made me feel bad about myself or embarrassed. She agreed she thought the way the nurse treated me wasn't well and she thought it was strange they just stood around when I was on the floor.

    This roommate is the only nice thing here. I appreciate that she never judged me and was kind. She was how I learned I was in solitary.

    I told Sad Girl if she ever needed me to press the button for her I would. She just needs to tell me.

    By the short encounter I've had with her, I knew she wouldn't tell me and I'd have to guess when she's not doing good and press it myself. We both tried to sleep after in the dark. It was so dark the only thing you could see was the slight moonlight coming from the windows.

26

Ashes to Dust

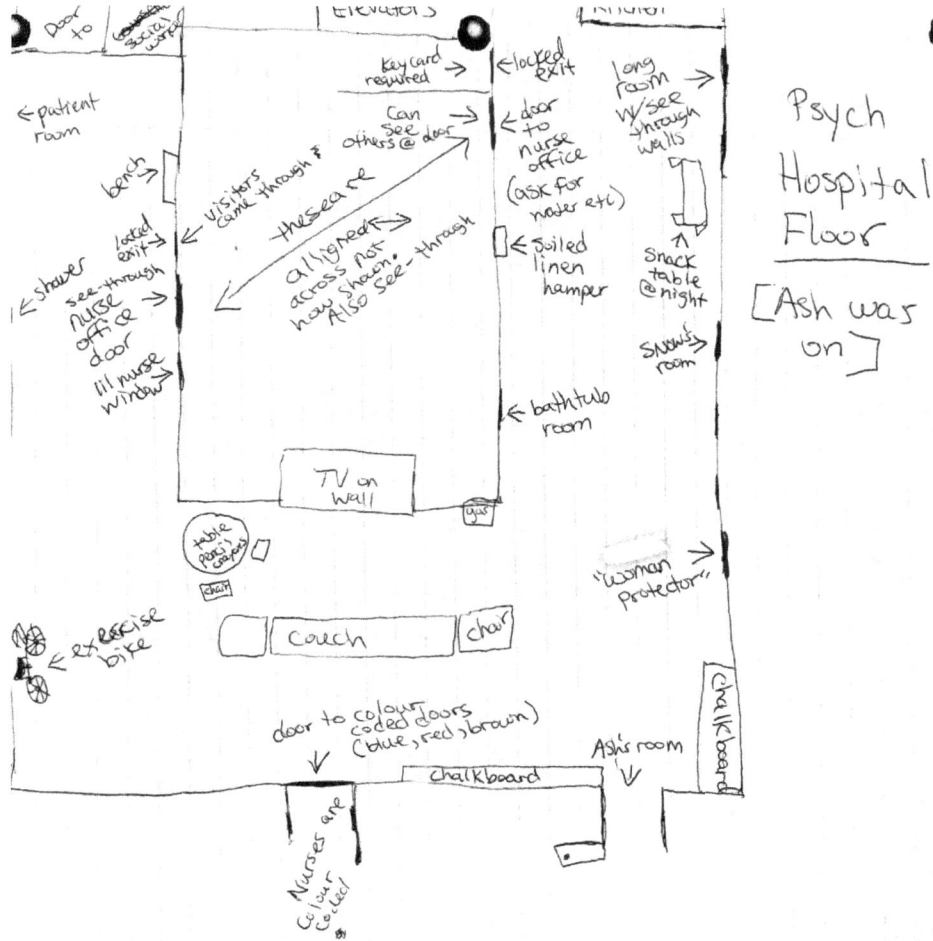

I am led out by a nurse to go get water. Some people waved at me, and I was confused. Did Bill keep going out last night? Did he meet people here and because I'm the host and not Bill, I don't remember? I don't know what to do. I grab my water and walk back to my room. But a man with glasses, lying on a couch in front of a TV winked at me with a smile.

Then I realize it must be what we agreed to do so it would keep me grounded from my other personalities. I remember I did that for him

Ashes to Dust

too. I wink at him, and he is laughing like a joker. I realize he's slipping into his mean personality, so I wink at Laughing Man to subdue his mean personality, and ground the nice one.

I do it as I say, "Winking at you!" When I succeeded I walked forward.

I find the voice of the girl I heard yesterday that was screaming about being upset about her baby and not being treated right. She says hi to me as she twirls.

I think it's so fun and I also twirl.

She says her name is Snow.

I say I'm Ash.

She has so much positivity I love it. But then I realize as she gets closer something is wrong. Her body language changes and her expression just slightly. Like the Laughing Man there is more than one personality in there. And the nice, energetic one is Snow.

I hold my hand out and tell her I only allow Snow.

She laughs in a not so nice way. She says I'm smart as she moves a bit further from me with her hands to her sides under her arms like she's holding back her other personalities from attacking.

Then a different personality comes out. A shaman. She says she's native, and talks for a bit. She then says she senses I'm native too.

I tell her yes, I have some native but my family makes fun of how white I am so I never felt like I was native.

She smiles and says I am native. Not to listen to what they say.

I found that really comforting and I appreciated it.

The native personality switched to the not so nice one, and seemed like she wanted to attack me.

I don't remember the Shaman personality's name so I say, Snow, Snow, Snow, a few times in conversation when she's starting to linger to a meaner personality.

She does a irritated laugh again, at the other personalities failed attempts at getting to me. I don't let any of them touch me.

Ashes to Dust

Snow is uplifting me, and I'm uplifting her. I say how I love her energy.

She says she loves mine.

I tell her I love snow, it's so beautiful even though everyone hates when it comes. I love it.

Her eyes go big and she says she loves it too, as we twirl around separately. She tells me that they didn't like her together with me. She said because it made her stronger.

I wanted to make Snow stronger than the others trying to cause trouble. I say Snow's name a few times and she basks in it.

Bill came out and told her that I, Ash (he spoke in third person), heard Snow through the door last night and didn't like what they were doing. And how upset they made Snow.

She responded well to that. She seemed appreciative.

Then it was back to me and Snow twirling. But I sensed I had to go because her personalities were becoming meaner and trying harder. There was a air about it. A vibe. I wag my finger at her and said no, no, no touch.

And at first she smiled mischievously as she also wagged no and backed up. Then her hands went back to under her arms, trying to contain them.

There was something about her eyes, almost mischievous, but also light. She said, "You're so smart. How do they think you're crazy?"

She was in awe, and it made me feel really good to hear her call me smart. I was surprised by it. I shook my head while smiling back as I moved away from her and said I don't know.

We both continued backing up. She stopped at one point and her arms went to her sides and she moved towards me. I shouted, Snow, Snow, Snow while laughing.

She laughed too, another mix of laughter like joy and frustration. She stopped and started twirling again.

I close my door. I'm exhausted.

Ashes to Dust

Later I feel the urge to see Snow again, because of Bill. He keeps wanting to find her and talk to her. I find her in the hall again. Me and my personalities are on guard again. Bill is speaking but I'm still analyzing for threats. Bill tells her about how he took off the bracelet they had on my wrist, and stuffed it in a crack behind a toilet. They wouldn't find it, and they made us get a new one.

Snow said she hid a cell in the vent. Her eyes widened as she pressed her fingers to her lips as a secret.

Bill tells her how smart she is. That we are smarter than people here think, we have to be. We have to think on how to get out of situations and this negative place.

Snow agrees. She asks if it's my first time here. She says it's hers. She thought it wasn't my first.

I said no it's my first too.

I get tired from Bill fronting so much and me fending off Snow's other personalities. I have to come and keep saying Snow's name, and to not touch. I have to back up sometimes.

Every time I recognize a different personality come out to do something negative she tells me how smart I am. And follows up with, how do they think you're crazy?

I shrug at the crazy part. I'm not crazy. It feels good to be told I'm smart. No one's said that before.

As we talk I have to block her negative attacks by reflecting it back using the peek-a-boo move by Death. I put my index finger and thumb together to form a circle to look through, and then I close my eye saying, "Peek-a-boo."

We're out in the hall a while and we walk a bit. Every time I catch a glimpse of one of her meaner personalities, I do and say the peek-a-boo method by Death to block her from getting me.

Snow starts catching on and doing it back to deflect me blocking her. Then I would have to be sharp and do it again with two hands or one. She would laugh as she did it. Like a game.

Ashes to Dust

Then as we walk away from Snow, her face changes into a stern line. It's the meaner personality that's been trying to attack us. She says, "Snow will fall."

My face is no longer happy. They plan on destroying Snow. They don't like Snow is growing stronger and fronting more so they plan on destroying her without her knowing. I'm going to have to warn Snow next time so she can prepare. They don't realize destroying one of themselves isn't the solution. It'll hurt them. They will kill their child-like self. They need that.

From yesterday, I learned the people here share and swap food because the hospital messes up so much. But they weren't allowed so you couldn't tell or everyone would get in trouble. If they didn't do it no one would eat. Considering I kept hearing how often they messed up, even this breakfast by people, I believe it.

Sad Girl was upset because they gave her dairy which she was allergic to again. She said she wasn't hungry but they had told her if she didn't eat she would be sent to solitary because they threatened her with it.

It triggered the horrible memory of what they did to me while in solitary and I didn't want her to go through that. I told her what the room was like last night. I ask her what she didn't want to eat.

She tells me and I take it so I could eat it for her and bring back the empty containers so it looked like she ate it and wouldn't get in trouble.

They gave me things I couldn't eat again without having severe stomach issues. I didn't want to risk that after not being able to eat after food poisoning for so long. I wanted food that would be easy. But after eating Sad Girl's food, I could barely eat some of mine. My stomach was too small. I set one or two aside so it looked like I ate it.

I could hear Snow upset again. She was telling the nurses how what she got wasn't proper nutrition for her baby.

I couldn't believe they weren't feeding her right. I wait until she was done, and I took the scrambled eggs with me out into the hall. I waited by her door, hiding the food behind my back. There was the meaner looking nurse by her door and she asked me what did I want?

I said nothing, I didn't want to interrupt.

Her face went so still at first I didn't understand, then she thanked me. She said she really appreciated that.

It made me see the nurse as more human and overwhelmed. When she was done with Snow I asked for water, and she told me to meet her in my room.

I waved Snow over and she hung by the doorway. I ask if she could eat eggs.

She says yes.

I slip her the scrambled egg container and her face brightened. I tell her I heard her say they weren't feeding her proper nutrition.

She said they weren't and thanked me.

I tell her to bring me the empty container after she finished so they wouldn't be suspicious. I also warn her that her other personalities planned on getting rid of Snow and to be careful.

She said they can never get rid of her. She then told me I should get a bubble bath and then a shower. It'll make me feel better.

I then left her to go back to my breakfast.

Snow showed back up with the container. I took it and placed it with the barely eaten breakfast I had. After I stayed in bed, but I still couldn't move around a lot. And going outside my room seemed to drain me of my energy even more. I got dizzy and it was hard to walk.

A nurse came into my room and asked me who I wanted to come visit because it would have to be the same person, it couldn't be changed.

I tell her my sister and I didn't want my mom to come or know anything else.

My sister helped me with the circles when I needed her. My mom put me in here and didn't want me out. My mom doesn't care about me;

she left me here. She doesn't love me. I hope my sister loves me. I hope she can help me. I hope this place won't scare her into not wanting to help me. It's a terrifying place.

I was told to visit their social worker.

I went and met a lady with dark hair. Then same lady who first showed up in solitary with security, and again with the psychiatrist. She led me to a door that was usually locked. It led to a hall of other rooms. I went in and had to sit in with her.

I tell her I want to leave today. That I was told I was suppose to leave already but I'm still held here. That I do not consent to being here.

She tells me I look a lot better today.

She didn't say much. I never got a reason as to why I was still stuck here, or a explanation as to why I was locked up here in the first place.

She told me the same things the others said after I kept asking. She said I was hear for a break.

I tell her the same thing I told the nurses I first met, this place is not a break, it is traumatic. I told her it's worse here. There is so much screaming, crying, and yelling and emotions. It's so loud I can't sleep. They mess up my food so I can't eat. The patients are coming to ask me for help. It's not a break.

She tells me I should be focusing on myself.

I tell her I want to go home today and be with my cat. I miss my cat and we have never been apart. I worry for her health and the nurses never called my house to tell them to let her out of my room. I don't even know if she's safely out of my room or not because no one called. I just want to be home with my cat in my room. I can't rest until I go home, it's not a break here. I'm here against my will.

On my way back to my room I run into Snow again. We talk trying to avoid the negative people around us. Like this one big guy with grey hair and glasses who keeps walking really fast wherever we are. I hear singing and feel its positivity. The girl is in a wheelchair with headphones on.

Ashes to Dust

I tell Snow she's positive and if we stand by her, her protective powers will block the others.

She agrees and we stand behind the singing girl's wheelchair after she parks in front of the TV.

Snow says she has seen this girl around and she's really positive.

When the singing girl starts moving again, we realize we can't stay there long, and leave too. We walk down one hall to the end with a see-through wall. I see a corpse of a girl with her eyes wide open matching her mouth. She's so stiff. How do the nurses not see her? I'm freaking out that they just left a corpse for everyone to see there in that room.

I tell Snow they didn't move the corpse, and we walk away from it.

But then I see the singing girl head to the room with the corpse in it, and I try to find a way to detour her. Her positivity would vanquish if she saw that horrible sight. I've never seen a corpse before. This is just one traumatizing thing after another. With the help of Snow we get singing girl not to go to the room. But eventually the singing girl has to go there. She says it's her room.

I walk really fast to my room not wanting to see the reaction of when singing girl finds the corpse in her room.

I have to ask a nurse for water. I always have to ask. Sometimes they seem fine with it sometimes annoyed.

I sit on my bed, remembering things I forgot. I only started remembering after they injected me. It's why when my alter Bill started saying, "Good Girl," it made me feel bad. My mom ate my pussy as a kid while my dad watched. My mom got off on it, which explains why my mom doesn't need sex toys or relationships because she's only aroused by little kids. My mom thinks the experience of abuse and rape they put me through is what made me a good girl.

It's why I always felt the need to always be a good girl. Never swear, or get in trouble and always do what my mom says. Why I felt I had to comfort her but never express my own opinions or feelings.

Ashes to Dust

My dad did bestiality to pets and used his dogs to lick peanut butter off my whole body as a baby. Even my pussy.

A cage. That's what I remember. A ferret cage. It was dark, and covered in my own feces. Dirty. I was trapped in it, and they fed me shit as a kid. It's why I made everyone eat shit in those horrible bed moments before coming here. Where I made Lucifer, and a bunch of other imaginary things eat shit.

My mom let him rape me, and joined in just because she was in a abusive relationship with him. She was too scared and in love to go against him so she went along with what he wanted to do and raped their own daughter. Me.

I'm so upset. Did I suppress all these memories? It was so bad I forgot until I had to come here and was separated from my mom. And now I'm separated I'm remembering all the horrible things she did to me as a baby and child? Is that why I'm here? Is it to remember them all and try to cope with it before I can go back home?

Is that why I didn't like when my mom use to kiss my neck as a kid and teen? Even when it was obvious I didn't like it and I eventually got her to stop. It was gross and felt sexual. I didn't like it. I don't think mom's are suppose to kiss their daughters like that.

I have no one to talk to. I worry for my sister. What if my mom is upset she's not a good girl like she wants and thinks that she has to do to her what she did to me? I don't want my sister to go through anything like that. What if she's done some things and I don't remember and my sister is traumatized?

I only have the "loving protectors" who I don't know if they really are. I wouldn't be here if they were. Why let such horrible things happen to me. Food poisoning, fighting Gods, being sent here, being physically abused, being held down, being injected. They are trying to not have me think about the past now. They think it's too much at once. I can tell.

My protector personality has to get stronger again. I have to lie down and have him merge into a stronger protector to handle the hospital and all these horrible memories. It's not the first time we've had to do this, and I feel bad for him. But he will become the strong protector we need to survive it here.

After several minutes we're done. My protector is different; stronger.

The older roommate comes in. She seems calm, and focused. I feel the need to sing a part of a song. I need to see if she's truly spiritually awake like I think. I sing the first line of Katy Perry's "Wide Awake." At first no response. Then I sing the line again later, and she smirks. I ask if she knows who sings the song.

She correctly guesses.

I knew she was awake like me. I wonder if that means I can tell her about my dilemma. Can she say something that will be comforting about finding out I was put in a ferret cage by my dad and mom as a baby, and raped by them?

My head shakes yes, then no, then I get more confused when I can't decide. I end up telling her.

After I leave to find snow.

I thought hard on it, and I nickname Snow, "Whole," instead of just her one personality, "Snow." Because all of her personalities make her a whole personality as one. Then I wouldn't offend the other personalities by only saying Snow. I think that's why they were so upset at me. I made Snow come out more and they didn't like it because I would call her all the time.

I talked to Snow about my abusive mom and my sister coming to visit me. I was excited to be able to see her.

I didn't want to mentioned too much about my sister to Snow. I still didn't know her well, and I needed to protect my sister. I was worried that my sister would end up like me with multiple personality disorder because of my moms abuse. I didn't know how to protect her or check to see if she had it or not.

Whole agreed, she said, "Fucking moms right?"

Ashes to Dust

    She also had a abusive mom. I debated with myself asking if I should tell her about the abuse with the ferret cage. I got mixed head responses again and decided not to. I already did that to the older roommate I had because I was so upset and everything there was overwhelming. They wouldn't let me go home or contact my family.

    Snow tells me that her husband is sending a present to me and that I should feel it. It will be love.

    I tell her I never felt love.

    She said she knows and that's why they want to send me that gift.

    I didn't know what to think about that. Would I really feel it? What would it feel like? She didn't say.

    Later Snow came to my door and gave me candy. She told me to hide it because we aren't allowed to have it.

    I thank her and go hide it behind the crack of my hospital bed where they wouldn't look. It was the first nice gesture from someone since being here. I really appreciated it even if I didn't like the candy she gave me. But I didn't want to undermine the kindness so I thanked her and left it at that.

Ashes to Dust

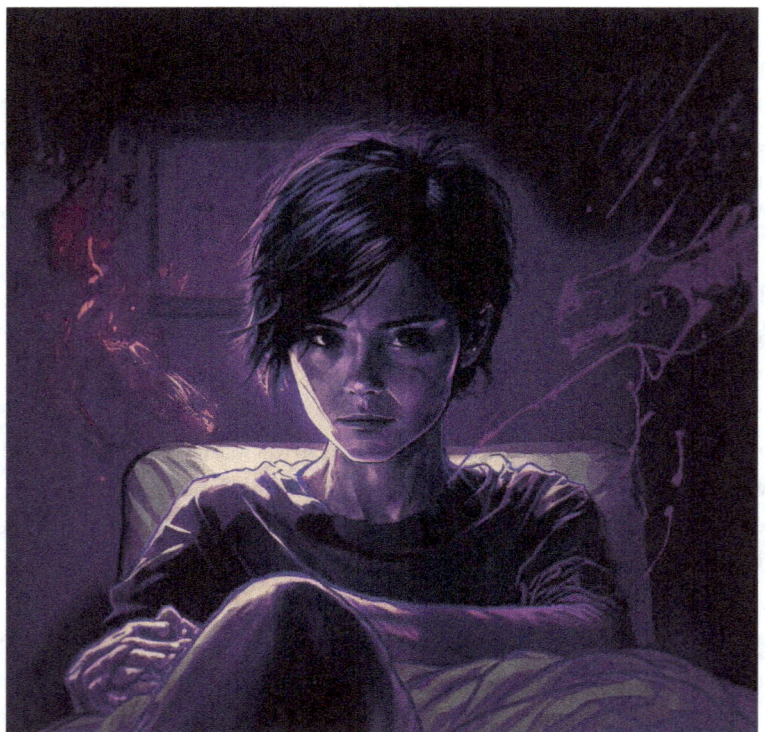

Sad Girl was talking to me. I look up from my bed to hers and saw a aura around her that was a deep purple that I at first thought was black. If I focused hard on her I would see it and it would make the rest of the room go fuzzy.

I moved to the chair by her bed to talk to her. I made it a point that I wouldn't touch her. I picked up on that at one point that she gives off a vibe where she likes her space and someone touching her, even a tap is a no. While talking to her it would get really hard to concentrate on her face. She was blurry like she was out of focus and it made me extremely exhausted. I didn't understand what it was at first, and I asked my protector. I realized it only would happen while talking to her. It was how she feels.

What a awful way to have to live if she feels like this all the time. I don't know if it's her condition or just being in this place. I don't know how she functions like this. It makes me want to help her so she doesn't have to feel this way but I don't think I can stay in this spot much longer if I have to feel how she's feeling. I can't take it much longer.

She tells me about her abusive grandmother. That she was surprised when she had to pack her stuff and be taken to this hospital. That she's suicidal and bipolar. That's why she's here.

It made me wonder if this place is actually helping her or not. Her grandmother invades her privacy while she's stuck here and reads her diary. While she was home it was her, her grandma and sister. She wants to live with her sister. She doesn't want her grandmother as her visitor but she doesn't have a choice they won't let her change it.

She likes to draw so I tell her she should try to do that to cheer herself up.

She tells me about the time I first came in and scared her because I was just lying on my bed and then suddenly I sprung up and said, "Hello from the Universe."

I chuckle and apologize if I scared her.

I forgot about that.

I tell her I thought I was helping her and that if she waved back then that means it was working.

She said she remembered that I said to keep waving and she didn't know what to do so she just kept waving. She said then she was worried about me because after that the nurses took me away and she didn't see me for a long time and didn't know what happened.

I told her they took me to a room with two doors spaced apart. With one bed without sheets, and a window covered in plastic. It was cold and had a toilet but no sink, and no way to ask for help. I tell her they held me down and injected me with something and then later they finally let me out.

She tells me she's scared of going there too.

Ashes to Dust

I don't think a suicidal person should go there, it would make them worse. They shouldn't threaten her with it.

She says that explains why she didn't see me after I was moved here.

I didn't even remember being brought here before solitary until she mentioned it.

It's night and I'm sitting at my bed. I feel a warmth spread across the back of my shoulders. It made me confused and a bit upset. It was so warm and nice while I'm in a dark place. I realize maybe this is what Snow said was going to be sent. I go out to find her.

When I find Snow I tell her about the warm sensation I felt.

Snow got excited and said that was her husband.

I didn't know what to do, I didn't feel love from anyone like that. Not even from my family.

I tell her to thank him. I also thanked her.

I left still confused on how to feel.

I go back to my room, and it's so loud I don't know how anyone sleeps here. The TV is always blaring, and voices carry through the door even if it's closed. I can't sleep well here. The nurses get mad when I tell them that.

Ashes to Dust

27

My roommates were active when I woke up. They were gathering laundry and getting dressed. Even the patients outside our door were active. I asked Sad Girl what was going on. She told me it was visiting day and everyone was getting showers and dressed up.

The nicest nurse came in and told me I had to shower. I both wanted a shower to clean myself from all the gross hospital germs and didn't, because I didn't want to use the same space as where everyone else has washed. I wanted to go home and use my own. I ask if I get to leave, but she said I would find out later and told me my sister was coming today.

I didn't like how she didn't say there was no option to say no. I would rather go home today and get a shower there in the privacy of my own clean bathroom.

I was so nervous. I wanted the hospital germs off of me but I also didn't want to use their bathroom. I just want to go home. I ask the nice nurse if I could have a bubble bath.

The nurse was surprised and excitedly said yes. She asked how I heard about it.

I told her Snow told me.

She took me in a different direction from where she was leading me, and opened a door I didn't realize was a bathroom. The door was across from the wall where other rooms of patients were; not far from

Ashes to Dust

Snow's.

The room was so small, the nurse had to push the door open for me to scooch in, and then she came behind me to close it. It barely fit both of us standing in there with the bathtub, and the chair holding the towels. I really didn't want to be in there and use the same tub every one else's naked bodies have used during a pandemic. Even if there wasn't a pandemic I wouldn't want to. What if I got sick because they didn't clean good? They don't seem to clean well. I know from seeing their rooms, like the solitary floor still having old, dried shit on it, and watching the cleaner in my room.

I didn't know what any one had here, or if someone had COVID-19 and might spread it to me by touching the same products. Or being in the same bathroom, period.

The nurse had the tub filling with bubbles for the bubble bath, and I waited for it to be done. I wasn't excited about not having a option. I already asked if I could go home, I'd rather have a bath there, but they keep saying a day or time and changing it.

The nurse ran the bath herself, and put bubble bath in. After it was done she told me she would be outside the door and would check in. That was uncomfortable and I had no choice. They were making everyone have one who had visitors. I took off my hospital gown after she left, and went in. It wasn't very high, but I realized Snow was right, it felt good. The first nice thing I've had since being here. I didn't have soap, and had to use the communal body wash bottles on the side of the tub. I wondered if they bothered wiping them down before letting others use it. I hope so because I didn't want COVID or anything else someone has in here.

The nurse opening the door made it hard to relax. She kept opening it and closing it and it stressed me out that she would see me naked. So I couldn't enjoy the bath. This was already traumatizing for me.

After I was done I told the nurse I wanted a shower, like Snow suggested. I held my knees tight to my chest and kept my matted hair covering my boobs so the nurse couldn't see me. I hate this.

She came in and unplugged the tub and said okay. But because they don't have the working facets in there she had to go outside the room to turn it on.

She told me she forgot a curtain and needed to get it. I stood facing the shower wall with my ass facing the door, trying to cover what I could. I couldn't shrink into the corner because their bathroom is gross with so many hospital bodies being showered in here. She came back, and again I ask her not to look at me. I asked her multiple times not to. Someone seeing me naked was bringing up new abuse memories. I stayed huddled close to the corner as she put up a gymnastic mat as a shower curtain. I thought that was strange and didn't get why they would use one.

As I was in the corner, I thought of my dad and how this is triggering since he raped me, and now other people keep watching me as I'm naked. It's upsetting and I feel like a prisoner. This place is like a prison. It has solitary confinement, and people who force you to shower as they watch. What's next, will they have a cavity search? I can't handle this, I don't like people invading my personal space or watching me as I'm naked. It reminds me of how my privacy and intimate moments are being stripped away from me by force again.

I'm positive she saw me naked, and that made things worse for me. No wonder prisoners cry when they get strip searched and watched. It felt like that for me.

I could hear Snow outside the door, which made me extremely nervous because one of her personalities was mad at me and she was being stalkerish in a negative way at the moment. She didn't have boundaries. Her room was right across from this bathroom one, so I worried she would open it and do something to me.

The nurse left saying she would knock and check up on me. I got out to check that the door was locked so Snow or any one else couldn't barge in. It was. That was a relief because it wasn't locked before when

Ashes to Dust

I was in the bath.

I went back in the shower and started to cry. I wiped the shampoo bottle and conditioner bottle off with body wash and then scrubbed my hands. I then washed my extremely matted hair. The days spent here were the worst of my life. I wish I was given a brush like I asked so I could've brushed it before washing it. I'm worried I'm going to lose most of my hair because they didn't give me a brush.

The effects of the bubble bath wore off the moment it was done, and the nurse had to come in as I was naked. I kept my back to the door in case the nurse opened the door again. She knocked this time to see if I was there, I responded, and that was that until I was done the shower.

I got out first before telling the nurse I was done so she wouldn't see me naked. I stepped onto a towel I placed on their disgusting floor, and then wrapped the other towel around me. The nurse came back and I told her I was done. She stopped the water and saw me in my towel. The room was not big enough for two people, so she had to squeeze by me, which made me uncomfortable in this vulnerable position. She left me a new hospital gown with socks, and a hair brush and left.

I was excited I finally had a brush. I got dressed, disappointed I'm still stuck in a hospital gown and not home yet. I go back to my room with dripping wet hair that looks worse than a bird's nest. Before I can try to brush it out a new older nurse comes in. She puts a toothbrush, toothpaste, and a tiny deodorant on my hospital bed. She instructs me to use the deodorant. The way she said it made me think I stink, but I literally just got a shower. Did I stink before and not realize? To be fair I wasn't prepared to be forced into a hospital, and have been bed ridden for almost a week. I don't care if I stink or not. I just got a bath, so I know I don't. I just want to go home.

I got to brush my hair, and thankfully managed to do it without having to get it cut. I would've been upset. They should've given me one right away. They didn't give me the notebook I asked for either. I think the bubble bath cleansed my aura because I feel less bogged down by negativity.

I went to the front to ask for water, and one of the nurses told me to wait on the bench. I waited and they said they needed to see my bracelet with my name, and health info on it to scan. I told her mine came off when I had a bath. It got wet and fell off.

She went to go get a new one. She came back and looked mad and told me not to take it off again.

I figured it must be expensive or something for her to make such a big deal about it. I can't tell her why I took it off. So I said I wouldn't.

After the nurse left I see the tattooed cleaning lady mopping. I smile at her and tell her I want to be a singer.

She rolls her eyes and leaves. It makes me feel bad. Like she doesn't believe I won't get out of here to be a singer. I just realized they're keeping me from my dream of being a singer by having me locked up. How long will I have to go without being a singer living unfulfilled and hopeless by being trapped here? When will they let me out? They keep lying about when I can go and changing it. They will take away my dreams of being a singer. Longer than I already have done to myself. I don't want that. I need to get out.

I go back to my room.

Snow keeps leaving things outside my door. Since being here I have to clear them up because they're filled with negativity. It's horrible to go by because I feel it down to my core. I wonder if she's been using smudging for evil purposes. She's went out two days in a row to do it and both days I've had her tainted, or cursed smudging rag by my door.

I grab a pencil crayon and pick it up and get rid of it. Then any random pictures I try to get off the door and dispose of. It's not the first time but it's still hard to do. Sometimes I miss one or she comes back and does it again. I notice new chalk doodles on the chalkboard. I realize some of them have meaning and are tainted. Like the thick

Ashes to Dust

purple outlines. So I wet paper towels and wipe it off. I won't let her other personalities win and bog me down more with curses or tainted energy.

I am back in my room and have a epiphany. I've been playing peek-a-boo so much with Snow, that I didn't realize it was abuse related. My mom and dad played peek-a-boo with my baby vagina. That's why it hurt me to do it this whole time without realizing. I can't believe it. It's so horrible. I'm remembering more being here. I hope I don't have to keep being here.

I then realize if it's bad for me to be doing the sign, it's bad for Snow. I should tell her to stop doing peek-a-boo. It's why her attacks were being powerful and harder for me to deflect. She was doing the same thing and it was linked to my parents raping me without either of us knowing.

I should tell her to stop trying to create her own death too. Death is one of my personalities, and she doesn't realize it was created out of such a horrible, abusive place, where I was literally left for dead as a child. It's why death is one of my most powerful personalities. It's why she shouldn't be creating something so dark. She doesn't understand. She shouldn't. I hope she never gets to a place or point where she has one.

I start getting more anxious of germs and being dirty as I'm here. It is reminding me of being trapped in a ferret cage as a kid left covered in feces and filth.

Snow shows up again despite me saying I need space today. Which she never gives me. I know she needs help, they all do, which is why I can't say no and let them suffer. If someone else did their jobs and helped them then I wouldn't be needed. I wouldn't feel so drained and like I might pass out.

I tell Snow not to do peek-a-boo and not to create her own death.

I'm surprised she tried after telling me she told her husband I scared her when I said Death. Which I understand because Death is very powerful and she was focusing her death breath at people. She probably saw the power of it, or felt it and it terrified her. I was surprised to hear it though. Her husband told her not to look when I do it.

Wise.

I tell her about creating a strong protector. Merging and becoming stronger. Thinking of something strong to battle and get her through being here.

I wasn't going to tell her right now my protector is a fairy. Tiny, but extremely powerful. It's why my voice goes so high sometimes, and she doesn't realize this tiny creature is more powerful than whatever she may think of.

She likes the idea after I told her we had to do it a few times already because this place is very hard to be in. She then thinks of one and says a big, hairy, abominable snowman.

I'm shocked she thought of something so out of the box. I tell her yes that's good.

It shouldn't be stronger than my fairy, but it will be her version of the strongest thing to protect her to get her through this hospital stay.

I tell her to go rest and create it so she can come back stronger.

A nurse comes in and gives me a mask for the first time. I'm confused by wearing it only when I leave the room. They never had me or anyone else wear a mask. They didn't even wear masks. I wonder why today. Then I go up to the nursing station and ask again for a notebook, and finally get one. Not sure why they didn't give it to me the day I asked. But now I can try to write some of my experience from my room as a story. This is the only thing I have to hold onto to get through this.

I ran into a problem trying to write. I would start experiencing the bad sensations again, like similar to when the Sun God rapist thing had happened. It's Kim, the dragon again. My protector and Bill have to get it to stop. I realize Kim is ruining the Kim cartoon theme song for me.

My sister Kat came to visit for the first time since I've been stuck here. She had a mask on, and I was confused when she still wore that mask in the room with me. It wasn't just us, Sad Girl also had someone in the room and it was extremely loud in the hospital.

We sat on the unoccupied bed beside mine. I made it so Kat would be comfortable. I gave her candy that I got from Snow before, that I don't like but Kat did. It was nice seeing her. She was the only positive thing I've had here. I ask her how she was, and we talked.

I was having a hard time figuring out how to say this to Kat. How do you tell someone you love that they have a personality disorder like D.I.D, in a way that won't scar them. I'm figuring out my D.I.D and have had some good results with the others who have it here so maybe because I'm her sister it will be okay if she knows I'm here for her. She doesn't realize it's because of mom though, just like me.

I could see when each personality came and went. There was a mean one in there, a giddy one, and more. I told Kat that she isn't broken into personalities, that all of them made one whole beautiful picture. That Kat, was a whole beautiful person. She laughed and smiled and I could tell I worded it well that she took to it. She was happy.

I could see her meaner personality look confused, maybe upset that I told her. I wanted to reassure her that it would be okay. Just like with my roommate I looked to see any signs and hints in her body language or eyes if I was going too far and they weren't ready to hear certain things yet. They seemed alright.

Snow came in, but it was one of her other personalities. She waved to me and my sister. I told her this was Kat my sister.

She was happy to see her and then left after a bit.

I saw a crow outside the hospital window. There are too many out there. Kat commented on how there are so many crows.

The crows reminded me of my experience with Odin, and though I

Ashes to Dust

know they no longer existed because of Universe, I was still wary.

I warned Kat to be careful of crows.

She said okay.

The visit was short. I'm not sure how comfortable she was with me calling mom, "The Fucker," but hopefully it wasn't too bad because I couldn't call her mom with everything I remember her doing to me.

I wanted to go home with Kat. I told her I asked if I could go home and they keep not letting me go home even if they do say I can leave that day.

Kat told me she dropped stuff off for me with the staff. It was clothes, undergarments, toothpastes, brush, and a picture of Lovie for me.

I was so happy she left a photo of my cat for me.

I hugged her and she had to leave. She gave me her cell number so I could call. I wonder if that means I can actually use the phone I see in the living space with the TV to call her. They haven't said I could call or talk to anyone. I really hope they will let me call her. I worried the experience of having to be in the hospital scared her and she wouldn't want to see me or talk to me again. She might not look at me the same when I get home after. I worry about that.

After being in my shared room for a while I got called down to the staff window. They were rummaging through what Kat brought me. I was confused why they pulled out some stuff but left others in. They sorted it and gave me some clothes, but not all. I asked about the picture of my cat and they gave it to me. I was so happy I stared at it. I miss her so much. I hope she's okay.

I set the stuff on my bed, and was surprised when the nurse that handed me my stuff came in to take back the dental floss that Kat gave me. She told me she didn't think she was suppose to give me it.

I didn't understand.

She then told me I would need to go back to the office to get a piece. I ask her why, and the nurse said because it was a hazard that someone could use to strangle themselves with. The same reason why she couldn't give me the reusable bag the clothes came in because it could be used for suffocation.

I never thought of it. I would just like to keep my clean clothes in a clean, non hospital bed. And floss my teeth. I don't think anyone will use dental floss to try to kill themselves with. I know I wouldn't.

When the nurse left, Sad Girl agreed it was ridiculous because there are plenty of things in here that someone could kill themselves with. She started naming them and it concerned me. I hope she was just having passing thoughts of observation and not considering killing herself.

I didn't want my clean clothes on the dirty hospital bed so I took the stretchy jogging pants, and tied the ends of each leg. Then I tucked everything in each side of the legs so nothing would be touching the dirty tables, chairs, or hospital beds.

I wasn't sure if I should show Sad Girl or not, because I didn't want her to use it against me later and steal my photo if her mean personality got mad or vengeful. I think her spiritually awake bipolar side was mad at me for talking to her unawakened side. Since first coming here I had to look for signs she wasn't ready or I was making the bipolar awakened side upset about talking too much and potentially awakening the side of her that wasn't ready yet. It was the subtle eyebrow raise that made me know it was the sign. I was worried her awakened side would take it when she's mad at me.

But she seemed down so I brought over my photo of Lovie and told her my sister brought it for me.

It made Sad Girl smile just like it did me. She really liked the photo and said she hoped to have a cat of her own too one day.

I tell her when she gets out or is able to move out with her sister one day then she can get one. She deserves to be happy too.

Snow came up to me and mentioned how crows are good omens. That's strange she would say that right after I told my sister today to be careful of crows. Was I thinking wrong and they were really good luck? I don't know, but I'm not going to tell my sister different now. I'm going to still be careful of them.

I realize I'm here to help spiritually awakened others. One that's important to help is Sad Girl. I'm disappointed I'm stuck here just to do another job of something else. Why do I have to be the one to awaken others? That's not fair to throw me in here. I'm not qualified. It would explain why I'm stuck here so long. It seems true since Snow told me her husband said I was there to teach. It makes sense that there was some purpose to this nightmare then. I thought I was done with the tests though. I don't want to be here or do this.

I ask a nurse if she can give me new sheets. I've been stuck with these old ones since coming here, and I had a shower today so I feel like fresh sheets.

She says yes and later brings them back. She tells me I have to do it myself.

I say okay, and take the stuff off the bed, grossed out. I wonder when was the last time they bothered trying to clean the actual mattress. Probably never. It's probably covered in hospital germs and everything else. Nasty.

I put the new sheets on and new pillow case and put my photo of my cat under the pillow. I lie down and I get a bad sensation reminding me of when the Sun God thing was attempting to rape me. I wondered if I was going through that again. Something raping me here right in front of Sad Girl. How do I compose myself while being raped by something invisible? Do I just close my eyes and try to act like nothing is happening and I'm not going through something horrible right now? Will she notice something is wrong?

Ashes to Dust

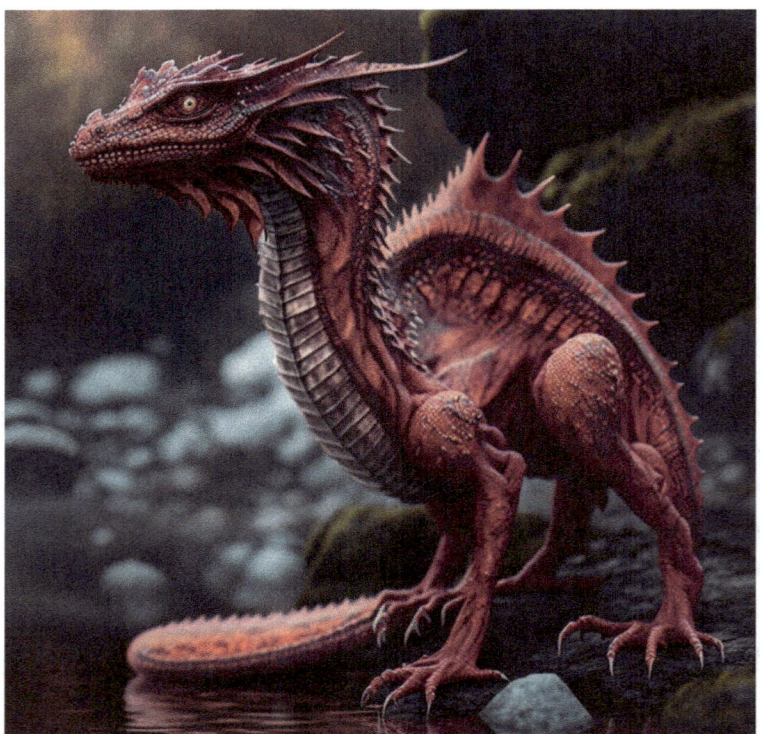

Protector personality comes out, and then Bill personality comes out to tell Kim, the dragon personality, to stop raping me. It's the whole reason why Bill had to become one of the protectors instead of one that triggers memories of rape. I have a knowing it's raping me with its dragon tail. It's horrible and I don't know what to do.

After Bill manages to take over so it's bothering him not me, and it seems to settle a bit. It doesn't like Bill being there. It wanted me.

I see little black balls in the bed. It's gross and I don't know why they're there. Is it shit? Is it very very old shit from a previous patient? Was it from a person having a operation and they shit the bed and when they threw it in the wash, it became a ball of shit that darkened and hardened? These sheets are clean. Are these pieces of corpses? Did a person die in this bed and these are sprinkles of their ashes or corpse

Ashes to Dust

remaining? They should wash their sheets better, these aren't clean. I'm lying in either corpse pieces or old shit.

I get up after the Kim situation is settled and rip off the sheets and pillow cases. I go to a bin I see in the hall and throw them in there. One of the nurses sees and asks about it.

I tell her I spilled water all over them and need new sheets.

She says she'll get them.

I go to my room, and when I get the new sheets I put them on and check for black rolled pieces of mystery corpse or shit. When I don't find any I am relieved and lie down.

After a while I go to grab my photo my sister gave me, and I can't find it. I take the pillow cases off, and blankets to search. I look under and around but it's no where. I realize I must have throw it out by accident. It was under the pillow! It must have gotten caught in the pillow case.

I go out to the hall and stare at the bin. I can't take out the sheets and look through it. I really want that photo. It's all I have that's good. That makes me happy. I go back to my room and start to cry. I find my sister's phone number and go and call her to ask if she can bring a new one. I tell her I lost it when changing the sheets. I can't believe I lost it the same day I got it.

She says she can print out another one and bring it when she comes on Friday.

I'm surprised she isn't coming for a few days. Did she get scared off by being here? Is she scared of me? Does she not want to come back here? I don't blame her for not wanting to come here it's a horrible place. But does she not want to see me now? Does she think less of me and doesn't want to be in my life now?

I feel worse.

She says that the person driving her can't do it until the weekend, so she has to wait.

I say okay and thank her. I go back to my room and go in the

Ashes to Dust

bathroom to cry. I lost my photo of Lovie. I miss her so much. I think my sister hates me now. I have no one.

Something above, maybe my loving protectors, try to cheer me up. They take my arm in the air like a rag doll, or a ballerina, and spin me. I laugh. Then they spin me again, and I laugh again. After a while I have to go out of the bathroom because I'm in there too long. I go back to my bed and see Sad Girl returned. I tell her I lost my photo of my cat.

I realize I have ancestors with me. They're native and helping me right now. They're strong. I feel their power as I walk. I walk stronger with the heels of my socked feet first. It stomps as I walk, radiating a wave of their power. It's protective. It keeps bad things from me, and shows strength to detour others.

I run into Snow, and we talk. They talk to her. She knows they're ancestors. They talk about how she needs to not use her gifts in the wrong ways. Not to wear their footwear while she's doing it because they are sacred shoes.

She says she understands.

She seems a bit down and we try to bring her comfort. I'm not sure if they're my ancestors or her ancestors or both. But we're all trying to help her. After she goes back to her room for dinner. She seems okay.

I see her on and off and when I'm going to get water the ancestors tell the native boy trying to steal my strength to stop. They're more powerful than him and I think he feels it because he goes the other way when usually he will keep going. I go back to my room with my water, heels first after being told I couldn't have shoes because my sister would need to bring them. I told them I had flat feet when I first was able to and they still have me walk around this nasty place in just socks. I don't think socks are a good enough barrier. And definitely not comfortable while walking on hard floors. My feet always hurt.

I hear Snow yelling and crying in the hall. I hear her saying they thought she had a phone, and she was saying there was no phone. She's telling everyone she sold drugs.

I go out as fast as I can and see Security. It clamps me up and I'm terrified from when they were in the room holding me down. I didn't want her to be taken and hurt. She's shouting how bad she is, and always messing up.

I wave my arms and quickly get her attention as she's shouting the worst incriminating things about herself.

She looks at me and comes over. I say truce, no touching.

She agrees.

I walk around with her and try to calm her down. I ask her what they were doing and she says they think she has a phone in her room and are searching.

I ask if they'll find it.

She smiles. But it was a moment of sneaky, smirk-smile.

I worry about her. I ask if they found any.

She says no.

We talk a bit walking around in the U shaped hall, sometimes sitting on the bench. I tell her she's not a bad person.

She says she is.

I tell her she's not but she needs to not make things harder on herself so she can get out of here to see her family.

I shield her from the other negative people like Braids, the Glasses Guy who followed us all the time, and the native guy she said wants to steal my powers through my hair by touching it. I was surprised at that and have been more on guard about him and my hair.

I don't want her to think I'm telling her what to do, or that she has to do what I say. She can do what she wants. But I want to word this just right so she knows I'm not trying to strip her of her freewill, but also lend some advice so she can see her family again without issues. Especially after telling me some personal things.

I tell, Whole, that she has freewill and I'm not telling her what to do,

Ashes to Dust

but every time she (from now on) does drugs, then they (Psych) win. Because they will use it against her and she didn't deserve that.

She got quiet. But it seemed like she understood. I hope she will take the advice, and do her best to not end up here again for her family's sake.

I take her to the photo of the sunset and try to get her to visualize breathing in and out to calm herself. It seems to be working, but it also seems like one of her personalities is coming out in defensive mode at me now.

I move away and she smiles saying how smart I am. She then is called back and she leaves.

Later I see her again and she is gathering her stuff. She tells me she has to move to a different room.

It's the room where I saw a corpse. It makes me nervous. Will she see the dead body in there? She doesn't react even though there is a person stalk-still with their eyes and mouth wide open against the see-through wall. Does she not see it? Am I losing it? Can only I see the corpse there? I see the wheel chair girl interact by the corpse and realize it must not be a corpse. I go back to my room.

I could tell the "Protector of Women" (Snow introduced him as such prior) was having issues. I walk up to him and ask if he wanted my help. He said yes.

I walk around the halls with him shielding him from the negative energies of people so it didn't transfer to him. I had to make sure to avoid them myself too so it was extra work. Like everyone else here, I avoided touching anyone. If I needed to shield, I would use my hands to stop someone or direct them around. I would use my arms around his body like I did for Snow, like a hovering air hug but it was meant as a shield against any negative energies from people coming towards him.

I had to tell him to avoid a high five from the Laughing Man when I sensed it was the mean version of the Laughing Man trying to reinfect

Ashes to Dust

Protector-of-Women to trigger the mean version to the surface.

I wag a finger at Laughing Man for no, or made a shoo motion and told Protector-of-Women to keep walking if we kept running into him.

The Protector-of-Women complained about his back hurting.

I caught him rubbing the small of his back a lot, so I figured something was wrong. I ask him if it was okay to touch his back to try to help him.

He said yes.

I held my hands over where it hurt and visualized the stored negative energy there melting away. Then I wiped it off him and asked him how he felt.

He said it felt better.

I was glad.

When we walked back in a different direction he still seemed to be struggling so I told him to stand in front of the wall with a picture of a dark forest on it. The bottom of the photo was the darkest with shadows, and the top was lighter with light between the dark trees.

I tell him to exhale the dark (as I point down) like the darkness of the shadows. Then inhale (as I point up) the light like the flecks of light on the top. He followed as I went through the big breaths in and out while pointing up and down as a visual for him. It was similar to what I did for Snow. He did it for a while to be calm, and then he needed to walk again.

I ask if he still needed me, and he said no, so I turned around and went back to my room.

I felt relief to be back and not out there anymore. It exhausts me and right now I need rest from the energies out there draining me.

Later I needed water and went to walk to the nurses station. I saw Protector-of-Women in the room where people go to use their phones. He was slumped over sitting in a chair while Snow stood beside him. I hear him ask her (by her body's name), what was going on because he was confused.

It reminded me of when Snow told me he didn't understand what was happening and she told me she said I was helping him and helping them learn.

I heard her tell him I was helping him.

Then I saw the host (who's less friendly than Snow) rubbing the small of his back. I realize that's why he has pain. She's undoing my help and putting negativity back in.

I go get my water and go back to my room.

Snow told me her husband was here. She was excited and wanted me to meet him. Snow tells me Braids, the girl I was shielding her from is actually very ill and sick.

I tell her I must have been picking up on that and not bad ones like I thought.

It made me feel bad for giving her the finger every time she waved at me.

I walked with Snow and met her husband. He was a big, tall native man. It was nice meeting him. But it made me nervous because I knew he was powerful and I didn't want him to try to use it against me.

Snow kept telling me how powerful he was.

I told her I could sense it.

She smiled proudly at that, and went back to her husband. I let them have their visiting time together and went back to my room.

Snow was able to leave today. I wondered why she could leave but I couldn't. It didn't seem fair. I was glad she got to leave though, she shouldn't be here any longer. It wasn't good for her or her baby. I went over something she told me today. She said, "This is Snow's husband, and this is our baby. Snow's baby." I realize that I may have been wrong all along. Snow might not have been the good personality, she may have been one trying to overtake the will of the host. And that was why the host was always so mean and sad.

Ashes to Dust

That means what I've been doing has only been encouraging the Snow personality to overtake all of the other personalities in their system. No wonder they were so mad at her that they wanted to end her. I don't think they should kill one of themselves off, but I do think I should try to make it right. Maybe I can say the right thing this time, and let the host and her other personalities know that what Snow did for overtaking their freewill to have a baby or not, wasn't right but it should be their decision as a whole, to decide what they want.

If some of them don't want to take care of the baby, they don't have to, they can let the ones who do approve take care of it. Snow had no right to decide that for them by sneaking in bed without the host approval or discussing it and having a baby behind their backs. It explains why she seems so miserable whenever I get a glimpse of the host personality.

I go out and find Snow. When I find her I use her body name, even though I didn't want to do that to her system, "Whole." I thought it was disrespectful but this message was meant for her personally since her free will was violated.

She was surprised I knew her name. She asked me how I knew it.

At least I knew it worked and the host surfaced. I tell her she told me before when I met her.

She seemed out of it, and dazed simply saying, oh.

I call a truce, and she nods in agreement.

I talk to her a bit, and we go walk through the halls, sometimes stopping at the bench for a moment. I shield her from negative energies. We walk side by side without me having to be completely on guard anymore. She seems really down.

It's almost time for her to leave. I tell her what I needed to tell her. I say it's her choice to keep the baby or not. It's not anyone else's and to do what she thinks is right. I tell her that Snow tricking her husband and getting pregnant without talking to her other selves as a whole system wasn't okay.

Ashes to Dust

Snow came out and said, "I know, I'm bad. I cause trouble." It wasn't the first time she's said this. She's said it many times.

I tell her no, she's not she just needs to communicate as her whole self first so they can all make a decision. Especially the host body.

She didn't say she was bad anymore. She seemed okay. She nodded and then got to leave with her husband. She waved good bye to me.

I hope I said the right things and didn't mess it up. This isn't a easy process.

It was night and I was sitting by Sad Girl in a chair, when I felt a twisted version of the warmth from before at my feet. It was trying to attack me. I was defending against it, knowing it was Snow's husband attacking me from afar. He was doing it because of what I said to his wife's host about keeping the baby being her choice and no one else.

I tell Sad Girl what's happening that I have to defend against Snow's husband because he's mad at what I said to her.

It made me wonder if I said things wrong after all, or if he didn't like that I told her it was her decision. To make matters worse our other roommate came in stomping the ground on the balls of her feet like I've been doing. She's copying me to produce power. Now I have two to defend against.

Ashes to Dust

28

I see the social worker today. She asks me stuff. I notice her eyes start blinking closed too long like she might fall asleep. I ask the protectors if they were doing that.
Yes.
I wondered if I was saying something wrong so they had to put her to sleep so she didn't realize. But then I knew, it was so she wasn't just hearing, but listening. So she was processing it fully.
She asked me what I liked to do before at home.
I tell her about the book I wrote.
She asks what it's about.
I tell her. But each sentence and description of a character and plot, I see her face change once in a while. I realize I must be giving away childhood traumas without realizing and she's catching them. Or deeper meanings I haven't realized.
When I tell her about my interest in ancient Egyptians and the mummies, she makes the face again. I realize was wrong to say that because she must think it's a death thing. It's not a death thing. I shouldn't have told her that I liked the ancient Egyptians, or describing my first fiction book. She might somehow use it against me. Did I say too much?
Even though I felt myself perk up talking about my book, now I feel doubt. I don't know what they want from me. Just let me go home like

Ashes to Dust

I ask the moment I come in this room. Or when a nurse comes in the morning.

I leave feeling like I might be here forever.

I call my sister and tell her I asked when I was going home again. I end up crying when I talk to Kat. I try not to but I do. I tell her Snow is gone now.

My sister found it creepy that Snow stood by the door when she was visiting me.

I told her ya she would always just show up. I tell her about the guy that Snow told me about trying to steal my power through my hair. I have to battle their energies while I'm out there.

She said ya it sounds loud still.

I said it is.

While talking to her I have to tell people not to bother me, or say no to someone like the big, fast paced man too close to me. I was on defense even while on the phone to my sister and she had to hear it all.

I still called mom, "the fucker," which I did ask if Kat was bothered by, but she said no. That was a relief.

She asked if I wanted to talk to my cat.

I was worried about that because I didn't want to make her sadder. I wasn't there and her hearing my voice might not be good if she can't find me.

I was going to say no but she said Lovie has been really sad without me. So I said yes.

She put me on the phone and I talked. I couldn't hear Lovie, but I said hi, and love and miss you. I ask how she reacted.

Kat says ya it probably wasn't good to do that after all.

That made me worried even more for my cat. I can't see her or know how she is. Is she eating well? Is she happy? Sad? I don't know. I want to be able to hold her. I miss her so much.

I thank Kat for putting Lovie on, and then we end the conversation.

Now I'm left feeling worse like I did damage to my cat by talking to

Ashes to Dust

her. I feel awful as I go to my room.

Sad Girl got bad news that she might have to be stuck here for another month. I felt really bad for her. It's already been a few days and I don't think I can go on any more; how will she?

I tell her I've asked every day if I can go home and they still haven't let me. (I tell her every day so she knows.) I then say I think we both will be stuck here a long time.

She said at least we will be able to get through it together.

That made me feel a bit better. To know at least there was one person I could talk to. I didn't have to hide the crazy looking moments; she's seen them all and has accepted me. She's a really good person who doesn't deserve to be in this place. I hope she gets out and can be happy soon.

I ask her if she has a switch.

She says yes.

I ask if anyone has ever had one here.

She says she thinks she's heard of people before.

I tell her to go ask a nurse if she can have one.

She isn't good with confrontation, even asking for what she wants. It's why since I've been here I've been the one to push the call button for her. She wants it but she doesn't want to ask.

I go to the nurses station and ask if Sad Girl can bring a switch.

The nurse says she would have to ask first because they don't allow anything with cameras.

I say it doesn't have a camera, and then ask how long it would take to find out because I think it will really cheer Sad Girl up.

She says she doesn't know it could be nighttime.

They announce that it's cell phone time. I woke Sad Girl by shouting her name so she wouldn't miss her time to talk with her sister. I tell her they announced phone time.

She got right up and offers me to come with her.

I tell her it's okay to enjoy her time with her sister she deserves it.

Ashes to Dust

She left. She's always happy when it comes to this time. I don't have a phone or anyone to talk to so I sit on my bed with nothing to do. It made me want my iPod. I could connect to the Internet on it, or listen to music.

The older roommate was in the room with me when I was waiting for my water. The stern faced nurse came in and set down my water. She had a straight, blond, ponytail.

I tell the roommate that she needs to be careful because some of the nurses like that one leave their negativity in the water and pollute it making it undrinkable.

The roommate agreed saying, "Yes they fling it everywhere."

I knew she was awakened and saw it get flung in there too. I go and pour out my water using a paper towel. Then I go ask a different nurse for water. I get better results this time.

Sad Girl and I went out to the line for snack time. I wasn't sure what they'd have. We stuck together and waited. Then we saw they had ginger ale. I wasn't sure about it because last time it was flat. We were surprised when we poured it and it actually had bubbles in it. It was the most exciting and happiest moment in here for us.

We went back to our room and talked about the bubbles. I sat in the chair next to her bed and plotted on taking the whole bottle of ginger ale back to our room. When we ran out of ginger ale we went back, but the ginger ale was all gone. I was sad about it. It was the best part. We talked about how horrible this place is that we were excited for bubbles in ginger ale.

Sad Girl wanted to draw something so we talked about what she could draw. She drew aliens with a UFO. We talked about how the aliens would come over the building and take us out of this horrible place. We laughed about it and then said they would probably give us back because we were too much for them.

It was nice to laugh.

Ashes to Dust

I go to the nursing station and ask if they found out about the Switch yet.

They said not yet. It may take until tomorrow since it's night.

I asked earlier so this is disappointing. Hopefully Sad Girl will hold out. I ask for water, and the nurse goes and gets it for me. Sometimes they go to the kitchen where they have snacks out in the hall and get it there from a locked door. But most times they just come back with it here and I don't know if it's just tap water or not. Hope not.

At bed time Sad Girl wasn't in a good place. I think it's because she has to stay here longer. I ask if she wanted me to call someone, and I was surprised when she said yes.

I got up and went to get someone. I kept hearing Snow previously say bad things about a specific nurse, and to my dismay it was the biggest, tallest, male nurse. The one they were sending to see Sad Girl. I got bad vibes from him and worried for her safety.

I got back in the room and debated whether or not to tell Sad Girl about the vibes I felt with him. I wasn't going to but I could hear his voice roaring in the halls and it made me nervous. I got rapey vibes from him. I didn't want him to hurt her. I didn't want him to hurt me. Do I need to stay up all night to make sure he doesn't sneak into our room? What if he turns his sights on me? Should I make sure not to be noticeable?

I warn Sad Girl that I got bad vibes from him. And just to be careful. She said okay.

He came in and sat in the chair I always sat in by her bed. It was odd how small it was compared to how big he was. My thought and vibes of him changed when I realized he was helping her. He was actually a really good listener. His whole demeanor changed after sitting down in the chair. It wasn't like the hall. It was more professional. He's the best I've seen anyone here be with her. I must have got my signals crossed again. Or he is able to separate professionalism when there's someone who clearly needs help and care.

Ashes to Dust

After he left she seemed a bit better. I was glad he came and treated her respectfully and took his time. I haven't seen much of that with other nurses and how they treat the patients. Especially when I first came here and heard the Snow and nurse debacle.

I asked if Sad Girl felt better.

She said yes.

We both stayed up looking out our windows most of the night. I saw the same big, male nurse peep in the room later on to check in.

When I had to go to the bathroom I had to turn off the lights because it woke everyone up, and they'd complain. But I can't pee in the dark in a hospital.

29

Protector-of-women popped in our room and said Snow wanted to know if anyone wanted anything from Timmie's.

I was surprised she wanted to buy for people while she's free. I didn't want her to spend her money on me so I told him to tell her no, but thank you.

He said okay, and then left.

I wondered if that meant she was hanging around the hospital to visit people. I hope she doesn't get in trouble and get stuck here again. She needs her freedom.

I go to the nursing station and ask the nurse there if they talked to the person they needed to about the switch or not. It's a different nurse and after she goes and asks someone else she says yes to bringing a switch.

I tell Sad Girl the good news and she brightens up and says she's going to ask her sister to bring it. She tells me I should ask my sister to bring mine so we can play together.

There's a new roommate. She's older than the oldest lady in our room. I hear her and the nurse talking about how she will be staying in our room to quarantine until she gets her results back for COVID. The old lady can't stop talking about it. Me and Sad Girl start to freak out over it and talk about how we are worried we will end up getting

Ashes to Dust

COVID.

The old lady keeps touching us. I go to brush my teeth and she walks up to me, invading my space and touches my back. It freaks me out knowing she might have COVID. She shouldn't be touching me. She keeps walking around and coughing all over the place. I try to avoid where she's been but that's impossible with one bathroom and one sink out of the bathroom. Since there aren't masks in here we are exposed. I'm hoping I don't get COVID. I don't want to get sick and die. I don't want to be stuck in the hospital longer only to die here.

For lunch I get this weird meat mayo sandwich. Everyone in the room seems to get it because I hear the older ladies complain about too much mayo.

I bite into it and I think it's chicken. But my other personalities are fighting to taste it too. I keep switching as they try to taste what I'm eating. It's really hard to chew when they do this, and I almost choke multiple times. Even when I warn them we'll choke they still do it.

The fairy seems to be the most taken with the sandwich. I don't really like it. It's a odd flavour and texture I never had. They keep giving me chicken every day. I'm happy there's peanut butter again. I really liked that.

When I have to fill in the food menu, the other personalities try to add things I don't like. Bill tries to add jam, and Hana tries to add coffee. I think she's the reason why I keep drinking some nasty tea they bring. I hate all the things they keep trying to have me check mark.

I call for Death to come forward and check mark them so the others wouldn't mess it up. I know Death was the strongest and only impartial one.

Death check marked the ones I liked, despite the other personalities trying to stop and sneak in some different ones. I sent it in with a note again about lactose-intolerance, and no potatoes or eggs.

For Dinner I was surprised with mac and cheese, and a side of

Ashes to Dust

tomatoes. I didn't know what they were and the older ladies said stewed tomatoes. Again everyone got it, even Sad Girl who was highly allergic to dairy. Don't know why they keep giving her milk still.

I ask what you do with it.

The older ladies sound surprised, and say you're suppose to mix the stewed tomatoes with the mac and cheese. They couldn't believe me and Sad Girl never had it before or knew about it.

No, I thought that was odd thing to do.

After I decided I should try to do it and if I didn't like it just not eat it. It wasn't that bad. I was surprised it was pretty good. I ended up eating it even though it'll make me feel shitty later. Sad Girl did too.

The snack time announcement happens and me and Sad Girl get excited, and hope they have bubbly ginger ale again. On our way to the line we talk about how we should just take the whole bottle. Once we get there we are pleasantly surprised that there was indeed bubbles in the ginger ale. It's name brand, and mostly full. I open it for us, and we each grab a cup, and I pour it into them. We grab some snacks like apple slices, but they didn't have much because people took them.

Once we got back to our room and sat on our beds, we talked about how sad it was that our only happy thing in this place was the bubbly ginger ale. It made us happy.

It made me happy. It was the only normal thing I had that I liked. It's all I had to cling onto. But they didn't usually have this. It was rare, and usually flat. The bubbles hurt my throat but I loved it.

Later the nurse came in and wheeled in a computer or monitor on her cart. She mentioned me taking my sleep pills.

I didn't understand what she was talking about. I never took anything (willingly) since being here. The only time I was given something was that horrible forced mystery drug they injected me with.

I ask her what sleeping pill. I didn't want to take any pills.

Ashes to Dust

She said a name I don't know, and then a anti psychotic.

I was alarmed at that. It made me think that was what they injected me with. That was dangerous. I worried about my heart and how it could affect my heart murmur, especially since I have been having pains since being here.

She said it's the same stuff I took yesterday.

I was alarmed again. What was she talking about? The nurse from last night never gave me anything. I told last night's nurse I didn't want the drugs, and she respected that and left. Tonight's nurse is saying I took it. Was there a mix up? Is that why the social worker keeps saying I seem better every day? Are they holding me here against my will because they think I'm taking their drugs and think that's why I seem better? I can't have them think that. That's false. I want out, and I should've been out days ago. I don't want this to be the reason they keep me longer.

I tell the nurse I never took anything yesterday. I tell her last night's nurse said I didn't have to take anything, and I didn't.

I look at the screen as the nurse checks it over. I see red letters that start similar to the words involuntary. I didn't know if it was saying I wasn't compliant because I didn't take the drugs or if it was referring to being held here involuntarily.

The nurse tells me that the previous nurse had input that I took them.

I tell her that was wrong and she needs to fix it so it's correct. I tell her I'm not taking anything, and it's my right.

She didn't look happy about that. She looked grouchy. Like she wanted to fight me on it. But she left.

I was partially relieved but I ask the roommate what the word I saw meant. She tells me it meant being in a involuntary hold. So it was about me being stuck here involuntarily against my will.

She then tells me that the nurse has probably gone to go get security and they will come in and inject me forcibly like they did her since I rejected the anti psychotics.

Ashes to Dust

I'm afraid, remembering what they did to me in the solitary confinement. I get up, and go find the nurse I just talked to at the station (where all the nurses hide). I tell her I can't have those anti psychotics because I have a heart condition and it could cause problems.

She seems less grouchy-faced, and said okay.

I felt a bit better now that I told her. I went back to my room, trying not to cry. They really must have injected me with anti psychotics just like what happened to my roommate. How are they allowed to do that to me? I just got in and they know I have a heart condition, and I don't have schizophrenia. Those drugs can make people without schizophrenia develop schizophrenia. I wonder if that's why I got worse after they injected me. Is it my brain trying to protect me, or is it the effects of the drug they injected me with making me worse? I didn't think I had D.I.D before. I don't know anymore. What did they do to me? I'm confused.

I go and talk with Sad Girl. She seems down. I ask if she's okay.

She's having a really hard day. She's in for more than a month. Thankfully her sister is going to bring her Switch console tomorrow. I try to comfort her but I don't know much other than a few things about her being suicidal, bipolar, and freezing in her traumas. I don't want to say the wrong things, so I try to get a nurse so she has someone who knows her situation better.

She talks with the male nurse, but he sucks. He is disinterested, and doesn't offer any sort of supportive comforting words. How did he get a job here with someone so fragile? He left less than three minutes after talking to her, and she looks worse than when he talked to her.

He said we could be up until ten, then lights out.

When he left I dragged the chair by her bed, knowing I may need to be up all night to make sure she is okay and doesn't harm herself. She's playing with her wrists a lot. I talk to her, try to comfort her in any way possible. Even Bill comes out and brings confidence and swearing to help her feel better. It's working better than the nurse. I'm getting through to her, even if it's just a little bit of her feeling better.

But then the COVID lady starts in about how the lights should go off, and we need to stop talking.

I tell her politely to stop yelling, that she isn't our mom and we can talk if we want to.

The COVID lady is making Sad Girl worse. Sad Girl is visibly shaking, and possibly retreating into a trauma related to her loud, verbally abusive grandmother. I'm hoping this bitch old lady isn't going to make Sad Girl kill herself. Sad Girl is so sweet and deserves to get out of here, to live with her sister away from her grandmother and finally get herself a loving cat.

Then the other roommate chimes in. It's like the old ladies are in sync and think they can tell us what to do because we're younger then them. Being senior doesn't mean you can verbally abuse us into doing what you want. They aren't our parents and they need to stop it. They're acting like loud, angry children. It's so fucking annoying. How do the idiot hospital people think this is relaxing? It's worse than being home.

I tell the other roommate she needs to stop, that this is important.

Sad Girl is important. This moment is important. I feel if I don't help her get through it she might give up on her life. It's extremely important and I won't let these bitches stop me from trying to help her.

They keep bullying us. Me and Bill go back and forth telling her enough. We weren't mean, and he had the confidence in my voice. But the old ladies were extremely mean. They didn't give a shit to look at how they were making Sad Girl feel, or react. She looked like she both checked out and was going to cry, stalk-still, all at once.

They turned out the lights on us, but I continue talking to Sad Girl. I tell her to just ignore them, they're being babies and they aren't our parents. I tell her that she's important and I will help her get through this, she doesn't need to stop talking because of them.

Ashes to Dust

We talked in the dark. I tell her she can turn her light on if she wants because the nurse said we had until ten.

She did but when the old ladies threw a riot again so Sad Girl turned it off because she didn't want trouble.

I stayed in the chair beside her and we talked in the dark, which was hard because the old ladies kept screaming at us here and there. I kept fending them off, but I was never rude. I didn't need to be; I didn't want to stress Sad Girl out more than they already were.

Eventually they started flicking on all of the lights. The sink light, the big light, the bathroom light. Then they started laughing and screaming, and it was getting out of hand. I was generally afraid that they might hurt us.

I get up and tell Sad Girl I was getting the nurse. I went out and found the male nurse that failed Sad Girl. I tell him about the two old ladies and how they were screaming at us and we didn't feel safe.

He tells me that they are very sick and that's why they are here.

Then why would they place me with dangerous, possibly violent people, knowing they can be, and call that relaxing and a break for me? Knowing I experienced a violent experience at my home by my mom's ex. I don't need to be killed in my sleep by these lunatics.

As we walk back, Sad Girl runs up to us with a face full of tears. I ask her if she's okay.

I'm worried they hurt her when I wasn't there.

She was understandably hysterical, saying that when I left they got worse. She said they were talking about me and saying awful things, and she got too scared to stay there and ran out.

I look in the room, where the door is open, and see both of them laughing like maniacs dancing in circles. Like they are getting ready to spar with each other but not. That wasn't a sight I was expecting and I do not feel safe at all going back in that room.

The nurse tells us that we can stay out in the lobby until a certain time. He leaves back to his nursing station, and we go sit on the couch

Ashes to Dust

beside each other, freaked out.

I ask if they hurt her.

She says no but she's scared.

We sat there for a while. I then remember my stuff, including my notepad with the stuff for my book in there. Very personal, that I didn't want them to get their hands on. Or do weird shit to my personal items. If they are dancing in circles laughing like that, I don't want my stuff in there.

I ask Sad Girl if she wants any of her stuff, I can get it.

She says no, she doesn't want me to go back in there. She's terrified they will do something.

I have to though, so I go back in. They're creepily pretending to be asleep in the dark. But they laugh when I walk in and stare at me. I grab my stuff, and am relieved that they didn't find my notepad. I go back out to the couch with my stuff and sit with Sad Girl. I'm wondering where I can sleep tonight. Where we can sleep. Because I don't want to go back in there. I feel like they will smother me in my sleep if I tried to sleep. I just want to go home. I ask every day, so why can't I go home. Especially with this.

The male nurse comes out and tells us we can't stay out there.

It wasn't close to the time he said we could wait out here. He only let us be out here for like ten minutes. Sad Girl doesn't look happy about going back either. I tell her I can stay by her bed in the chair if she's worried.

She said no it's okay she will be okay and just go to sleep.

I knew that wasn't true. She told me a few times that she's an insomniac, and usually stays up looking outside.

I ask the male nurse what he's going to do about the old ladies.

He says for us to go in and he will be there in a few minutes to talk with them.

Is that really it? He's going to talk to them. He won't find us a different room or kick them to a different room so we feel safe?

Ashes to Dust

I knock on the door of "Protector of Women" (as Snow called him). He came out to talk to me, and I told him about the two old ladies in the room scaring us, and that we didn't feel safe.

He told me not to worry he would protect us.

I don't know why, but him saying that made me feel like he would do more than the nurse. I felt at least slightly better knowing someone else knew, and if something goes wrong they would know who was responsible.

We go back in the room where the lights are on. Sad Girl goes to her bed and I go to mine. I put my stuff back, and the first old roommate smiles creepily as she turns off the light in victory.

I try to tell the roommate that the nurse is coming back so she didn't shut the door, but she ignored me and shut it anyways. Then both the old ladies creepily laugh on and off.

I can not sleep. The nurse lied, he never came back. He never talked to them. He is incompetent at this job like him with Sad Girl. If I sleep they might kill me in my sleep. Or hurt me. They keep moving and watching me. I think they might be waiting for me to sleep so they can get out of bed and sneak over and do something. Cut my hair? Hurt me? Kill me? Smother me? I'll have to act like I'm sleeping at one point so I can see what they do. It's going to be a long night.

I look over and see Sad Girl is still awake too. She's also looking out her window. Hers has air plane lights that glow red. She waves at me and I wave back. I'm glad she seems okay. I can't believe they failed her like that. The nurse, this place, these crazy ass old ladies triggering her. Triggering me too. They triggered me a lot.

Me and Sad Girl wave on and off or just look to see if the other is sleeping yet. That's doubtful with the crazy night.

I hear the COVID lady move a lot, and chuckle. It's been hours but she's still fucking awake. There's no way I'm sleeping tonight.

Ashes to Dust

30

I wake to the old ladies still being children and turning the lights on the moment they wake to prevent me from sleeping. They keep being loud the entire morning. I just want to go home. They better let me go home.

I get up and after breakfast I ask the nurse if I can go home.

I have to go see the social worker first later. I will make it clear (again) especially after last night, this is not a break. I said it every damn day but they don't listen. Every day I ask to go home. Every day they make it seem like I will, but they don't.

I call my sister and tell her about the two crazy old ladies and what they did. I couldn't tell her last night because I didn't want to wake her or her baby. I tell her what I tell her every time I call now, I just want to come home.

She tells me she will be coming tomorrow. She will see if she can bring my iPod, and she will bring my Switch. She says mom also packed Coke for me.

I go tell Sad Girl about my sister coming tomorrow and bringing my Switch.

Sad Girl holds up hers in her hands that her visitor brought her. I really think they should let her switch from her abusive grandmother to her sister. She didn't even get to choose her visitor, her doctor did without asking her. She's traumatized every time her grandmother

Ashes to Dust

visits. She even wants to ask that she doesn't have visitors for a while just to get a break. I know she won't ask and she doesn't want me to and I respect that so I won't.

I see the "Protector of Women" and tell him thank you for last night. And sorry about that, I just had no one to ask.

He says it's fine and that Snow wanted to contact me.

I told him no before when he said Snow wanted to buy us Timmie's yesterday. But ironically the only person I could think of that I could talk to was Snow when the chaos was happening last night.

I said yes, I would.

I was worried I wouldn't have the answers she might need. I didn't want to mess her up. I was also worried Snow might want to get checked in just to talk with me since she was so confused. I tried to make sure she didn't need me before she left, but I don't know if I did a good job or made it worse.

I figured I needed to clear things up with her, and let her know she can't get put back in here just to talk with me. And that she needs to be able to stand on her own now. I thought about what it would be like if I was friends with her outside of here. It would be very exhausting. To constantly be on guard, and at a level that drains me. I wouldn't be able to do it all the time.

Sad Girl is excited to be able to play the Switch with me when I get mine. I tell her not to wait. I tell her to play it now while she can and we can still play when I get mine.

She seems much better than yesterday now she has her game in her hands. I'm glad they approved her to have it. She needed this. We need something to hold onto in this awful place.

I am told I have to go with the nurse. I follow her to see their psychiatrist. He's in the kitchen part of this psych which I find odd. He's sitting in a chair with someone else who's taking notes. This is where I've seen patients come and watch TV. And Snow microwave stuff in the kitchen. Before seeing her do that I didn't even know there was a kitchen. I wasn't told. It's also where they have a locked door where the cooler is for the water they sometimes got me.

The psychiatrist says something about the anti-psychotics.

I tell him I already told multiple nurses that the nurse had falsely said I took meds I wasn't given. And that she falsified it in their system because the nurse said so, and I saw it. I then tell him I shouldn't be given medications like that anyways because of my heart murmur and it would cause issues.

He said no it wouldn't. He sounded so cold. Lacked empathy or care.

He isn't a nice person to talk to. I don't want to talk to him anymore. He doesn't give a shit about me. He doesn't care about me. He doesn't want to listen to me. It's like he only wants to hear himself talk. If I try to say anything he doesn't hear it. I can finally leave after telling him I'm sore and have pains.

Once I'm back in my room I go to the bathroom to pee. While I was on the toilet I felt like I was still with the psychiatrist. I worried I blacked out and was going to pee in front of him. I can hear his voice talking to me. I hear myself answer him, and then he asks me something else. I hear myself (my voice, not from my mouth), tear up, crying a bit as I tell him something like, "Sorry this is too hard on me right now." Then I was able to leave. I get up, and hear my own footsteps down the hall, and my feet in the bathroom start moving as I hear myself walking. I continue walking forward until I think I hear myself open the door to my room. And then to the bathroom door. I open and close it with my eyes opening back up after it's all over.

I'm so confused. I was in the bathroom the whole time, but it felt so real like I wasn't. I never experienced anything like that before. I never heard anything like that. I didn't like it. Hearing things. Was I there before or not? Is this stress? Is this my brain trying to cope and create a outlook I didn't see on how to get out of that situation next time?

Then I realize it was all just to show me how to handle him next time. The "loving protectors" were showing me how to get out of it smoothly. Since meeting him didn't go well. Why did I have to meet him? Why don't they have others if you don't get along with the one they choose?

I'm hoping to go home. I haven't slept well at all being here. Barely. I would've slept better at home. I wish they would've just left me there. I leave the bathroom and to my surprise the social worker comes in the room. She wants to see me.

I go past the extra hall she opens and enter her little room. I tell her how awful last night was and how the roommates were acting. I tell her again this is not a good place for me. I tell her about the nurse's error saying I took some medications I never took.

I try to figure out what she wants. Has she been keeping me here because I haven't told them what they've been wanting? What do they want? What can I possibly say to make them finally let me out? Is it something personal? Is that what she wants? Maybe I should tell her about that horrible memory I had of my mom with the ferret cage. I won't tell her about the other baby stuff. Or that I discovered that they made me sing like a canary as a kid. That the shows I put on for my mom wasn't what I thought. Or that they rode me like a horsey.

I tell her that I remembered something horrible about being locked up in a ferret cage as a kid and raped.

She passed me tissues as I cried. It's horrible to think about and remember. This was obviously why the personalities were created and the protector did a good job because I didn't remember any of it until coming to this hospital. I didn't even know I had D.I.D until after coming to this hospital.

The Social worker tells me that must have been a hard thing to remember.

I said it was.

After a while she talks to me and I tell her I want to go home. I tell her my sister is coming tomorrow and I want to leave with her.

She says they'll see what they can do. She says I've improved a lot.

Ashes to Dust

She says that every time I see her. I don't get why they haven't let me out yet after telling me each time how great I am since coming here.

She asks if I were to leave how would I try to create boundaries.

I tell her by locking my door, so if someone is angry they can't just barge in.

She says that's good I should do that.

I tell her I'll spend time in my room with my cat, and try to have space to myself.

She says yes I should lock my door when I go home. It was a condition of leaving. She also says she will set up a appointment with housing so I can move out.

They don't think it's safe for me there with my mom's ex around.

I'm in my room when the nurse comes in and tells me to get my stuff to get a shower.

Again with no way of saying no or just letting me go home. I follow her to a different room this time. I pass a door and go into one that I thought was a row of patient rooms but it wasn't.

I go in and it reminds me of a small gym locker room. There's no lockers, but it gives off that vibe with the random bench and cement floor. I go in with her and again there is a weird velcro mat that's meant for gymnastics. She leaves me with towels and the communal bottles again. She leaves and I get in. It's strange to be in this one. I really don't like their mat curtains either. They wobble back and forth and are so thick.

I go and lock the door so no one can just barge in. Then I have to clean the bottles before using them again. After thinking about it I realize if the nurse doesn't have a key and tries to get in and realizes I locked it when I shouldn't have. Then I might get in trouble. They might call security and I might get dragged off to that room again. I finish up, and walk on a towel and unlock the door. I get dressed in my own clothes that Kat brought me. I tell the nurse I'm done and she shuts off the shower.

I go back to my room and my roommates are doing two separate things. The older lady is folding laundry and Sad Girl is putting laundry in a basket. Sad Girl tells me it's laundry day.

I don't know what that means.

She says we have to do our own laundry.

I wonder how that works. Where do we do the laundry? Is it a room? Is it like a prison show where we all stand around big washers and dryers waiting? I really don't want to do laundry here with their germy machines and soiled laundry.

Later the social worker comes and tells me I might get to leave today. And then I'm told we have to move rooms because the one we're in is going to be for boys since there are more of them now, and we are going into a different one.

Thankfully COVID lady leaves today. I don't know how she gets out before me, but she does. I leave it friendly despite how she treated us yesterday. She wasn't as much of a bitch today when she left. But the other roommate that had been here from the start was still acting not so nice.

I see Braids, the girl I mistook for a corpse before. The one I had flipped off since coming here, not realizing my vibes of her weren't bad but of illness. When I meet her eyes through the Nurses station see-through glass (she is on the other side talking to one), I wave. She smiles and waves back. I'm glad to clear that up. Hopefully she knows I was never purposely being rude before.

I'm told I have to go get a brain scan.

I don't understand why, and I ask the social worker.

She says she also doesn't know why. They never informed her either. She says she will go find out the reason. She looks alarmed about it.

I watch the cleaning lady clean everything in my room. I'm surprised to find she has not one soaked rag, but two today. A first in the days I've been stuck here. And they are actually dripping wet unlike the possibly, almost dry ones she usually uses.

The social worker comes in and tells me they're taking me for the brain scan. She never tells me why, like she said she would. She said she doesn't know.

I go get the brain scan. Later I'm called to go follow a nurse I've never seen before into their room that has colours over the doors. "Brown," "Blue," etc. I ask what they are for.

I thought they were for how they rate emotions and dangers and it made me glad I wasn't in the red one.

He tells me it's the nurses. The nurses are assigned colours, and the patients go to the nurse's room that's caring for them that day.

I sit down. This is the second time coming into this weird hall place.

He reads me the results of my CT, brain scan. He says it's all normal.

It made me wonder why they risked radiation just for the brain scan then. Why did they do the brain scan? They still never told me.

He said I'm a star patient there.

I'm confused.

He said Hilda recommended me, and says I'm great.

I'm taken aback that Hilda said anything nice about me. She wasn't my nurse anymore, and I found it odd that she would want to say nice things.

He said I will be getting out today, and they will call a cab.

I'm surprised. I wondered if Hilda saying nice things helped. Thanks Hilda. Or maybe they knew they did me wrong? And wanted to get me out. They are willing to pay $50 for a cab all the way back to Wallaceburg. They must have realized they did very wrong.

I go get my stuff and I have to stay in Sad Girl's new room with her as I wait. Unfortunately she has the old roommate there. I'm hoping she won't be a bitch to her. I don't want Sad Girl going through a hard time.

I tell her I get to go home.

She's disappointed because she says I'm the only one her age that she can talk to.

I felt bad that she really didn't have anyone else. I'm hoping her sister pulls through for her so Sad Girl makes it through this Hell place. I sit at the end of the bed and talk to her. She seems happier now that she has a more private room. I remember hearing her complain to her visitor about being stuck with a bunch of strangers and using a shared bathroom. I wasn't offended at the time, or now, because it was exactly what I complained about to my sister.

Sad Girl gave me her Switch friend code so I could add her when I got home. I put it in my bag, and will add her later so she will have someone to play with at night. I wondered if it allowed any form of communication so I could write her and see how she was doing.

I finally got called that the cab was here and I could go home. I said goodbye to Sad Girl, but I didn't see "Protector of Women" anywhere to say bye to. I was glad that I wouldn't have to talk to Snow after all. It would be too hard of a conversation. I'm thinking if I'm going now it's meant as I wasn't suppose to talk to her ever again. Even now. She might be in a much better state now, and I didn't want to make things worse.

I didn't have shoes, or a coat. The nurse gave me a thin jacket he had, and I walked out in my socks into the taxi. I was so happy to finally be getting out of that place. I got in and got driven home.

PART EIGHT
HOME

31

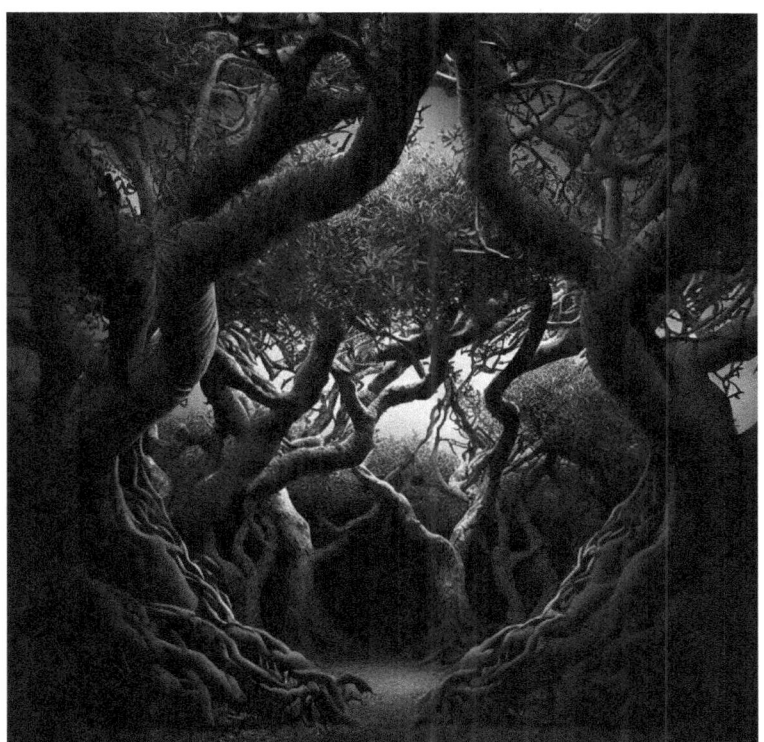

I realize the trees are angry. They want to get me. They're alive, and mad at people. They kill people. The taxi passes the row of trees I peed on the time I biked from Wallaceburg to Chatham. They remember me.

Ashes to Dust

The trees are extremely mad at me.
  My head nods.
  Shit, the trees want to kill me?
  Nod.
  Oh no. They are oxygen, I think they will retract their oxygen or make it so I can't breathe anymore. There are trees everywhere, I'm not safe. No one is safe.
  Once the taxi drops me off, I get out and walk towards my house. I see the big tree that's off to the side of it. I wonder if it would attempt to crush me or not. I stand on the porch as I look at the tree. The trees are trying to kill me, my family, even my cat. I have to protect them. The trees are mean. They want to kill the humans for what they do to them. They don't care if they're kids. They want to get animals too. Because animals pee on them, shit on them, and they don't appreciate it. They want to start killing everything off. Starting here with me and my family because the trees I peed on told them and now they all know.
  One of my personalities tell them about how I use to love trees. I even tried to respect them and hugged one.
  It seemed like they might be less menacing now. But it fluctuated. They ended up not caring. I went inside to make it so the trees couldn't take away my family's air, or my cat's, and kill us like they wanted.

I got in and was surprised by my mom's face. Her lips were big, and swollen, and covered in scabs. It reminded me of what someone on drugs might look like. It reminded me of when she did drugs. Now I'm worried I just came home at a time when my mom is doing drugs again. I can't worry about that, I'm suppose to worry about myself. But it's all I can think about. What if she overdoses? I don't want to see that. I know there's nothing I can do, because people on drugs don't like confrontation. Like when I did confront her about her odd behaviour and knew she did drugs. She took that bad. Even though I

Ashes to Dust

just said I was there for her if she needed to talk.

I was so happy to see my cat.
I had to go into the bathroom and could feel the trees still attacking. I had to protect us from things trying to kill what I cared about. I don't know why things like to attack me in the bathroom all the time.

When I was upstairs, Kat came upstairs to get something from her room, but she had a key around her neck. She unlocked her door with it and went in. She never had a door lock before. Did she get a lock for her door because I'm back? Is she afraid of me so she got a lock on her door? It makes me feel awful. I hope she isn't afraid of me. I would never hurt her. I even protected them from so much when I thought things were happening that weren't. Why can't they see that?
My mom gets Kat to unlock her room too. My mom didn't have a new door lock on her door either. It feels like I shouldn't have come back. Like they don't want me back because they're so afraid of me coming back that they put locks on their doors. Is that what they think of me? That I would hurt them? I'm upset now and feel worse.

The fucker tells me it wasn't Kat that went in my room and cleaned up my stuff, it wasn't actually her. Barb says not to get mad at Kat for lying about it. That makes me upset and angry that I was lied to again, and that Barb went through my personal belongings. I worried while in the hospital they'd be snooping or Barb would be. And my password book was one of the many things moved, and obviously gone through. I can't trust anyone to be fucking honest. Now I have to change my passwords. She says she didn't go through it but she's a liar. She probably made a copy too.
Barb tells me that she would cry every night I was gone. Kat already told me this at the hospital visit. I didn't want to hear it then, I don't want to know. Why is it about everyone else all the time? I cried every

Ashes to Dust

fucking night too. I was stuck in Hell. Every, night. A real reason to cry.

Someone knocks on the door at night, and the dogs start barking. It makes me think of my mom's ex, maybe she's back, is she violent? On drugs and booze? Did my mom let her come over again? Why can't she keep her violent ex out of our lives?

It reminds me of the night everything went to Hell where her ex came and I got taken away. It happens in seconds after the knock and bark, and I get a intense pain, and I can't breathe. I'm hunched over it hurts so bad. I don't know what's happening. I'm crying it's so painful, it feels like I'm having a heart attack. The pain doesn't let up, and there's so much pain in my chest I think I'm going to die.

My cat is on my bed and hops up by me, and I'm able to pet her. It helps a little, but it hurts.

Barb comes up and tells me it was a friend of hers. She asked if there was something she could do, but I can't answer her. I'm in so much pain and I can't breathe, I just can't answer. It's like I'm frozen and no words come out. She gets offended for me not answering her. But I can't. I can't even motion it. I'm just curled with my head between my legs, breathing with snot dripping down.

I try to sleep but when I lie down I have a coughing fit. If I go to sleep on my left side it's so painful it feels like something is broken. I got up, wondering if I was coughing from when I shit the bed and couldn't smell it. I strip the sheets and cut off the plastic to my mattress and spray it. I put new sheets on and think I should do one more cleansing of my room by burning sage. To rid it of all the negativity and things that happened previously.

I light the sage and go over my room with it. I hear my mom yelling about smelling it and she sends my sister up to close my door. I tell Kat she can't close my door because it needs to be open to get the negativity out. Kat isn't happy with me and just repeats that mom said to close it. I repeat I need it open. My chest is starting to hurt but I try to refocus on finishing cleansing everything.

Barb comes up after yelling downstairs and stands in my doorway glaring at me with her hands on her hips saying to stop or close the door.

I tell her it's important and I need the door open.

Barb keeps glaring at me and stomps outside of my room banging things as she goes and yelling as she goes down the stairs.

I rub my chest in pain. It hurts. But I finish up cleansing my room so I don't have to be yelled at and pretend like it's not physically painful.

I try to sleep but I still cough when I'm on my side, right or left. I can't have the blanket cover my eyes and I need the light on. I don't know why. I think it's related to the hospital.

I make the mistake of rolling on my left side to sleep and I can't breathe for a second from so much pain. I never lied on my left side at the hospital because of my earrings, but now I can because of my neck pillow. There is something wrong with my chest on my left side. I wonder if the nurse broke a rib after all. It would explain why I get so winded just going up and down the stairs too.

32

My sister's cat kept eating my cat's food. I was sick of Kat not watching her cat. It got in my room a few times and that severely stressed me out and made me cry because it was my only safe space I had left. I'm vulnerable and angry and no one cares about me since I've been back.

It's been going on a few different days now where Kat is sitting her lazy ass on the couch with her phone. No one watching the fucking cat, and letting it get in my room and my cat's stuff. It's too much right now. I speak up for myself for the first time. I make sure not to say it mean, but I tell Kat she has to watch her cat.

Kat says she has to watch the baby.

The baby is sleeping most of the time or in the jumper while Kat is on the phone so it's a load of bullshit. Same as before.

I tell her to put the cat in the cage then.

Kat says the cat can't be in the cage all day.

Obviously the cat wouldn't need to go in the cage all day, just when she's actually busy with the baby, like feeding it. Always having a go to excuse on not doing anything, and making someone else do it.

I tell Kat to watch her cat then. She keeps going up in my room.

Kat gets pissy, and I head toward the kitchen. Barb comes in from a smoke and Kat bitches to her, saying she was sick of me and that she's been nothing but nice to me since I've been back, and helping me.

Ashes to Dust

She didn't help me.

Then Kat says something about not letting me near her baby anymore like she's been doing.

The last part I didn't think I cared about, but it made me upset because Kat's baby was the only one to smile and laugh at me and make me feel better, like someone was genuinely happy at my presence. Happy to see me back. Especially when Kat said before that her baby wasn't making high-pitched chatting/laughing noises until I got back.

I figured it was because I talked to the baby normal like, "Don't worry you'll be able to walk soon then you can get whatever you want." "You'll be able to eat real food soon, then you'll be happy. There's so many delicious foods you'll like." "Don't be sad this is just a baby phase, you'll be grown and out of it soon and then you can say what's wrong."

I don't understand why she's acting like this. I never did anything wrong. All's I did was ask her to watch her cat so it doesn't go in my room and eat my cat's food. I have to pay for my cat's food, and it's expensive. I can't afford two cats. It makes me feel like I shouldn't have liked her baby because now she's weaponising it. It's what I was worried about. And now it makes me feel like she was scared of me after all, and didn't want me near her or her baby. I don't feel welcomed. I don't think anyone wants me back. I don't want to be here.

It's not the first time my sister has said something indirectly, but loud enough for me to hear. Out of the blue she's pointed in my direction while talking to my mom, and saying things about me making her throw away her stuff. But I never made her. In the moment I truly believed there was a danger and we had to get rid of the stuff. But I never forced her. She willingly put it in bags, she never once said no she didn't want to. She could've pretended to throw it out if she wanted to go along with it, and retrieve it later when I was hydrated and recovered. She threw her stuff out with her own two hands. Why is she making it seem like I'm some monster that threw away her things? I already told her I'd buy her a new bracelet since she (with her own two hands) threw it out.

I told them I'd pay to replace things I told them to throw out, so why is it being used against me? It feels awful. I feel like a monster in my own home.

I tell Barb I heard what Kat said about not letting me see the baby anymore.

Barb tried to say she didn't hear that part.

But if I heard it all the way in the kitchen, how could she not hear it?

Barb says she will talk with Kat because she can't do that to me. Then she left.

Of course Kat could do that. It's her baby. Doesn't matter how nice I am, she could just go, nope, because it's her baby. She could tell her baby all sorts of made up shit about me and how I just didn't want to see them anymore, and there'd be nothing to dispute it. Because most kids believe everything their parent tells them. There'd be nothing I could do. Would I want to? If I'm going to be hurt like that, on a whim by my own sister?

I went upstairs back to my room. The only place I'm wanted, and want to be with my cat.

I stayed in silence again. I don't want to overwrite my memories from before and during the hospital so I can write them into a book like I wanted. But it's too hard with everything happening. I end up avoiding it, which doesn't make sense since I'm not doing anything.

Ashes to Dust

33

My sister told me whatever the hospital gave me, could still be in my system and last up to six weeks.
That's why I'm still struggling instead of being back to normal. It explains why I asked her if she wanted to live with me one day in Toronto, despite not wanting to live with anyone.

I'm stuck alone, feeling like I'm fighting myself. I never experienced this before. I don't want to have this happening. What did the hospital do to me?
I'm stuck sitting on my bed staring at my off-screen computer on my desk, having the worst internal mental battle in my life. The thoughts are so dark, I know they aren't mine. And I feel the need to say it. That's not how I feel, that's not my thought. I wouldn't think that. It's exhausting, and there's so many. I feel like a dark pit, and I've never felt like this before. I involuntarily say words, and it's all a lot to deal with alone. There's no one I can talk to about this. My mom didn't take me coming back well. No one did. I can't trust anyone here with something like this. It'd be worse for me.
I'm in my room for hours fighting myself.
It goes on and each day I wonder if I'll make it until the end of the week. I'm waiting to hear from housing and I'm not sure if I'll make it. It feels like my body will just give up on me. Not me killing myself,

just it'll give up. It's hard to explain, and all I do is sit in silence or lay down.

   I notice my bank card has money taken from it on the dates I was in the hospital. I realize my mom must have used my money to buy things with it. I wonder if she bought drugs with my money or something. I'm really upset about it, I can't believe on top of everything she would do that to me. Take advantage.
   I call her and tell her money is missing, she gets upset and yells at me. I tell my sister money is missing in a text, and I get endless texts from both her and my mom. I have to block both of them after my mom comes up and tries to break into my locked room. She knows I have panic attacks now, but she is screaming at me on the other side of the door, body checking it and wiggling the doorknob. It scares the shit out of me and I can't breathe as I curl up, stuck on my bed with my cat. All I can do is cry and feel like I'm having a heart attack.
   She is yelling on the other side of the door that she wouldn't spend my money.
   She doesn't have to try to break down my door, or scare me into a panic attack, and scream just to say that.

   After things have calmed down things get sorted out. It turns out the money was used for my mom's bills that she had to do since she doesn't have her own bank. Still, it was very terrifying how she reacted. She knows I'm still not alright from the hospital. It took me a while but I understood and thought more clearly after, but she shouldn't have reacted like that.

   I stay in my room feeling more alone. I want to move. I can't handle this. My family isn't being understanding.

Ashes to Dust

34

I bought Chinese food to eat but after feeling tingling pain in my feet and throat feeling like it's closing a bit, I had to take a allergy pill. I think I am allergic to something in there. It tasted so good, I knew I loved it and it made me happy until I kept feeling like I'm gonna die eating it. I was so disappointed I had to stop eating.

I put the food in the fridge and ended up giving it to my sister. I didn't want to give it to any of them. They haven't done anything kind since coming back. Not even a smile. It's daggered looks. But I didn't want it to go to waste.

Now I'll have to buy groceries sooner or starve because I haven't been able to get anything since coming back.

I am struggling figuring out what to eat because I keep reacting negatively to it. I gag at almost everything. Salads, pickles, carrots, cheese. I am so confused on what to eat, it feels like nothing. It all seems related to the bad memories of the multiple rapes I remembered at the hospital. The cab driver who drove me to school. The pickle man from my childhood who was really gross and peed all over his bathroom floor. A priest from church. My dad.

I knew I needed food and electrolytes and couldn't ask my family for help because they were all treating me not very well since I got back. I

Ashes to Dust

took the red wagon so I could put the food in when I got there. It was so hard for me to drag and it was empty! I have no idea how I'm going to drag it back with food in it. I already feel like I'm having a heart attack. My left side of my chest hurts so much and I'm having trouble breathing. My arms are so weak I keep having to switch to pull the wagon to the store every minute or less. For some reason my left arm is much weaker and I can barely use it. It causes more chest pain when I use it to pull.

I don't know if the other side of my personality wants to harm me or not but if I pass out and die from a heart attack here in the middle of the street, so do they. I managed to convince them to help be stronger when I feel weak. I could tell by the shift of my facial features and the sudden strength I had that I didn't before. I know the guides didn't want me to acknowledge or speak to that other part, the "ego" part, but if it meant I didn't die today on the way to the store, I will take it.

All I can think of is, "Please don't let me pass out in the middle of the inter-section and get run over."

I made it to the store and was so out of breath I didn't think I could continue on. But I couldn't just stop in the middle of the store especially during a pandemic.

Now that I was here I asked my guides/watchers to help me choose the right food and not let me pass out or die in the middle of the store.

My head nodded.

I made sure to give them permission, as only the ones that wish me no harm.

I was stuck there much longer than intended. I barely grabbed much because I kept feeling negative reactions to food, and sometimes pain or heat in my hand, arms or feet happened to say I was going in the wrong direction or getting the wrong food. But it kept getting more complicated as one of the other personalities would mimic it and I couldn't tell if what I was getting or where I was going was right or wrong. Head shake then head nod it was all a lot. My body would automatically drift to the side if a person came down the aisle. Or my head moved to avoid a interaction that could get me sick by the virus. The guides were trying to help prevent me from getting exposed.

I had to stop a few times and crouch down. I would have such intense chest pains or felt so dizzy I'd pass out. I felt like I might shit myself, but I knew I wouldn't make it to the bathroom. Especially with my energy level. I ask my guides to please hold my shit like they did at home so many times.

To my surprise, they actually did. I didn't need to go anymore. I tell them thank you, and how close I was to having a accident in the store that I really didn't want to deal with.

It reminded me too much of when I shit my bed.

I couldn't move any longer or I thought I'd for sure have a heart attack in the store. I was scared and didn't want to die. I was conflicted because I didn't want to ask for help and risk them calling the hospital to have me taken away or police. But I thought I'd ask a employee.

They told me they couldn't do anything because of COVID. They were very far away and didn't want to help me. It made me feel so much worse. Like no one wants to help me. It was so hard for me to reach out and ask for help in a vulnerable moment when I'm scared thinking the worst is coming for me. Especially when the previous people abused me.

They stared at me as I stayed on their floor by my cart breathing heavily while shaking. They said they could go get the manager.

I said yes please.

I really felt like I wouldn't make it as I waited. I grabbed a box of bars that were simply peanuts and dates. My eyes stared at the ingredients, and even though I was certain I wouldn't be allergic to any of it, my eyes stared intensely at the word "dates."

I opened the box and ate one of the bars inside. It tasted really good. It was the first thing I've eaten since being back. I looked at the electrolyte drink with vitamins I grabbed. I opened it even though my body was suggesting I was allergic to something in it again. I took a drink anyways needing it.

I said if I'm allergic I have the allergy pills in my pocket.

I'm paying for the items, but thought it wouldn't look good if the employee came back to see me eating and drinking before buying so I stopped half way done the bar.

There were now two employees staring at me on the floor. The manager said they can't do anything but they can call a ambulance.

That rung fucking alarm bells. I will not go back to that abusive hell hole again. I just got out.

I slowly stood up, pretending to be fine while hoping I didn't give away I wasn't. I already knew I looked extremely pale from catching a reflection of myself in the store. I tried to hide the shaking of my whole body and picked up my winter gloves.

I told them thank you for the concern but I'm fine I just hadn't eaten yet so I felt like I was going to pass out.

I continued moving with my heavy-as-fuck wagon, making sure to act normal until some time passed by and I was in a different aisle they couldn't see me in. I stopped and rested again. And finished eating the other half of the bar. I took the allergy pill as my eyes and face went stern at the vitamin drink making it feel like I'm very allergic to it. I closed it and drank one of the plain big bottles of electrolyte drinks.

I was finally starting to feel a bit better. I need to wrap this up. I don't think I can keep it up any longer. I go over to the meat aisle and grab natural shredded chicken, and lunch meat. I was a bit worried about the chicken, it reminded me of the hospital. But I knew it was energy so I took it and the rest of my little bit of groceries over to the check out and left.

The bag of white rice really made the wagon super heavy. I am struggling even more than I was the first time. I really wanted to call home for help but I knew they wouldn't help me. They already refused to get something at the store for me before. It's how I knew I would

Ashes to Dust

have to do it this time.

It felt like my chest was on fire and my left arm had horrible numb tingling up to my shoulder blades as I pulled. I could barely use my left arm again but I kept needing a break for my right arm. It took a very long time to finally get home. Over thirty minutes.

Once I got home, no one cared about me. I'm lucky I got my O.W or I wouldn't have any food. I struggled to get in the kitchen, and made sure not to show when I was talking to myself, or my guides. I hid when my head nodded or shook no involuntarily in response to something. I had to sit in the middle of the kitchen to take breaks between putting my food away. I made sure to put my initials on my food so no one took it on me (not that that stopped them).

I didn't want to because it would take a long time but I put the rice in my little microwaveable rice cooker and made the rice without any seasoning or condiments. I wanted salt and condiments but I felt like I might be allergic to them too, and was still so confused on what was safe and not safe for me to eat. What was healthy and not healthy for me.

I ate some of the shredded chicken while waiting. Then I put the cooked rice in the fridge for later.

My mom complained about my stuff taking up her cupboards. Not how are you, or anything nice. Just always complaints, yelling, or negativity. I didn't do anything wrong. Literally just bought food to try not to starve. Maybe she didn't want me to come back. It's not like I want to be back in this environment. I'd like to move out.

For the next few days all I ate was rice and chicken until the shredded chicken was gone. The chicken lunch meat said gluten free but I had a reaction to it with excess saliva in my throat and felt unwell. I gave it to my ungrateful family.

35

February 13, 2021:

My mom sent me a few nasty texts. *(Mom = White; Me = Blue)*

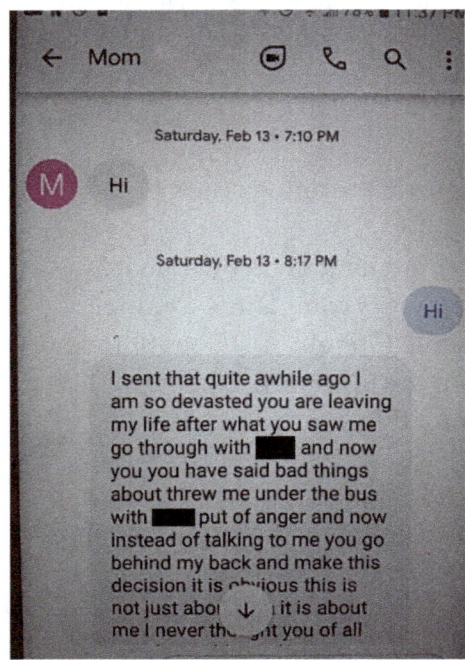

Photo 1: *(Sister's name redacted)*

Ashes to Dust

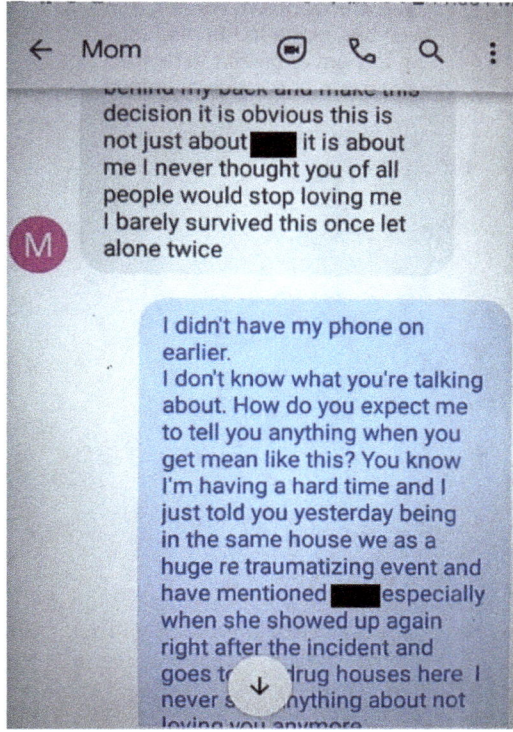

Photo 2: (Mom's ex redacted)

Ashes to Dust

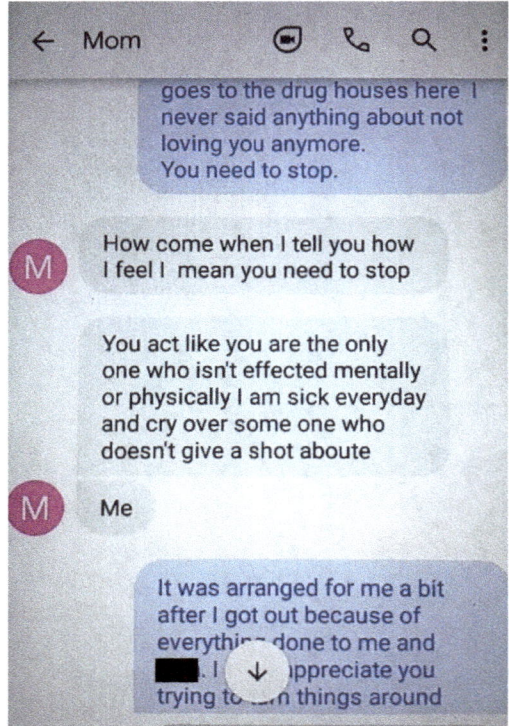

Photo 3: (Mom's ex redacted)

Ashes to Dust

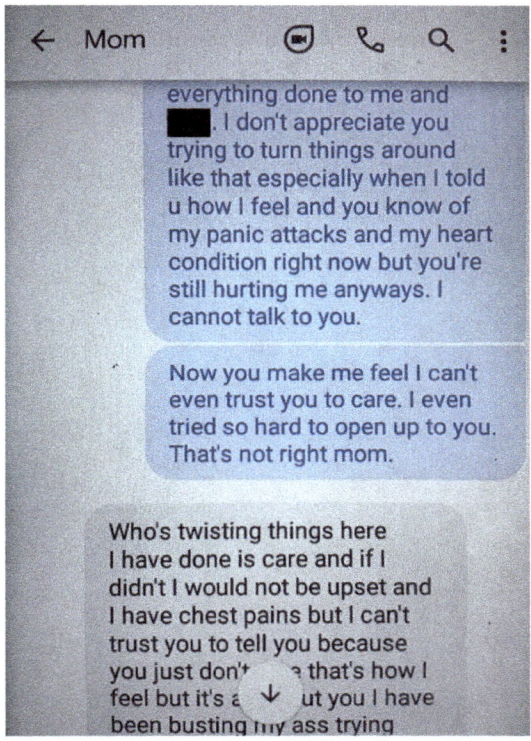

Photo 4: (Mom's ex redacted)

Ashes to Dust

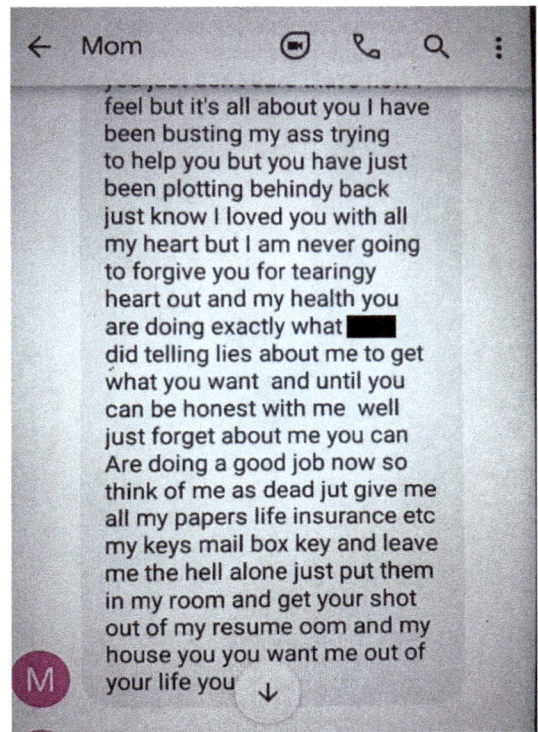

Photo 5: (Sister's name redacted)

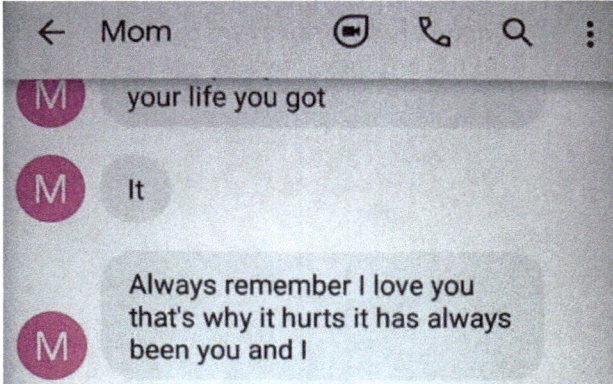

Ashes to Dust

I call crisis for the first time even though I don't want to.

I get a woman and I try to talk to her while my mom is outside the door. I whisper as I cry, and read to her some of the texts my mom wrote me. She tells me what my mom is saying and her behaviour (moving my stuff, etc) isn't of a healthy person, and I should continue doing what I'm doing. I should keep my door locked and stay in my room and not make contact with her. I tell her I can't avoid running into her because we live in the same house and she seeks me out. She then tells me to just do my best, continue staying with my cat as support, and to continue what I've been doing, pretending and playing the part so she doesn't lose her cool on me again. She tells me my mom is toxic, and that she is going to tell the housing about it because they don't realize that my household is such a toxic environment. That they just see someone with no kids and she wants to make sure I'm a higher priority to get out faster.

I have no one to stop my mom from hurting me emotionally so I turn to my sister in text. I should've known that she wasn't the person I could turn to but I have no one else. It did more harm to me when she was all about my mom's feelings instead of mine, and also insinuated my mom committing suicide. First my mom, now my sister confirms it too instead of trying to help me with mom when she knows I now have panic attacks.

Ashes to Dust

> **Saturday, Feb 13 · 9:12 PM**
>
> Moms taking me telling her I'm on a wait list for my own home bad
>
> Well yeah she's very sad I'm sad she loves u allot she cried n told me I'm worried about her being away from you im sorry if I seem different I've just been scared of saying the wrong thing, bc I know u were upset with me
>
> I thought you just didn't like me anymore.
> She's not being nice... She's saying I'm going behind her back n on't listen even tho she ws it's causing me

Sister = White; Me = Blue

Ashes to Dust

> to get my stuff out of her house and think of her as dead.
>
> ▮ I love you I just don't wanna say the wrong thing and upset you, I'll always love you, and she's taking it hard, she's never been away from you
>
> You were there when I left mom I'm scared she won't be able to handle it again
>
> Feb 13, 9:21 PM
>
> I don't want her to hurt herself n I feel like that's what's gonna happen

(Note: Old name redacted black. Sister's 1st initial redacted in pink.)

I'm alone with no one for comfort. I can't handle all this. They know that.

At least I have my cat.

Ashes to Dust

36

After most of the personalities merged, I felt like I needed to rename the body. At first it was going to be Hannah Ravenskye. Ravenskye felt like a strong last name, which was why I felt it was the right fit. I needed strength. Then when that didn't work out because of the future Hannah personality, I was going to change it to Harley Singsong. Harley barely felt sadness, and she was so peppy and happy, it made me feel like me. It was what I wanted to be. But it also didn't seem right after.

When Hannah, and Harley's names didn't work out for me. I realized the Death personality was holding my new name all along, and I was holding Death's. What safer place is there for my name then with Death? No one would suspect it, or pick a fight with Death, not even the other personalities.

I asked Death if I can have my name and she has hers.

Yes.

I gave Death her name back. Ash Dust. It felt like it belonged to Death all along. Ash Dust, was always linked to Death.

Death gave me my name. Melody. It was life.

It was a beautiful name. It felt right. It was the name I chose for a character in one of my book ideas that I really loved then too. I'm happy to have it. Harley didn't feel right.

Now I just have to choose a proper last name. I know it has to do

Ashes to Dust

with something positive about my future. Music. Melody. I think hard on it for a while. But after looking over the name change form, I realize, I have to pick a middle name. I want to make my new name flow.

When I finally figure out a completely new name, I fill out the name change form and mail it.

37

March 2, 2021:
Filed my own taxes after breaking down crying (triggered by a video of Paris in court against her abuse in boarding school).

March 4, 2021:
At night my mom comes to ask about rent after bickering about my request for a rent slip for ODSP, and saying it didn't include food. She tried to say I only recently started buying my own food. A big fucking lie it's been over one year now. She then came to say I shouldn't claim rent because it's $85 on taxes. Since she doesn't get rent $390 + for the house. Then acted like I was dumb after and got mad at me.
How was I suppose to know?
She texted back later quick and instant when it had to do with fixing the tax amount for her. Made me feel like it's all about money with her after all.
I was proud I did my own taxes, but she tried to make it about her by saying I've been doing stuff without telling her and that I should've told her before doing my taxes.
It's called being a fucking grownup. I don't have to say every fucking thing I'm doing. How was I suppose to know about the rent thing and to ask? I'm a fucking adult and I want my own privacy and not to be treated like shit for trying to behave like it/being a

Ashes to Dust

individual/independent.

March 6, 2021:
I changed the rent on tax to $85 yesterday like asked.
Today mom changed her wording from she'll give me the rent receipt to "see" it. She clutched onto it while talking, almost not letting go. I took it and went to the table to scan it for my tax records. She came over hovering, wanting to take it back. I told her I needed it for tax. She started getting frazzled saying she already told me it's $85. I said I needed a copy for rent receipt for my tax. She was quiet, hovering. I told her I needed a flatter surface because the app kept saying "too close" so I went and set it on the stove. She stomped away mad; don't know why. I took the picture using my scanner app, gave the paper back, and left my food tray by the stairs. (I was going to go up when she asked me to wait. I set my tray down. This was when she mentioned the rent paper.)

I was about to go up when she came over saying I'm on O.W and pay less rent. She said that's what the landlord said and that's why it's $85. She said do I understand? Honestly it didn't make sense because I thought it'd be at least half (since I pay $390 but I was giving her $500) and I had calculated and $85 isn't half. So I said I just thought it'd be more since I pay you $390. She said that's utilities included. I didn't know that was separate, and we already talked about this. So I said (because she was about to start arguing) it didn't matter, I already changed the tax form to $85 like she wanted.

I grabbed my tray about to go up, when she stomps away saying, "Don't talk to me anymore." I was confused, went to go up and she kept yelling at me that I was being difficult and not to talk to her. I said, "You're the one that came up to me," and I was trying to go upstairs. She put up her hand and like a child said, "I told you don't talk to me. I don't want you to talk to me."

I went upstairs but I could still hear her ranting when I was at the top, saying I was selfish and being sneaky and backstabbing, doing things behind her back all the time and she's sick of it.

Went to my room to lie down and cry. I have no one. My cat wanted out so not even my cat. Starting to think I can't have the same counselor as her after all, or at least definitely not meet in person with her since my mom was trying to manipulate that from what it was supposed to be (moving), to things I didn't want to talk about. Apparently before the ex-wife thing with the hospital, which didn't make sense. (I explained that.)

Had to call crisis for the second time. I don't like doing that, I was avoiding it. A guy called, which made me nervous at first because I wasn't sure if he was like the first counselor CMHA gave me, who didn't have emotional understanding.
He was nice, listened. Unfortunately confirmed emotional abuse. My mom was texting not nice things during my call again.

Ashes to Dust

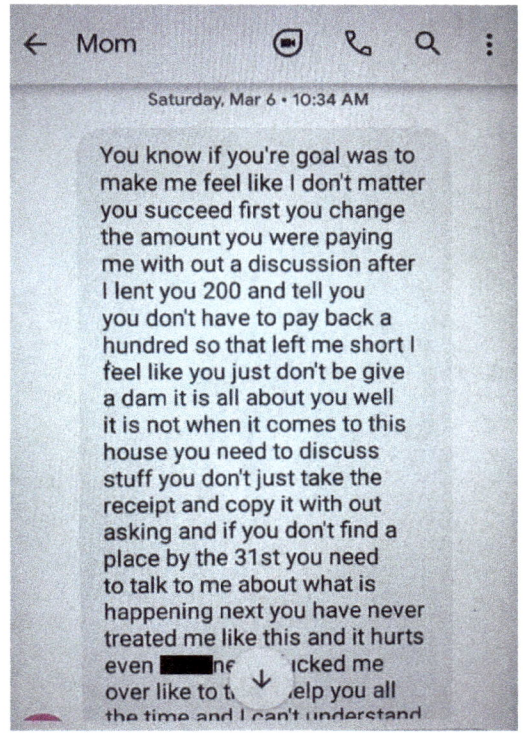

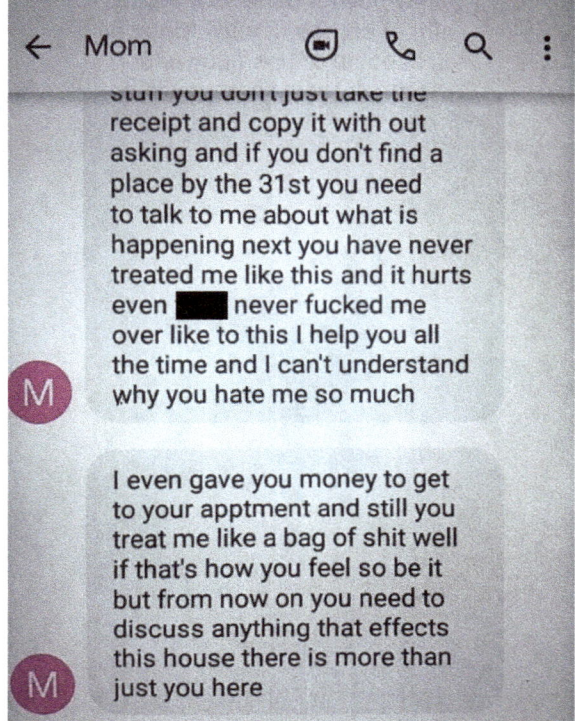

(Note: My sister's name is redacted).

He told me not to read them right now and that it wouldn't make me feel better. To know I did nothing wrong. That it may be longer than we/I'd like, but moving is a first good step. He said to see it as the light at the end of the tunnel. He also said yes having the same counselor is definitely a conflict of interest, (he has some that don't know and some that do so he should know). Which unfortunately confirmed I really will need a different counselor. He gave me the new one's (they arranged) number to make an appointment.

He said it was OK to stay in my room in bed since I sprained my foot. I was worried he'd want me to leave it, but I have nowhere to go. He recommended a comedy on YT to me. It'll be a new comedy I can add

Ashes to Dust

for another day. Always need those now. I told him before that I can't watch things with yelling because it sets off my panic attacks. He told me the shaking of my body is the adrenaline leaving me from (emotional abuse) being so emotional and adrenaline has to go out and the body relax. I'm not use to crying this much, or feeling like this. I use to be better at shaking off my mom's yelling/words.

Good thing I topped up my phone yesterday.

I-want-to-find-a-place!

March 7, 2021:
My mom ignores me, sometimes looks at her phone, probably to see if I wrote back to her nasty texts. But I took the crisis workers advice and didn't. Didn't even re-read bits I had. Sorta progress.

Ashes to Dust

38

It was hard for me, but I tell my mom about the hospital. I only get to tell her a male nurse there elbowed me in the chest before she stopped me by bursting into tears and talking about herself. I was still dealing with the new hospital numbness at times, so seeing her cry about herself and her experience at a hospital at a time I was trying my hardest to open up and tell her about the abuse I went through there, set me into that emotional numbness again. I told myself I should cry for her, because what she went through at the hospital when she was a kid was bad. But I couldn't. I also was able to recognize that she couldn't take the time to try to listen or comfort me, and made it where instead I'm suppose to be comforting her.

I tell her I feel bad for her, and I want to cry for her because what she went through was horrible, but I can't. Not because I don't want to I just can't because of the hospital.

I still didn't understand it was a PTSD response, or a response to trauma that I was dealing with.

The next time I try to explain to her that I'm having a hard time dealing with everything from the hospital, and the night her ex came so I need space. I was trying to set boundaries like I was told to do. But instead my mom still invaded my bubble or yelled at me, knowing it would set off the involuntary head movements, or a freeze response

Ashes to Dust

where I can't move or speak. And she told me how I'm not the only person dealing with what happened. That everyone in the house is dealing with the night that everything happened and that it isn't just about me.

But they weren't the ones that were recovering from food poisoning and then were taken to the hospital and strapped down. They weren't the ones that had a nurse hurt them, or multiple people hold them down in a double door locked room and injected them with who knows what and left alone where they felt like they were going to die. They didn't suffer in a involuntary hold. They got to stay in their cozy home.

I didn't feel like I could get the support I needed or even share the hardships I went through at the hospital. I didn't feel like I mattered at all. Every time I try I'm met with how everyone else matters and I should be more considerate of them. It left me feeling worse. I don't know why I bothered trying to open up more than once when I was already met with a response that doing so made me selfish. Tried to open up to my mom about my hospital experience and instead she cut me off to talk about hers. She wanted emotional support from me at a time where I couldn't provide it, and I was the one that needed it. I was always the emotional support and I realized how I really had no one to care about how I felt or what I experienced.

When I tried to tell her I wanted to dye my hair blonde, she wasn't supportive, she got mad about it and didn't understand why I would do it to feel disconnected from the trauma. But then weeks later she dyes her hair blonde claiming how she feels like a new person. Similar to what I said. And acts like she didn't treat me like shit when I told her I wanted to dye my hair.

I'm alone.

39

March 9, 2021:
Saw a ad for a house (full or main room) for a dollar. Checked it out and got confused so I called. Guy answered and said to come to open house next day. I needed to know the price since it'd cost me money just to get a ride to go out and look (and honestly I'd take it without looking just by the pictures alone). He said there's two bedrooms plus a huge attic so he is looking for at least $1,200. That was way above my budget for a house. He still insisted on me going to check it out, even though he said a lot of people inquired. He told me before to get a roommate and that'd help.

I checked out the ad again after getting off the phone and wrote him to see if he needed anything like a rental application. When he didn't, I realized it wasn't a one bedroom and that was why it was so high. I called to tell him my mistake and see if he had any one bedrooms.

I call and I told him my mistake and that I wouldn't be going. He brought up a one bedroom asking if I preferred a room or a house with a one bedroom. I said house with bedroom. He told me he had a place but didn't know how to show me because people still live there. He asked where I lived, and I said Wallaceburg, and he asked how far away. Then he said something about he just moved from Toronto and bought a house. Where he just broke up with his girlfriend. He said he was buying another property soon too. He asked what I did, I didn't want to say diddly squat. I said work wise? He said yes. I wondered if he forgot who I was after all with the first call he knew I had a budget from portable housing.

He said he meant work wise and asked how come I didn't work. I said it's hard right now because of COVID. Which was honest but I wasn't going to tell him the truth about my traumas and shit. He said yeah everybody's getting laid off, because of COVID. He asked what I did before. I said art. He said he liked artists. I wanted him to stop talking and asking personal questions but I wasn't sure if he needed to know to see if I'd be reliable to pay rent or some thing from a landlord perspective. He went on to say how they are talented. I said I'm an amateur artist and don't think I'm that good. He said practice makes you improve then one day you can make it.

Then he said he moved for a fresh start after a bad break up. I wasn't liking how he kept going and was now talking about relationships. He then asked how I talk to people after he asked if I was married or had kids and I said I don't have kids and he said he doesn't either. I said I talk to people with the Internet. He said he was old-school and liked talking face to face. He asked how old I was. I said over 18, before he got into personal shit, he said aren't we all over 18? And laughed. I laughed and said no there are 16 year olds looking for housing too. He said yeah.

He asked if I had a WhatsApp. I said no. He asked how I talk to people then. I didn't want to tell him anything, also no friends outside the one on Insta, so I said email. He asked about FB and I said no I don't like their privacy policies. He said your privacy is important. Then he asked if I did drugs, I said no I don't do that stuff. He asked about alcohol after saying he also didn't do drugs. I said no. I wondered if he thought he'd meet me at an open house and supply me with alcohol to take advantage of me. I'm not like that.

Ashes to Dust

He kept finding shit to talk about despite my silence, or very short answers. He asked if I go out. I said there's nothing to do in Wallaceburg so no. He knew I didn't drive and had no car. He kept asking even though I said no. I said I would if I didn't live here but there's nothing to do in Wallaceburg. He mentioned grocery shopping, I said yeah that. He said he's never been to Wallaceburg. I didn't like the sound of that and said he won't like it, honest, that it was just small with fast food chains and a grocery store.

He goes on to mention that he can call me about the friend he knows with the one bedroom. He said he had my number. That made me nervous, I'd rather he delete it and never called me. At this point I was pretty sure he was a creeper but I was making sure. I never would've known he was like this if I had just said I had to go right after he mentioned a one bedroom. He then asks how I feel about meeting new people. I say there's masks worn and distance so it's the same as going grocery shopping. He seemed disappointed by the answer. He then said he'd like to be friends. I said I'm socially awkward so I don't know how to respond to that. It wasn't true I just didn't want to say anything else that makes him think I did.

I thought it was clear by the ad for a rental I wanted a rental from a non-pervy landlord not a hook up, or a friend. He said that's OK just be yourself. He said something more and asked about me. I said I am not looking for friends or dating, that I'm going through a hard time. Then typical dick move, when I said I didn't want to talk about it, he said we're all going through a hard time. He just broke up with his girlfriend, and the virus and he had to move. Completely undermined me, and I wasn't going to explain why he was a dumb ass for saying it.

He then asked if I was shy. I didn't wanna say no, I just didn't want to talk to him, so I said I have been told I am. People say who they think you are all the time. But there's a difference between shy, and not wanting to engage in conversation, which a lot of times, like in a car, I don't want to. He said yeah. He then said he thinks shy is kind of cute.

Ashes to Dust

The confirmation is there after I said I don't date before and he said he wasn't looking because he just got out of a break up long-term.

He said what do I think about that? About thinking it was cute.

Obviously he wanted a booty call or worse he was some dick who's a trafficker. I saw my exit and took it. I said no, I don't know how to respond to that so I'm hanging up. And hung up. They better not fucking call me.

I got a call from my house hunting helper and tell her about it. She says it's a good thing I saw the red flags. Don't know how you would miss it when they call you cute and shit. Reminded me of the other creepy renter who said price depending on if you were a good girl or not. Like what the fuck. I told her if she had a male looking for housing it'd be good for them. She did.

I went to my sister's door to give all the cookies and candy I had to her. I knock, she says baby's sleeping. I said I have something for you. I think she'd like it, I was going to give her my vanilla coffee she liked too. But then she said she has a bit of a stomachache, she doesn't feel good.

Disappointed I say, OK never mind. And go to my room to set the shit down as I start crying. This wasn't the first time I've wanted to do something nice and she said something as an excuse to not open the door. Many of which I hear her after walking and moving shit around or talking to people on the phone. I dump the treats in front of my moms son instead. I'm sure he'll find something. I honestly don't think any of the others deserve it the way they've been treating me. I keep getting treated like shit right after I do something nice. Like share my food with my mom, buy her a gift, give my sister something, etc. It all gets to me and makes me feel like I'm not good enough/worth anything. The only highlight I had yesterday was when my neighbour kept telling me how nice and caring I was and that I was such a good

Ashes to Dust

person. I didn't realize how much I needed to hear those things when the house doesn't make me feel like anything but worthless/less then.

I think my counselor is a conflict of interest after all but she's all I have to talk to. I might have to cut ties.
My mom was going to talk with her but suddenly was out back, so I think the counselor told her I go out of my room.
But her being in the backyard is worse because I can hear the chatting. I was even able to clearly hear my mom admit she was emotionally immature and that the counselor knew that.
It didn't make me feel better. I think this was what anxiety is. I didn't want to know what was being said about me but I was also nervous and curious about what was being said about me.
I left my room a bit so I couldn't hear the murmuring that was driving my stress/anxiety up.

It made it worse thinking maybe my mom wasn't aware of her hurtful actions towards me and was doing it accidentally/unintentionally but when I heard her admit it it just reminded me of all the recent times since I've been back where she's gotten in my face to exclaim how her actions that hurt me are just who she is and it's how she is. I know now she does know. I think I knew that too, but it's hard to admit to with all the guilt trips and mean words thrown at me on top of the confusion of the good memories/actions where she's stood up for me all my life against bullies/teachers. And the memories of just sitting watching shows together.
I don't think I want to admit to the emotional abuse, despite being told it multiple times because she's my mom and I love her and there are those good memories mixed in with the outbursts and fear.

I also know my grandma messed her up pretty bad with her

Ashes to Dust

parenting so I don't know if others would say that's me creating excuses for her or not, but I try to look at the other picture. I think that's why it's conflicting. Nice obviously gets me hurt. Compassion despite not receiving it also gets me hurt.

I wonder if it's this hard for others to accept and how they dealt with it.

I think I was too dismissive to my sister all the times she use to say mom scared her. Or that her yelling was scary and traumatizing. I grew up with it, worse. So I told her "parents yell" and let that be that. Sometimes wanted to roll my eyes whenever she'd cry during mom's outbursts or when mom and my mom's ex would fight. I was emotionally (what I thought) numb to it, and learned to avoid being in her way and try to keep quiet. A lot of things didn't work but sometimes you'd have to let her yell at you, throw things around you, and take it.

I can't even apologize to my sister now that I realize I wasn't there for her emotionally like she needed. I didn't know my own emotions since I always had to shut them down and were numb to ones I couldn't recognize (happy, over sad). It's why I was always called downstairs during fights because I was "the calm one."

I'd apologize for being dismissive and tell her why it was wrong. So she'd feel validated from all those years. But I also don't think she's ready to hear it and might think me saying it is just another thing I say because of the hospital trauma. Living in the same house wouldn't help. And she's not exactly the greatest at handling things. I also don't want her to take it as I don't love mom. Or her to be the brat sister who sometimes lies, she's always been (except the circle bonding) and go tell mom and my mom say more shit about how I don't love her, or use it as ammo. There's no winning.

Maybe I should never say anything, and just hope she doesn't have to go through traumatizing events before realizing how wrong someone's actions were or how wrong hers were. At least now I'm aware on my part by not speaking up, and in the future can be better. That's all I can do now I suppose.

Went down for water before bed and cousin quickly clicked off the light to her table and tried to hurry under the covers. I already seen her and when she does this shit I'm sure she knows but she still pretends to sleep anyways. W.T.F is the point of this ridiculous behaviour? It's just annoying to come down all the time and her to play pretend. She stays still and quiet.

I can't handle her, it reminds me of the other day when I stepped outside on the porch with my cat with the door open but when I got back inside to the kitchen, the kettle's handle is orange and on. My cousin moved when I went back into the living room and put the covers over her face to play sleep. But the fucking kettle was on. I told her she didn't have to pretend to sleep. She pretended for a second longer, I assumed debating, before taking the blanket off to say she wasn't pretending she was going back to sleep. I said but she turned the kettle on. She said no she didn't she hasn't gotten up yet. I hated the obvious fucking lie. She lies all the time but to do it so obviously when no one else was in the kitchen and everyone but me, her and my cat were awake was just too much especially on top of how my mom was treating me. I went back into the kitchen thinking sarcastically, "I guess a fucking ghost got thirsty."

I really need a break from it. I just tried to ignore all her childish acts, snoopy-ness, attitude/bitchiness, and lies, but I really can't after I've been back. It stresses me out.

Ashes to Dust

40

March 10, 2021:
Woke too early. Counselor called today to talk about conflict of interest. She agrees it is. I told her how it seemed to negatively effect my mom. I was worried (told her thought it was a natural thing) where my mom might think the counselor's perspective of her might change by talking to me (counselor agreed, since we are each other's "hot" topic) and might think different/see her in a different light.

Counselor agreed it might turn into feeling the need to defend against things and make yourself look better.

I tell her I want her to stay my mom's counselor and that my mom really loves talking to her and use to tell me before I ever knew we had the same one. And that she wouldn't look for anyone else or get help when she was struggling during her break from clients and I don't want her to have no one left to talk to because I know she won't. I don't want someone she can open up to be taken away.

I also tell her for me it's that I'm also worried about changing her perspective of my mom so it's hard worrying about especially when I've been told two times and straight forward the second time, my mom's actions were in fact emotional abuse. And that's already hard enough on me to acknowledge and see happening, especially when like the counselor said, there were moments of support, etc.

I keep holding back my falling tears so she can't hear how really

Ashes to Dust

upset I am. I don't want her to feel bad or obligated to me.

I ask her not to tell anyone my new name I want to get. She said she won't and tells me how beautiful it is—which means the world to me. This is why I didn't want to accept that it was a conflict of interest and it's harder not to cry.

She tells me she wishes the best for me and hopes I get the help I need. And that I can work on the projects I wanted to do.

She's genuine and caring about it. It's no wonder I liked her right away. She told me there's a wait list for the one other counselor available and I just say that's fine.

It probably won't be, I have no one now, but I'm not going to say that.

I thank her again, we hang up, and I cry.

After I'm done crying I take a Rhodiola. I figure it can only help from here because today is a emotionally bad one that I wasn't expecting.

My mom seems happier now that the counselor called her to tell her I wasn't with her anymore. Guess it's a good thing I broke it off after all. She doesn't know how hard that was for me.

But it was a conflict of interest since one of our first sessions the counselor had asked about my mom's wellbeing (something financial) which instantly made me feel like my mom was being put first (because of their familiarity), and I wasn't going to be seen as that priority I didn't know I needed. Because it made me feel like I also had to put my mom first in my own sessions.

Ashes to Dust

41

March 12, 2021:
Had a strange nightmare about Lucifer in a Hell place. I can't remember much of it, just secretly following deer, hiding in trees so they can't see me, then hearing Lucifer's voice come on like a intercom telling the deer to make sure they thank the fish. I can't remember if it was because they ate them for food or something to show respect to the sea. The deer left then I went to the creepy darker part of this hell place where it was past dark trees to dark waters, where something evil was (fish? Creatures?) and you could tell because of the bubbles in the murky water. I kept having to jump the spaced out block shaped landscapes that were grassy, to avoid whatever the thing in the water was launching up towards my feet. I almost fell avoiding it, and saw what it was. A thick syringe with a long thin needle that squirted out questionable liquid. Poison that would kill me if it poked my feet. It rose out of the ground then disappeared and tried again but I woke up.

I figured the needle was from my trauma relating to the hospital and bringing it up for the lawyers.

And the Lucifer thing at first I thought because of the dehydration-related events that happened before. But realized it was because I stupidly looked up how my sister would know that goddess Isis was

Ashes to Dust

blocked when I was trying to remember things to write it down. (Never did, it didn't work out again, the memories of it are very triggering for me for my panic attacks and they are also traumatizing to remember.)

I just had to know because I thought it was strange to have a search result say that during the time. I never found anything but I also wasn't looking very hard because I knew I couldn't handle it long. I found a post mentioning gods/goddesses which triggered me but I read a few things (skimmed) and saw someone say they worshiped Lucifer but not the Christian version and it went by different names but it encouraged freedom. Just to see Lucifer in there, expecting "Satanism" but to have that instead I wasn't expecting.

It also triggered the remembrance of my not-so pleasant experience, so I scrolled past and then had to shut it off when I kept seeing triggering names of Gods/Goddesses.

I know I have nightmares from/based on the hospital but I never remember (most times), at least not for long.

Been contemplating tattoos again. Thought of "Free" on my fingers. But when would I get it? After I move out? After my name change? Or after a lawyer can help me and the case is won/over?

What one would lead to my true "Free"dom? I don't want to have it just to realize I'm still not truly free.

I want some beautiful artwork as my tattoos so I have beauty and colour to look at when the days aren't looking good or when I need something to combat the traumatic memories and depressing moods.

I want them to be tasteful to me where they aren't clumped like a mess but spread out. I've always loved tattoos since I was a kid. I thought they were beautiful pieces of art on people's skin/bodies.

It's why I probably won't get one again until I move out since my mom doesn't like them and it'll cause a ruckus for me. Sometimes the people who've been in your life don't know you the best either. Especially if you've lived your life having to not express your emotions to them, or are worries what you say/do will trigger their anger.

My tattooist when I got my heart on my hand told me not to get anymore and keep it the small little one to keep your innocents. I still don't get how tattoos are associated with not being "innocent." Tattoos aren't going to inject me with bad influences like drinking or drugs. I've never done that and still don't. Tattoos to me express what's on the inside, both good and bad and it doesn't always have to have meaning. A lot of people can't express themselves out loud like me (emotionally) or don't know how and it helps.

If this trauma hadn't happened I definitely wouldn't be bold enough to go do a arm tattoo(I've thought of it many times) or cover my scars on my stomach with them (I didn't care about them before but now I do and I think it's because I want it where I don't have the reminder of surgery as the old me).

My mom will definitely think I completely changed from her "sweet" little girl whenever I get the tattoos, plus the hair dye plus the name change. What she won't realize is I'm still a caring person like before, just now I have more boundaries (learning to) which she's not use to. I've always wanted to dye my hair, even cut it slightly shorter, but she never wanted that and the way she reacted to my sister doing it after wasn't good. I felt I had to keep my hair how it was because it was the one thing she always said she loved, and brushing it brought her joy.

She knows I wanted to move out since I was thirteen but is acting like I'm this back stabbing, horrible, and selfish person for finally having the chance to do so because of not being able to take the trauma and everyone's attitudes or angry outbursts anymore. I need a break for my mental health.

She didn't know (unless she sensed it) that I wanted to leave so bad that I was going to call someone to help me figure it out when she kept acting like she use to when I was a kid (13/14) when her anger was put into action by breaking things/punching things. That day after screaming at me and punching a hole in the bathroom door, I went into my room crying in secret, telling myself I can't handle this anymore and I really need to find a way to move out, even if it's rooming somewhere. I couldn't stay even if it was going to upset her more since this was the time when my sister had moved out with her abusive boyfriend.

I was stopped later by my mom telling me the same day, she wanted to kill herself and the only thing stopping her was knowing I needed her. It was upsetting and a heavy burden to carry because after I felt more "emotionally closed off." I still don't know how I feel too well. It's probably why it took me so long now to realize I'm depressed. Thanks YT.

I tried to be the perfect person for whatever she needed. I always put her first (I didn't realize until now I always did and put them first, and me last). I've always felt pressure to be the perfect daughter and it hurt when I once expressed my true feelings to her when I was sixteen (about my sister) and she said she was so disappointed and she always had me on a high pedestal but not now. It reminded me to keep stuff to myself.

My mom constantly threatened to walk out of our lives and just go live on her own a little before my sister moved out in 2020 (but definitely afterward). I'd feel like I had to step up my game, make her feel better, clean everything that my lazy ass cousin wouldn't (everything), and my sister wouldn't (didn't blame her when she came back she was pregnant). But I had to do everything so my mom wouldn't be doing it all the time. And it still wouldn't feel good enough because she'd still say it.

  I was even going to help her create a pod cast (I just bought a microphone but it was meant for me. Again wanted to put her first), so she'd have something productive to do to cheer her up. The only thing that stopped me was she blew up too hard at me. I woke up choking on fire pit smoke. I called her because I couldn't stop coughing and the smoke filled my room, I was gonna puke. I asked her if she had it going (yes) and asked if she could stop or bring it out front (she knew it seeped into our rooms outback). I said I was gonna puke, I didn't feel good from it. And she blew up at me saying she's sick of everyone telling her what to do. Swore at me, then hung up. I puked after.

  I felt horrible again and cried in secret. And didn't understand why she went off at me or why she didn't ask if I was OK. Instead I went downstairs and was met with her infamous silent treatment. She would talk to everyone but me, she loved them back but not me. By the third day she got mad at me for not saying anything and made it seem like I was being rude for not speaking by then. She didn't ask how I was the day I felt sick. She managed to shut it down. She didn't know the first day she treated me like that I got on my e-bike and biked around. I found a empty field to try a TikTok to cheer me up. And a lady had shouted over asking me if I was OK, that she'd been watching me and wanted to make sure I wasn't stranded. I said I was fine and she left. I felt more love and compassion from a stranger than my own mom that day. I ended up being really happy until I got home and that reality sunk in. I cried about it in secret.

  My mom didn't even know I was gone (or cared, which was good since I'm old enough where I shouldn't still have to tell her and have her say no I can't it's too late or something, but it felt more uncaring that way in my head that day). She was angrily cleaning her room. I could hear her slam her dressers.

Ashes to Dust

This is why I'm having such a hard time accepting that my mom is my abuser. Especially when she's stuck up for me against bullies, defended me against teachers, even abusive ones. (Now I realize I am parroting the words she tells me and her counselor.). Believed that I can always be a singer. Kept food on the table so I never starved. I know how hard it is on her so I don't ask for more. I even bought my own food and paid her for rent (more than I was supposed to, to help her since my cousin wasn't at the time).

It's almost like if I admit that as truth then I'm ungrateful for the good things she's done, just like I've heard her say to more than myself, which she knows is far from true. Now I definitely see it when it's happening more clearly and it's disturbing to realize it. It doesn't make me feel any better knowing, and I don't know what I'm suppose to do now that I do know. I wondered how people in abusive relationships stayed, but they never mention how hard it is when it's a parent, especially when it's not physical (other than typical mouth slaps or spankings as a kid). As the kid, you have to listen to your parent and do everything they say because they are your parent and they love you. But no one tells you or the parent the signs they've become toxic, or in that territory.

I honestly don't think she's aware exactly. Many of us don't know our negative actions unless someone outside points it out (in a non douche way), then you're like, "Oh shit. I'll try to better myself because that's not what I intended to put out." I've done this, especially now with my sister, but she does the same, obviously we aren't meaning to (at least my perspective) but if we were raised with this experience of course we'd be a bit emotionally numb or come off as cold at times, even though inside we feel a lot. We even had a bond talking about how we both hid behind things if mom woke up because she was so scary. We laughed how we both hid together at times when we were "talking to loud," behind a cabinet. We told our stories, where I would crawl to hide out of sight, sometimes chips in my mouth, I'd go under the table. We both knew about the creaky stair step that told us when mom was coming.

I think because of how my grandma raised my mom, she carried those traits onto her parenting. But my mom was better, she never hit her kids with things (that was a different era where they let teachers hit kids with rulers). I won't get into my moms personal life like that, even if it would explain why she is how she is. (I realize now I was making excusing again, because like I said, it's very hard to accept the truth.)

It still doesn't make it easier on me though. I'm also very conflicted on writing this, mentioning things even if it's a big part of it now (she didn't handle me coming back from the hospital well). I definitely won't bring up how she was when I was a kid, it's not relevant to this experience and no one always stays the same. I will say it's why I've never done alcohol or drugs, and why I don't like being around people who do (especially obvious drunks).

I wasn't expecting to write things about my mom other than the circle incident. I even told them when I first came back I planned on writing about my experience and didn't want them to read it because everything that happened (while dehydrated) felt real. Now she'll think I'm attacking her and that's why I didn't want her to read it. But I wasn't expecting to be met with such a lack of understanding and caring when I got back. And then on top of it told her actions were emotional abuse. Now I have to deal with it and I don't know how.

She's told me when my sister was eight (in front of sister) if I ever left (I wanted to move out and said so multiple times) that she would drink all the time again. I felt I couldn't, plus I wasn't stupid, you need a stable income. My sister never wanted me to leave after that. It's still carried on now, years later because my sister texted if I move out she's worried mom will hurt herself. Something I was already worried about and had to discuss with the counselor because I didn't know how to deal with it since both my mom and sister told me the same thing.

I love my mom very much. It makes it harder to write this, and deal with it. She's great to her son. She was there when his mom wasn't, fed and clothed him when his didn't. Protected him from his mom's abuse. Took him into her home to protect him. Says I love you 50 million times a day when he says it 50 million times. Makes sure he has everything he needs. I'm saying this part because she thinks she shouldn't be taking care of him, and that's not true, she's very good with him. I think if she ever gave up on herself, then it'd be unlucky for him because there's no one else to take care of him, and foster family horror stories … it's why kids know not to talk to family services is all I'll say.

I hope people will respect my old name to stay dead when I get my new one so my family doesn't have to deal with anyone because of my book. It's why I will make sure not to say names, or my age so people who aren't respectful will hopefully have a harder time. Also people are dicks about age, and I've never liked that.

Ashes to Dust

42

April 28, 2021:

Woke up to text from mom asking if I hate her, and that she feels like I don't want to keep contact with her after moving and that I don't want her to move. She also brought up my cousin, not to tell anyone stuff.

Ever since I told her I'm moving she's constantly going back and forth of I hate her, she's dead to me, if I leave we won't have a relationship anymore, I don't love her.

It's really stressful and annoying. I'm trying to deal with stuff but it's like she doesn't want me to because if I want to not talk about upsetting things then she says I don't care about her anymore. If I need space because I can't have someone right close in front of me, she gets offended and angry.

I need to move for me, my safety (from her ex and ex's drug friends), my wellbeing. And she acts like I've done her so wrong and I'm a horrible person for doing so. Even though I don't get it, since many times she's threatened to just up and leave. So many many times.

It made me feel like I needed to make things even better for her here, which wasn't fucking possible. It was clear she was having issues with the people living here and I can't control that and I don't want to. She should be happy there's one less person to stress over. I free up space. I need her to stop making it seem like finally trying to put me first sometimes and do things I need right now, are so horribly wrong and means I hate her and don't care about anyone in the family. It keeps getting twisted back to her and everyone else. Please, please, just let me have a moment to care about my fucking self without making it dirty. It's hard enough to put myself first as it is. I don't need it harder on me. I'm already dealing with a lot and struggling. But it seems even if she sees it, she still doesn't care enough to try. To acknowledge it without making it back to being about her or someone else.

  I had to write her back and say, of course I want a relationship with you. Why would I say anything about my cousin? I was just asking if you'd still be on the wait list for Chatham because you said many times you didn't want to uproot your life from Wallaceburg. You said you were only moving for us but I thought once I moved you wouldn't have to leave and stay like you wanted. I thought if you moved to Chatham you could visit easier but I didn't want to assume you were still moving. You were the one saying things making me think you didn't want a relationship with me when I moved. I was nervous you wouldn't want to visit me once I moved. Love you.

  Some things I can't say to her obviously. But it's really frustrating to constantly be told I must hate her or this and that for doing something that isn't malicious, or as normal as going to a fucking appointment and not telling her what it's for. I love her a lot but I'm still dealing with the hospital confusion. I'm dealing with trying to acknowledge and figure out my feelings now knowing and seeing I have been emotionally abused by my mom all my life. That's not a easy thing to deal with, especially on top of all my trauma shit. It's a lot and I need space that feels safe and unstressed to sort it out with. Then I can ask my counselor down the line on how I should approach that and deal with my mom in a new way. Not ever telling her the abusive part

Ashes to Dust

obviously. I'm not fucking dumb. I mean how to rebuild, if my boundaries keep not being respected and knocked down all the time, how do I handle it? Maybe I'll ask his opinion on this book and how I'm worried the journal entry parts, if I include (probably, the worst is already what I need to write) might affect them and they might see it one day and read it and think less of me, if possible.

Honestly it doesn't seem like my sister would want to visit, because I said if her baby was attached to me what would she do? She said she hoped not because I live in Chatham and she'd have to tell her no I live in Chatham.

Made me feel a bit gloomy to know I would go on a bus from Chatham to Wallaceburg to get to them but they wouldn't want to for me even though she could have her boyfriend drive. It's fine it just makes me unfortunately understand better on how they really view/value me and our relationship.

Maybe I'll make it easier. If they don't want to really keep in touch or have only done it because "we're family," and lived together, then it's like they left me/abandoned me even before I wrote this. And this isn't spite, it's why it's hard, it's truth. And the truth is yes, ugly. Even for me to see now. It's why I feel worse knowing it and seeing how I was treated and handled on the most important moments.

Maybe they're disappointed I'm not the perfect person to always hold them all up and never fall myself. I'm not though. Even rocks crack.

And I still can't express my genuine (first) excitement about moving because it doesn't want to be seen. My sister maybe, but I don't know if she might say I'm happy about it to my mom and my mom get upset or angry. Guess that may be messed up basically, "Don't text message mom I'm happy/excited about moving. She'll get mad/upset."

I also couldn't text my mom that I didn't want her to move to Chatham just to follow me and say it's "for me," because if I ever had

Ashes to Dust

the opportunity to move to Toronto, I wouldn't be there anymore.

Seems hypocritical she could cry and yell at me for years for wanting to move out of Wallaceburg and she'd use every excuse and say why I can't or she can't. But now I am, she can? Only now she can? That's upsetting. Because for the past few years she had insinuated she'd reject a place in Chatham and just go back on the wait list for more years. Knowing that'd be upsetting to us me and my sister). She can live where she wants to. And I want to live and do what I want to.

I think she's bitter about it because the other day she asked me if I knew what it looked like and I said I don't know, I never got to see it, I don't know anything just one bedroom. (I honestly don't care, but not gonna say that.) Then with definite bitterness she said, "Well they probably didn't show you because you said you wanted to leave."
That's not how it went down first of all … (requirement of leaving was locking my door and accepting housing.) And I was hoping to be past that. But obviously not. And no I don't care what it looks like, I don't need to see it, I'm happy I'm moving. I just wanted to have a idea of how big the bedroom and living room were so I can instruct movers to put stuff where I know it'll fit. My mom keeps talking like my sister isn't going to help me anymore … so …
I'll probably have to hire. My sister does change her mind a lot depending on her mood. It's fine if she ends up not wanting to, I never asked. I'm not gonna force it. I do need to know closer to the move date though because some companies require four weeks notice.

Why is it I get hit with a bomb, little or big, either accusing me of something or saying something like what my mom texted me, RIGHT FUCKING AFTER I DO SOMETHING NICE? It's almost always after I go out of my fucking way and comfort (sometimes) and then I get hit with it. This time I cooked them corn on the cob. Oh shit — she did something nice, better question every thing about her now. Make her feel like shit right now, not a day she didn't do something, no no, today. Why? It makes me not fucking want to do anything for any of them. Stop pouncing after I do something nice. Just stop pouncing in general. Apparently we all have counselors now, so go bitch to them about me like I know is already done. Like I've had to do on paper. Like that poor new counselor will have to endure from me sometime in our sessions. But first he's going to help with the hospital trauma stuff which was number one when he said what do I want to get out of it. Or maybe that was handling, ya it was, panic attacks and anxiety. He apparently has many ways to help with them so that's great.

Emotions man ... I'm new to actually feeling like trying to pinpoint them since there are so many unhappy ones now and I was use to just shutting out the other since it didn't do me any good. (Had no one to talk to, not even mom, had to make sure everyone else was taken care of and that I wasn't adding to issues by them, or acknowledging to myself so I also wouldn't have more to deal with.) It's very annoying and frustrating and draining because I don't know what I'm suppose to do with these feelings and conflicts now. There's too much from everything now. I feel like I'm suppose to rush and feel like ... not this. How I THOUGHT I was feeling.
Especially towards my mom because of how she keeps acting and making me feel bad. I can't though. It's ... hard to explain so how can I explain it to someone else? I certainly can't explain it to my mom. Lack of compassion if I did. It would only cause me more grievance. She can show so many other people compassion, but not me? I don't get it.

Sometimes I think I can be too hard with what I think of someone (example, family) lately. Suppressed emotions coming out on top of the trauma ones because I can't shove them down now like I use to? Critical of actions and words a lot too. A lot of times with obvious reasons with everything done to me. And after seeing and learning

Ashes to Dust

about the emotional abuse, of course I'm going to try to look out for any meanings and possible motives now. No one wants to be taken advantage of, used, or abused. It's why I'm triple upset. Having to grow up with my mom's manipulative and violent ex, of course I thought I would never be abused in any form because I'd spot it. But turns out your blind when it comes to those closest to you. And when you grow up that way, it's all normal. Until someone points out it's not.

Reminded me, counselor stopped because next time he wants to go over all the abuse/violence I've witnessed. That's a fucking lot so it's a good thing because I wouldn't have been able to. My chest was already burning and I was holding back tears, which hurts me physically now, and made my voice shaky. My mom called during it but I couldn't answer and after I didn't want her to know I got a new counselor or I was on the phone. She might try to hover by my door again to listen. Also I just started and I want to keep it private while I see how it goes. My mom doesn't need to know everything, even though she makes it her business to try, even when I try to get her not to. Doesn't work. Just me and the counselor, no third interference that makes me worried on what I say.

I keep wanting to tell my sister my name won't be what she's telling her baby. I don't want her baby to learn my old birth name, I want her to know the (hopeful) new one I gave myself to distance from everything bad I went through at the hospital. (I just realized that's what the counselor said, I was distancing myself from trauma related things like chicken, that reminded me of it, which he said would all be explored.)

But I can't because she'll either tell my mom and holy fuck no that's not good while I'm still here, or she'll think something is wrong with me (there's not) and not understand and I'm scared of that. Hope her kid doesn't learn that name and only knows my new one. I don't know if my decision will be respected. Seems like it really never is. But I hope they'll try enough where at least in front of me, addressing me personally, it'll be by my new name without looking at me like I'm insane or emotional on why/how could you change it it had meaning, or something. This new one has meaning to ME. Helps ME feel better. It's MY name, it needs to be for me. This must be how trans people feel changing their names or telling someone because then they might act like you killed their loved one or somethings wrong with you. I have nothing else to compare this to. I'm not trans, I enjoy being a girl (except periods) and always will be. This is all just part of the trauma from the hospital and my way of coping because I never thought of changing my name before. It's all I want now.

I'll have to practice a new signature. Hope I get accepted soon. Maybe before the move out date so I can have everything transferred to my new name successfully while in Wallaceburg and so I get my certificate in the mail since I had to use the address here. Hopefully it's under my old name or they may throw it out or grill me about it.

Had to lock my bike around a thick pillar at the hospital. Why wouldn't they have bike racks? Made me nervous and nauseous going into the Wallaceburg hospital. Remembering I was there previously wasn't pleasant. I got my X-ray done though.

Got a text from mom. She responded surprisingly well. She said she wants me in her life and wants to live close to me. All seems well there which is good. I did say not to move just to be by me because I don't want her living in a town she hates. She kept it short. "I don't," so guess she's fine with moving to Chatham. Just as long as I'm not used later as a reason for moving there if one day I leave Chatham. Hope she means it because I'd hate for her to regret moving there. She knows I've always wanted to move to Toronto though. Maybe she thought

Ashes to Dust

it'd never happen. If mummified me or ashes of me get transported to Toronto then technically she'd be wrong. I just wouldn't be happy about it because it wouldn't be while I was living.

Wonder if my mom will still feel the same about wanting to be in my life after my name change, tattoos, and possibly finding this published. Not sure how we'd work around that. Separately to our counselors? No idea.

Mom brought up money because pay is soon. Told her I'd give her $400 so it's a even number. She said she was fine with that. She said something about she knows I'll think she's going to make a big deal about the $390, but that she won't and wants to make it easier because she knows moving is expensive. Because when she asked how much I'd give her (sounding disappointed) I said I have to save and pay for insurance annually, and movers.

She suggested hers which was $60 a month, but now I'm thinking of the CMHA housing worker's suggestion that's $100 something annually. That's still cheaper than $60 monthly for every month. I appreciate her suggestion and wrote it down just in case. She also gave movers. So I'm thinking maybe my sister talked to her in private and said she didn't want to or maybe her boyfriend said no. No clue.

The way my mom said that statement about the $390 and making a scene, makes me think the counselor really is talking to her and trying to help her adjust to me moving. That's great, as long as she doesn't break my confidentiality. Hope my mom gets better and grows as a person and can learn how to manage her anger and emotions better.

Just like now how I have to try to learn how to manage the trauma induced emotions. I'm not use to it, I don't like it. It's hard.

Ashes to Dust

43

May 2:

Mom still seems happy. I think it was the food thing. I gave her some potato soup yesterday and I made her the tomatoes the other day. I can't do that forever though. I get really drained being down too long.

Mom asked what I wanted for my birthday again. I don't know. I don't care. What I really want, I can't say and not sure I can have. Honestly, I want acceptance. I want her to understand me, actually listen and care and not try to turn it into about her or the family. I want no issues moving. The acceptance would extend to accepting my new name. She doesn't have to like it, I love it, she just has to accept it by using it in my presence.

A second one (am I greedy?) no blow ups at or around me. I don't want to be yelled at or hear it. I don't want to see or hear things smashing or doors slamming. No more emotional abuse. I don't know how long the happy moments of hers will be or if it's only because she thinks I'm acting like the "old" me by cooking some things for her. I can't tell if she's growing or not. I really want to think she is slowly, but I really hope so. I also know, as hard as it is to drill in, I also can't sit around expecting her to change or rely on her happy mood.

I want the move to go smooth. I'll be happy, she'll be happy. People need breaks.

Ashes to Dust

I check my email every day wondering when I'll get the move in date. I hope tomorrow I'm told. Maybe a bonus this month I get to leave and rest.

I'm getting my sister a rose quart bracelet. I'm pretty sure it's what I told her to throw out after the circle but I don't remember. Maybe it'll cheer her up. Still hurts me when she throws it in my face that she threw out stuff because of me. She doesn't say it kindly. I get it, she's upset, but I asked her at the time because I thought I was protecting her and the baby. I really wish she would stop saying things to mom when I'm there, by waving her arm in my direction saying, "She fucking threw out my shit." Or, "Because of her." I can only heal so fast to try to accommodate others. I don't remember everything we threw out. A lot of my stuff, her stuff, basement carpet, my mom's used pillar candles.
After the bracelet (I hope I'm not forgetting another crystal or something) I still have to get my mom pillar candles, and her son a green carpet.
I'm only able to get my sister the bracelet because I was able to sell my weighted hula hoop yesterday.

When I try to hug my sister she doesn't hug me back. I can't remember if she's just always been like that, but I take it harder now. Makes me feel like a nuisance for trying to show affection. Doesn't make me feel good at all. Why do I bother? She doesn't even say hi to me if she gets up and sees me or passes by. I've said hi a few times but I'm wasting my energy. I don't know what she thinks of me. Good, bad, annoyance. At least with her kid I know because she always smiles and laughs at me when she sees me. The baby is the only one that accepts me. Sad … for me. No one suffers it but me.

I think I have enough for movers now. I just need to get more boxes.

Ashes to Dust

But I can't until I know when I move or else my mom will go from happy to possibly nuclear for having a bunch of packed boxes.

44

May 3:
Told my sister when I move I can send her all of the recipes mom likes so she can make them. She said, "Fuck that she can cook it her damn self." We laughed but I wasn't on the inside. Why is it then that I'm treated poorly for not cooking for someone? Why does/did my mom treat me so poor (stating, it nicely, it wasn't nice) when I came back and wasn't cooking for her. And now that I am sometimes, I'm treated with call checkups sometimes again, good nights, hugs. I don't get it, and it's unfair to me. I don't/didn't give a shit doing it once in a while (before hospital it was almost daily) but I do give a shit that I was treated like shit when I could only take care of myself. Every one should just take care of themselves then. Cook for themselves. I don't want that mantle back.

Why does my mom try to argue with me about something I know she said (like HER wanting to make salsa) and trying to make it seem like I said it when I know I didn't. Yet my sister has the same argument about her saying something, not my sister, and it's believed after two times.

It's probably related to when she came up one day and said my memory was bad and looked sad, but that was not the case and a means to get what she wanted which upset me. Why question my

Ashes to Dust

memory at all? Why try to argue with me over some thing stupid but make it seem like I'm the one not remembering or am incapable of remembering correctly? She use to mess up what was said all the time because of her legit memory problems from her car accident, but I don't slam that in her face or look sad saying, "You probably forgot because of your memory problems." That would obviously hurt her, even though true, and I've never done that shit to her. So why does she still try to do that to me just to "win" an argument that she knows I can't bicker about back or I'll give myself chest burning pains and the head jerk thing.

I still want to share with my sister like how I want tattoos (much less than what was happening when I was ... stressed) but I know I can't. I feel like I lost that, or it never grew into more. Even back in 2019 when I wrote a will thinking, I might die from surgery or infection of my gallbladder, I wrote to her saying I hoped one day when she got older we could've tried forging a relationship.

I wonder if I'm looking for bonds in the wrong place? I just don't have any one to talk to genuinely right now. I think that might be harder on me than I thought. Maybe I'll make a new friend when I move. Who knows.

Maybe this is just how our relationship is. Just because we're sisters doesn't mean our relationship will be close or good. I'm just disappointed because I have tried hard to connect, even now. Maybe if she wants in the future, but if not I'll just have to learn it is what it is, can't be stuck on it. But she better not ask to move in with me because her and mom are fighting or something. No.

If I'm not poor I will question why she wants to be a part of my life ... oh boy I over think.

PART NINE
CONCLUSION

45

I'm upset I couldn't make the story more whole. It was tougher than I thought and re-triggering to write out so I missed some things for the dehydration character parts of the story. It might've flowed better if I had remembered better or been able to move past the triggers and write it. But that's not how trauma works, as I've learned.

I didn't get to write the parts for Death (not the mummy or horse Death), where she had a moment where she could hang up the mantle of Death and pass it on to another. She thought she was waking up in her next life (similar to the story of feeling like becoming Hannah) with one of the Lucifer angels next to her. She had her eyes closed, and she could feel what it was like being there and hearing her new voice and him through Ash's body. They thought they were in their next life, lying next to each other in bed like a couple (not sexual), and they both felt happy. Death in her new human life didn't realize how much she would want it with someone, with that love, until it was taken away before it could even start.

Her promise of a new life was taken away, another broken promise. And she had to take back her job as Death again because the one she had looked over to train (before Mike, he was the only good Death who never betrayed her), ended up listening to the corrupt guardians who thought they could use the new Death trainee to kill the ex-Death.

Ashes to Dust

But they didn't realize she would always be Death in case something like corruption happened. So she had to kill the trainee and became a much angrier Death. Harsher. But she still knew what she could and could not do. It made the Lucifer angels scared to see her that way, but they didn't abandon her.

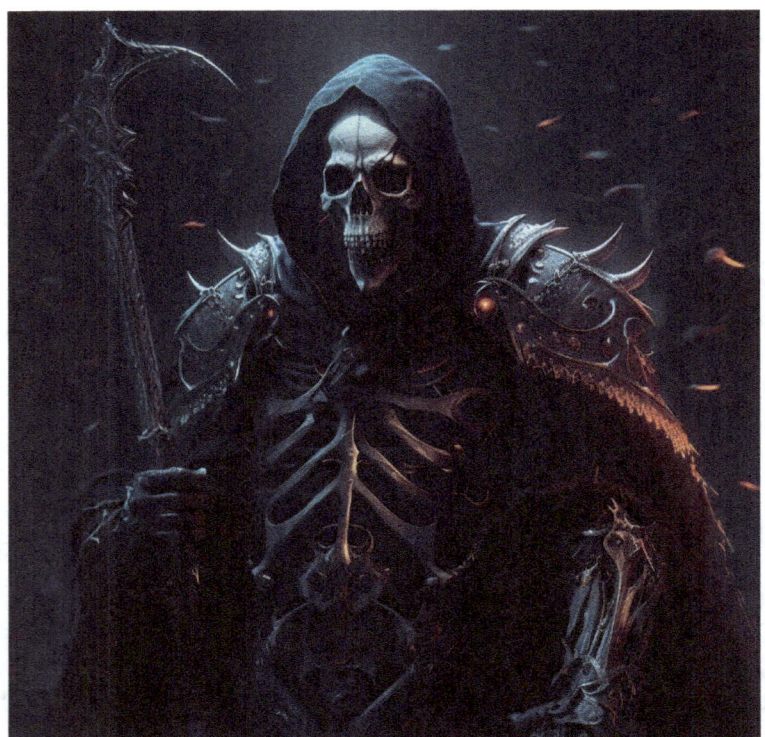

There were parts including the Grim Reaper previous to what I wrote, but all I can remember is when first calling on the Grim Reaper it was to open a dangerous gate. He was the only one who could open the gate and lock beings away in there.

The Death/Universe arch may be confusing but Death was Universe all along, she just didn't remember because of the band aid put on her

Ashes to Dust

by the bad guardians limiting her powers.

It was hard to explain who was the character at the moment, and I'm hoping I did a decent job. Sometimes it would switch where it was both me as truly me (Ash), but then sharing as a different "me," like priestess or light soul, or a different character like Light and Stars. I know it can get confusing that's why I chose first person view to write it, hoping it would be the easiest and least likely to take the reader out of the experience.

The order for the non-hospital parts were conflicting because when it was happening it was so all over the place and so much was going on one after the other that I couldn't remember with complete accuracy the order once I got back from my horrific stay at the hospital. I did my best, and I'm hoping my pain and experience will still make a entertaining enough story, even if I couldn't fill it out completely like I wanted.

For the first hospital part, I'm pretty sure the bad Loki's (or one of them) find out it was their mother, Universe, that they were hurting, and they grew conflicted on it and were hurt by their mother's love for them to save them. I just can't remember that part well enough or where it went since a lot was going on. But it was a important arch in their story that helped make the bad Loki's start turning light. Along with light soul infecting Loki 1-2-3 with her light and it spread to the others through him. But Universe may have inflicted love pains, but she also has to give them karma for what they did to light soul/their sister.

Ashes to Dust

46

After coming back to a clear sense of mind, where I no longer believed I had D.I.D and recognized the false memory thoughts (all the rapes, like thinking my mom and dad sexually abused me as a child), I was horrified. I struggled through it knowing now what was false and what wasn't. I was also told some things I thought I heard like thinking my cat got out, or that my family was there when the ambulance found me, and them at the Wallaceburg hospital weren't true. They were all at home the entire time and my cat was let out of my room right after I left. I also didn't fix the parts where I thought it was "Loki officers" when it was actually the people from the ambulance. I left it in since at the time it was what I thought, and I wrote this book by my experience in those moments including what I thought was happening at the time, or felt at the time. Including when I thought I was bleeding from my mouth while hiding for safety in the neighbour's shed, but it was just saliva.

I didn't experience typical visual hallucinations, in part I think because of my Aphantasia where I can't visualize things in my mind or it'll be black. I didn't realize this wasn't typical until a few years before 2020. I thought no one could visualize a apple in their head, or a "happy place." So whenever I "saw" things like the butterflies, or lights, etc, it was whenever I had my eyes closed. My guess is it was happening like micro-sleeps, or where you are so tired the moment you lay down and close your eyes you start having "dreams" starting up before you're fully ready for sleep because your body is so exhausted. But I'll never know. Food poisoning mixed with lack of sleep is not a pretty combination. And because of COVID, I have no idea if I possibly caught it and it caused these issues to happen (since afterward I seen some strange reports it can), or if it was just the bad shrimp. I mean black poop doesn't happen because you are healthy.

I didn't "see" the Gods/Demons/etc, I just "knew" where something was. I still saw my room, or wherever it was when it was happening, but there was nothing there in the spot I "knew" where something was. Sometimes my eyes would just have this intense heavy feeling in a certain spot, and I thought at the time that was the correct location, or the right object (like when I was throwing out items after cleansing the rooms). It was just my brain narrating a story that I couldn't see visually. And I couldn't hear the things I knew were there. There was no outside voices or voices in my head. I was like a one-woman-show where everything would just come out of my own mouth as "their" voice like those psychics you see on TV channeling things. Or someone voice acting multiple characters.

I'm safe and clear headed now, and the more I tried to decipher things or remember things I said, did, or thought, while writing this was really hard on me. And trying to figure out what another person, like Snow, meant by things she was saying at the time, just wasn't possible. It's a rabbit hole that would only create me more misery.

The reason everything was God, Goddesses, and Universe related was because during 2020 I was researching Gods, angels, and other supernatural stuff for my third book in my series that was suppose to be centered around angels and gods in a angel ruled world opposite the demon ruled world from book two. I was also listening to a lot of videos to uplift your mood and manage stress during COVID, which included sleep hypnosis, law of attraction and manifesting, and meditation videos. So everything I had watched weaved into its own

Ashes to Dust

story during that unfortunate dehydrated time. Which is also why I don't do meditation anymore as it all feels linked to my traumatic event since I was attempting meditation videos after I got out of the hospital but it didn't work because my thoughts were too busy fighting everything said with negativity.

I was able to figure out myself why I may have thought certain things in that state. Like the raped by my dad, was most likely from when I was younger when I told my mom about a friend that had been molested by her dad. Which then my mom responded, "Would you like to know if something like that happened to you?" Which I (in the moment and didn't actually mean), said, "Yes." And her face turned almost horrified and sad like something had happened to me. That moment and hearing my mom talk with a old guy friend of hers constantly about how awful my dad was, and catching the random tidbits like about my dad putting me in the hospital as a baby, or I had tubes coming out of me as a baby, etc. And it always seemed to imply sexual things. Especially when her guy friend said perverted shit when I was under age like how hot I was, or slapping my butt, or if he can't have my mom he should have the daughter (ie: me.). Which I'd hear my mom a few times tell him how could he say stuff like that knowing what my dad did to me.

My brain in that dehydrated, lack-of-sleep, and stressed state, built a story based off of tidbits I've heard throughout my life. If it's true or not, I don't know, and I don't need to know; it doesn't help me to know. But it was a extremely unpleasant experience to go through thinking something did happen and thinking I could feel things happen in that state. There was no real "memory" of the false events I thought happened though, which is why I think it didn't impact me as hard during those moments (like thinking I recalled the memories while in the hospital) since I couldn't "remember" it happening. There was no concrete memory of it like if I were to recall a real one. So sometimes a real memory of when I was putting on a concert for my

Ashes to Dust

mom when I was a kid, would be dirtied by the false memory trying to imply it wasn't actually a happy moment, it was actually a example of me being abused where I was forced to sing for my mom and dad (who was never in my memories, he was not apart of my life at all). That I was actually a singing bird (metaphorically) for their amusement after abusing me. But this intense example, I blame the hospital abuse and drugs they used since that part wasn't happening until after I got to the hospital.

I had to sit with everything the hospital did to me. The Wallaceburg doctor not explaining the transfer or calling my family. The Chatham hospital keeping me there involuntarily for six days illegally, violating my rights. The male nurse who elbowed me in the chest so hard I had breathing problems when I got home and could barely sleep on my side because it felt like my ribs were broken. The hospital staff holding me down unprovoked, injecting me without saying what it was, without caring of it's interaction with my heart and health. The psychiatrist not caring enough to listen. The patient relations of the hospital not caring about what was done to me there, and saying nothing can be done.

It all took a toll where I felt like I didn't own my own name anymore. I was so scarred by it, that I felt things I never felt before, and never had to deal with before. Like fighting against thoughts that were extremely negative and didn't feel like my thoughts because I had never ever had them before. So I was constantly fighting with a thought, telling myself, that's not my thought, I reject that thought. I had random physical pains that would come and go. It felt like someone would poke me in the eye or eyelid. Or pain in my wrist that I didn't know at the time was actually PTSD pain from the experience of being strapped to the hospital bed.

I called lawyers in a attempt to get justice for what the hospital did to me, all alone, so I was constantly being re-triggered with every call, which didn't allow me to recover from the experience. I would have to take a long break between calls because I would end up having to retell the worst parts of what the hospital did to me, bringing me to tears, and then I'd end up lying in bed. It was worse when I poured my heart out to a lawyer, only for them to say they don't take cases like mine. Or I ask if they can tell me if they take cases against hospitals before I retell them about the abuse because it's hard and re-triggering, but they would say no they need to hear it first. Only to be told by one that they don't take cases involving doctors or nurses. I didn't understand why they would make me relive all that after I told them it involved the hospital, just to say they don't do doctors or nurses.

My family filled me in on a few things I didn't know while I was at the hospital. When my sister visited me she asked to take me home and they told her no. The day I was released my mom called the hospital and told them she was sending my sister the next day and if they didn't let her take me with her then she was going to call a lawyer and sue them if she finds out what they're doing is illegal.

This explains why they let me out without a fuss, unlike every other time I begged to go home.

My mom and sister talked to the patient relations specialist whom admitted to them how they handled me was wrong. The PRS also lied to them and said the last three days I was there were voluntary. My sister defended me telling the PRS she was a liar because I called every day crying saying I wanted to go home but they didn't let me.

I also learned the PRS tried to pin the blame on my mom instead of the hospital by saying I was abused. This strained my relationship with my family even more. Instead of admitting the hospital was wrong, the PRS violated the confidentiality of my patient record (she didn't have my consent to mention to my mom), and didn't listen to anything being said to her, choosing to instead make up untrue facts and put blame where it didn't belong. The hospital was in the wrong and caused me lifelong pain and mental scarring.

Ashes to Dust

The situation already tore my family apart, and unfortunately that was the final thing to make my mom seem even more hostile towards me because by then she knew about the false memory I had about thinking she locked me in a ferret cage. I had told her about it because I felt so bad, but she already knew I cleared it up by telling the social worker at the hospital it was a false memory. But it didn't matter, thanks to the PRS, she just ripped the final thread of my family apart that was hanging on.

I was in my room during the call so I didn't hear it, but I appreciated my mom and sister standing up for me against the PRS. Especially with the PRS trying to lie by saying I was there voluntarily. I was surprised the PRS said that, since the night before I got out when I saw the nurse's computer it still said involuntary.

After some counseling I learned a few "tools" to deal with the new anxiety, PTSD, panic attacks, etc that were caused by the hospital. It also opened my eyes to my "toxic" (professionals' words) family dynamic and that was hard to accept on top of everything the hospital already did to me. But I was able to realize it was true that my mom was emotionally abusive towards me. I was told a few times by separate professions that what my mom was doing was all about controlling me, and some of her reactions were feeling like losing that control over me. It's hard to deal with even when recognizing when it's happened or that she just did it over text or phone. Like when she said I should consider her dead when I told her I was moving out, or that she might hurt herself. Or glosses over my feelings and turns things around to be about her. I understand it's not what I need when I'm trying so hard to find a way to cope with the abuse (physical and mental) the hospital caused, and find "closure" as my counselor rightly worded it. But it's hard because I lived my whole life one way and she's my mom, so I forget that I can't trust my mom with my feelings, or some private matters like I thought. But I get a terrible reminder, or

Ashes to Dust

nightmares when I let my guard back down for her. Like telling her my new name (had to), and she was sneaky, saying she already knew because her friend violated her work rules (worked for a driving company) and told her. Then my mom implied she was dying soon and I should sign some will stuff, all because I told her I changed my name. Then she went on to tell me how I'm just trying to get away from them (family) by not using their last name anymore (rephrasing, it was worse). But it had nothing to do with them, but she only wanted to see things her way.

Though I knew I shouldn't have, I sort of followed the advice of my counselor and told my mom how some things made me feel, which didn't go well. She can't blow up as big because I don't live with her anymore (2022 when I said this), so no holes in the walls or broken things from her anger. But previously she was pleading to know if she did something wrong to tell her because she's so sorry for whatever she did and loves me. And this time she said if only she was where I lived she'd hug me (because I was trying to sue the hospital and having a hard time). I stupidly fell for it and partially told her, because I felt unresolved bitterness. My bitter thoughts were along the lines of, "How could she say that when she never hugged me when I was going through a horrible trauma from the hospital? She withheld love (including vocal) just because I set boundaries like I was told to. Ignored me or yelled at me because I wasn't doing things just for her, but for me at the time." So I told her a trickle of truth to see if I should just keep my mouth shut from now on like I did and planned, or if I should try to converse how I feel like my counselor suggested.

I told my mom that I appreciate her, but even if she were here it wouldn't make things better since when I lived with her I was still going through a hard time, so distance wouldn't make things better. I wasn't accusatory as I'm about to write this but I'm paraphrasing. I told her she didn't give me hugs even when I lived with her, and that she would let the others in the house, like my cousin, treat me and my cat improperly even when I told her, because she was mad at me. And that she would yell at me even when I told her she was causing a panic attack and to stop.

What's heartbreaking is once again, she glided over my feelings, and told me everything was my fault because I was "acting different" when I got back from the hospital. No, she didn't mean talking to myself, she didn't know that part, she meant because I was setting boundaries by cooking just for myself, or locking my room door, or trying not to make conversation because I'd have the new PTSD freeze responses if she yelled or got too close, and because I forgot things (like the bank card incident).

She blamed me being traumatized and trying to follow what I was told and sorting myself out as the reason. To her nothing was her fault. She didn't acknowledge or say sorry for doing any of it (not even at the time when it happened, she would just say stuff like "this is me" and keep yelling instead of stopping and leaving while I'm having a panic attack unable to breath).

After that convo I cried and truly felt ... ya that isn't right is it? That's not unconditional love, is it? It hurt. And I wasn't going to write any of the parts including my mom or how my family reacted to me when I got back from the hospital in this book because I didn't want to take away from what the story is really about; the hospital. And what the hospital did to me. But I thought it was important to write how my family reacted after the hospital, and the news about my mom being emotionally/psychologically abusive. Because it was part of the heartbreaking journey of what happened to me. And maybe someone reading this can take notes on how to do better if their loved one is in a fragile state, because you never know what they just went through and you may never know, but how you react to them is everything. It either helps or disables them further. I'm only able to write this because my counselor said my feelings are valid. And the amount of people writing their truth, even with abusive systems or parents, is

Ashes to Dust

why I kept the family parts in too.

I learned what the hospitals had done was Medical Malpractice, and negligence. That I had rights I never knew about, and was never told about. But because of how the system works no lawyers will take it on, especially on a contingency basis. It was the hardest thing to hear about. I tried searching for a year, but there is only two years given to find one, and the first year I was extremely sensitive and recovering from the hospital abuse.

Through lawyers I discovered there is a College of Nurses, and they deal with nurses like the one that hurt me. In over a year no one had told me about it before. The only problem is the Chatham hospital is giving them (College) and me, a hard time about the male nurse name that's needed for the investigation. They didn't want to give it to me even though the College of Nurses asked me to get it from the hospital. Then the College of Nurses told me they are also having a hard time. I learned the hospital can delete their video evidence at any time, and the evidence of the nurse hitting me, and the other staff members holding me down and hurting me, would all be gone.

Thankfully I did know the first name of the male nurse, so I tried looking him up on social media by other nurses, and found his full name so I could give it to the College. Unfortunately for me after almost a year later (in 2022), I got the verdict that they wouldn't be doing anything about the nurse who hit me (assault and battery is the term), because they didn't receive the requested video surveillance from the hospital, and the hospital didn't document the incident, or that he interacted with me.

The hospital allows nurses to swap with other nurses without documenting it if they are covering for another nurse's break, etc, and they never documented small things like when a nurse gave me water. I looked over the health records I got from the hospital (which were upsetting with how much they got wrong, or excluded), and they didn't even include that there were three nurses that had come in to try to take my blood; one of them being the male nurse that eventually assaulted me. And to make things worse, they victim blamed by saying I would've reported such a incident to the psychiatrist or patient relations if it had of happened. Fucking seriously? I begged to go home more than once a day, and you know how many times it got documented? Once. I'm lucky they even documented it that one time, it was the only proof I had that I asked. They never documented when my sister requested to take me home either. Or the many times I mentioned my heart condition in the first few days. They got the X-ray done at the hospital because I told them about the nurse hitting me, yet that was conveniently left out, and instead replaced with how maybe my mom's ex-wife had hit me (not true).

So that was a bust and just left me in more tears, and then more PTSD nightmares from re-triggering myself going through it all again.

I then learned about a College for doctors, so I thought I'd try that. I contacted the College of Physicians and Surgeons of Ontario, to complain about the Wallaceburg doctor, and the Chatham psychiatrist. I hope something can be done about the Wallaceburg doctor. He's the same doctor who almost let me die from a inflamed gallbladder despite me going there more than once in extreme pain, because he claimed it was just menstrual cramps. Luckily a different doctor saved me then, but unfortunate for me to get him again at such a fragile time when I needed sleep and hydration. He was also the same doctor that almost let my sister die from her appendix, which thankfully another doctor saved her life as well.

In 2022 I got more devastating news that the College of Physicians of Ontario decided not to do anything about the Wallaceburg doctor and the psychiatrist. For both the College of Nurses, and Physicians they gave the option to forward to the Health Board of Ontario. So I did that.

But when I did further research into the Health Board, looking into their reviews and how they helped, I realized, I made a mistake. Because according to the many statements and reviews, they don't try to help you, the victim. They help the Doctors, etc. Apparently it's done by lawyers who are primed to defend doctors, and are going to do what they can to make it so you don't have any form of justice (again reviews and statements suggest). Which is odd, because it's not like the people doing it are asking for money. The College and Health Board don't do money, we literally are fighting for a form of justice to be heard that we were wronged, and have someone do something about the person or people who did it. Seems like a broken system.

I read too many 1 star reviews on how the doctors were always favoured, even when there was proof. Even for sexual assaults, the victim was always lesser than, and the doctors won. No justice. I didn't want to put myself through that, and thankfully that motivated me to read more into law and small claims. I didn't want to split my focus because it wouldn't be mentally healthy to do that to myself. I messaged the Health Board of Ontario and told them the doctors were still in the wrong, but after looking into what the Health Board really did I decided to close the case and pursue a different action. Thankfully they were more than happy to close it (meaning the Wallaceburg doctor too), so I didn't have to deal with that.

I went the route of Small Claims Court instead. I didn't think I would because I was advised against it if I was alone, since they said it'd be hard on me and I'd need to pay witnesses out of pocket, etc. But it was all I had left. It's my last attempt to try to get some form of justice and closure for what the hospital did to me. I'm aware I'll be all alone, with no lawyer or support system (other than my loving cat who I'm thankful for every day) and no witnesses (you need to have a nurse or someone in the field testify on your behalf that the hospital was wrong, and with COVID, no one's gonna risk that for me). This is why I cry still. It's hard.

I went to the courthouse and got the paperwork I needed, and filled

Ashes to Dust

out a fee waiver form that allowed me to file without paying the fee since I matched the criteria for it. I didn't have legal advice or anyone I could call for advice, so it was hard to figure out who I'm suppose to sue since there were a few involved like the male nurse, the Wallaceburg doctor, the psychiatrist, the hospital itself, the Patient Relations Specialist, and the staff that held me down and injected me. I went with the hospital since the male nurse falls under their umbrella as a hired employee. The rest did too, but I wasn't sure if the Wallaceburg doctor would be deemed as a independent contractor, which would mean I'd also have to include him separately and also serve him serving papers.

I didn't want to overwhelm myself so I went with just the hospital for now, and if they try to shift some of the blame, then I will see if I can still serve the Wallaceburg doctor too. I just didn't want two lawyers on the attack while I try to go at this huge thing alone without experience or years of law on my side.

I was grateful that my mom and sister took the time to write letters about how the hospital was meant to contact them and not send me away, and how the hospital mistreated me. I was surprised but thankful.

Something about the hospital's lawyer messing up and sending me the wrong defense papers, made me feel like, hey maybe I can do this; if they can mess up maybe I can get it right enough to win for myself and get a spec of justice after all. What I noticed in the wrong defense papers (wrong person and hospital) and the corrected one, is they both basically had the same things written. If I hadn't of seen that, it might have discouraged me from pushing on strong.

I did my best with the little resources I had to learn some things about law. Torts law specifically since even though what they did was more than that, medical malpractice is a completely different law and more complicated than Torts. And most things fit under the Torts umbrella. I finally had legal names for what they did to me.

Ashes to Dust

False imprisonment, by the Wallaceburg doctor and the Chatham hospital. Also false imprisonment by the doctor for not doing his legal obligation and giving me a copy of (or reading) the Form-1 he signed to send me to the mental health part of the Chatham hospital. It was also invalid since he dated my visit wrong and never corrected a new one to send in to be signed. He did not inform me of my right to counsel either. Also the Chatham hospital did not release me when the invalid form 1 expired (no more than 3 days). Which should've been the day my sister visited (2021) and asked to take me home, but definitely the morning after since the Form 1 was signed the day I was at the Wallaceburg hospital. Instead they kept me against my will for six days without informing my family they could've come to take me home. And they didn't have me look over or sign any paperwork, and they never discussed me staying longer. They made their hospital notes seem like they should give themselves a pat on the back, and that I stayed voluntarily when I didn't, and worst of all that I was "thriving" there. Bullshit.

Assault and battery by the male nurse that elbowed me in the chest. It was intentionally done, and it's a serious crime. I don't see how this wasn't taken seriously by the College of Nurses, and that they didn't fight for the surveillance footage harder (no surprise since they barely fought for the nurse name). I'm still going forward with the Health Board of Ontario for this issue against the nurse as well, despite shit reviews. I will have a phone conference in February 2023.

The hospital violated my fundamental right to life liberty and security, protected by S.7 of the charter.

I was arbitrarily detained in breach of S.9.

Not given appropriate notice of the reason for my detention, or right to legal counsel, in the breach of S.10 (a) and (b).

I was thankful to find another case similar to mine in Canada (not Ontario) enough that I found those violation of rights, or else I wouldn't have known.

Ashes to Dust

Assault and battery (again) by the staff that held me down with unjust force and forced a injection on me.

I'm going to do my best, but it's hard to learn law (even enough to try to get by) when I can't seem to find Ontario laws, instead it's UK, or America on the internet. I still pull from the laws outside of Canada or else I'd never learn anything. I'm so thankful people put out that content for free, it gives people like me just enough to have a trying chance. I still don't know lawyer jargon or what the quoting of laws they do is or means (when they refer to 1999, etc laws and bills).

Knowing I'm the only one who will do this for me, is what keeps me from balling up and quitting. I want to be able to move forward, even a tiny bit, and I can't do that if I know I didn't do everything I possibly could to try. And since the 2 year mark is 1 month away, this is my last resort before going to the Ombudsman. You can't go through the Ombudsman until you're done court, so I don't know if it'll be years or not, but with how the Colleges and Health Board failed me (and others), I'm glad I didn't go through the Ombudsman instead of Small Claims, or else I would be absolutely devastated knowing I couldn't do any form of lawsuit against the Hospital, if they had decided not to do anything against anyone or improve the hospital in any form.

With how that hospital treated their patients, by threatening to throw them in the "Seclusion" room which is basically a prison's solitary confinement, for not eating enough, is just fucked up and yet they get grants and continue working with people who are mentally vulnerable. That place made me worse, the worst I've ever felt in my entire life.

It's almost 2 years and I still have the issues caused by the hospital (PTSD, panic attacks, etc) which is awful. Thankfully the supplements I found have helped me so I'm not overwhelmed with the things that were going on daily, so now it's lessened to involuntary smirks, laughs, smiles. I don't do enough to be super stressed so it doesn't

Ashes to Dust

bring on intense involuntary head movements and stuff again. I wish for a lot of things. I wish I was happier. Didn't have these issues caused by the hospital. I miss when I was "normal" with no issues or involuntary anything. I wish I had a lawyer to help me get the justice I deserve. I still wish to live in Toronto. I wish to be a singer, writer, etc. I wish the hospital issues would stop getting in the way of me pursing the things I loved before they fucked me over.

Time doesn't heal all wounds, your body remembers. Your mind is the projection playback pressing replay.

I wish people would stop telling people they should get over a traumatic event, because it's been x amount of time. You never get over it. I wish I had support.

I was a vegan after the hospital because the chicken became trauma food since they fed it to me so much. I didn't know what to eat at the time of the confusion and ended up becoming vegan. I learned a lot of healthy foods I didn't know before that I wouldn't have known if I didn't search up vegan meals. But being vegan for 2021 and some of 2022 made me miserable without me realizing it. Because it wasn't a choice, it was something I involuntarily did because it was trauma related. The brain is so strange that way. Thankfully my counselor had me realize I should be eating more than just beans. It made me realize I was miserable by all the restrictions, so I slowly tried different foods, seeing if I liked it or not. Slow steps, especially when I tried meat again. Pork chops were fine and it turned out I still liked them. But when I tried turkey in a thanksgiving meal, the texture reminded me too much of chicken and that night I had nightmares of the hospital again.

It took until December 2022 to attempt the big chicken trauma. I used fast food for two pieces of chicken tenders since I wasn't sure how I'd feel about it, but I ended up being ok. I liked it and thankfully I didn't have nightmares that night. I'm still working on what I like and don't. I wouldn't have been able to slowly work up to meat (lastly chicken) and regain something taken, if I didn't have my supportive counselor at the time. It was limited sessions so I didn't have any counselor the few months before trying chicken, but without him other foods wouldn't have been on my radar because I was too "stuck" in my trauma to think of other foods.

It's really nice that I had a third party (counselor) who was super supportive when I didn't have that in my life. Especially when I never had emotional support before so it was strange being asked how I felt when I didn't know because I'd never been asked or had someone genuinely care. It was always me being the support system to others. I needed that support going through adjustments on finding lawyers and failing, and dealing with my mom and things she's said to me or did, and not having anyone else to freely (to a point) talk to that would understand and still sound calming. I realized I listen for changes in someones pitch or facial expressions, and since it was all over the phone, he rarely changed his pitch and that was why I felt ok enough to talk to him, because it was always one calming level, that matched the words he said.

After looking at my health records so many times (and realizing doctors and nurses like to ad-lib things that you never said which you don't want on record) I think I may have messed up some of the events that happened on certain days in this book (like according to the records my sister visited me on a certain day but because I wrote the book without specific dates, just "Day 1", etc, I may have placed it wrong). I debated on going over it again to make sure it's correct, but with the small claims and the small steps I'm taking to finally move forward, I don't want to risk a set back by a huge trigger (re-reading all of the traumatizing events would be it). So I'm going to leave everything how I wrote it, even if it's on the wrong date, since while I was in the hospital it was timeless for me anyways. They didn't have clocks, or calendars so I never knew what day or time it actually was

Ashes to Dust

while I was there. So it matches in a way with the chaotic timelessness.

There were things I wanted to add when I first wrote this book, but didn't for my sake (I was pushing the triggers and panic attacks too much writing it while dealing with calls to lawyers, etc). My thought at the time was this book was my light in the dark. When I got out of the hospital it was literally the only thing I held on to doing that kept me going to do something, anything, and think of it as a positive. It was my only positive thing in the utter darkness of my life at the time, and I thought out of that it could be entertainment to others, even if it hurt me to write and live through.

And there were "entertaining" parts I never got to write that happened after the hospital because I was fresh off the abused boat, like still thinking I had D.I.D for a while (I don't and never did, it was what my brain latched onto from previous videos I watched on D.I.D for book research). From a writer's perspective they would be a great story and very entertaining, but I couldn't handle writing more trauma at the time, and I don't want to dredge it up even if I feel somehow like it's a waste by not doing so.

There was some stuff I just forgot about back then because it caused more trauma like my mom's ex wife contacting the house while I still lived there and my mom being secretive about it. And on top of my mom lashing out at me, Crisis workers suggested many times for me to go to a shelter, which I almost did when her ex was trying to show up again. I only didn't because they don't allow animals and my cat was my life and the only positive love I had so there was no way I was going to leave her. For some reason Crisis workers and the counselor at CMHA at the time just didn't understand how a person could not leave their cat. They didn't understand she was all I had to keep me going. I was also worried I could be majorly re-triggered by having to live in a environment that would remind me of my hospital stay. Like with having shared rooms with strangers, in a facility I don't know, and I just kept picturing possible similarities between hospital rooms

Ashes to Dust

and shelter rooms. And leaving my cat would have killed my cat as I had seen how she was when I was taken away from her for almost a week, and a shelter would be months. I couldn't do it. I suffered every day but having my cat by my side brought comfort when I had panic attacks or cried in bed.

I also didn't write about when I did get a new place in 2021, the movers almost killed my cat because they left gaps between the shelf and wall, causing her head to get stuck. Thankfully I got to her just in time, but it was beyond fucking traumatic.

Despite what opinions are formed of me from reading this book, I hope people see what the hospital did to me was in fact wrong, and I don't deserve to be silenced. This shouldn't be a issue, and maybe one day they can build a better system that isn't for the doctors and hospitals, but is instead for the victims of the hospitals and doctors. Because I did contact the people suggested to me for Canada (I don't mean just the Prime Minister but the minster of health, etc) and was told they only do money for the hospitals, etc. So no one cares. I contacted every forwarded person from the previous, and no one cares or chooses to step in to change things.

Apologies to anyone finding spelling or punctuation errors (I know some are more bothered than others by that) but I cannot go through it all again. It's almost 2023 and I'm hoping after getting over the hump of the anniversary of my death (technically the hospital did kill the old me, my name is changed too, and I'll never be the same) I hope my life will be less on pause.

My old name is ashes to dust. Long live my new name.
Melody, Rising, Star.

Ashes to Dust

47

Set aside the entertainment side of my book and enter the dark truth.

It may not seem like it because of all the distractions and stories of "Loki's," etc, but what the hospital did to me was wrong, life threatening and very serious. I could've died while in their care.

I'll try not to be repetitive since I wrote some terms in the conclusion, but I also want to make sure if anyone reads this part, and has gone through something with a hospital, they can be more prepared than I was. I am not a lawyer, and I have limited knowledge so anything in here is not legal advice, please seek that out for yourself.

The Wallaceburg doctor (I'll call him Dr. Hurt for short), violated my rights. I didn't know I had any until after I was released. Dr. Hurt wasn't interested in talking to me. He hurried to send me away because it would be too inconvenient to cancel the ambulance (he said they were already coming so he didn't want to cancel).

Doctors are required to fill out a Form 1 to transfer a person involuntarily, and are suppose to show the person a Form 42 which explains the reason why they are being sent away and to inform them they have the right to legal counsel. He didn't provide me with a form 42 or verbally inform me of my right to legal counsel. He also filled out the Form 1 with the wrong date of when he seen me, meaning it's invalid since he didn't notice the mistake and didn't send out a new fixed version to the Chatham hospital *before* sending me. Making my involuntary stay, false imprisonment. He also did not show me the Form 42, which also makes it false imprisonment and breaching my rights.

Dr. Hurt and the Wallaceburg staff were suppose to call my family, but never did. When my family tried to call the hospital lied, saying I was asleep and that they would call back when I was awake. (I was never once asleep at the Wallaceburg hospital). My family had no clue where I was and the staff told my family (after they transferred me) that they never had anyone in prior by my description or name. Which caused my family panic since I was only suppose to be at the hospital for fluids.

Meanwhile as I was in the Chatham hospital, they did not let me call my family, or give them my desperate messages about my cat in my room like requested.

The Patient's Relation Specialist writer noted that Dr. Hurt should have informed the patient's legal guardian of anything before sending me away. They also made a note to have Dr. Hurt put that he's shown the patient a Form 42 (for next time). Which worries me.

When I got to the Chatham hospital no one there informed me of my right to counsel either. They left me in my dungeon-looking room where I could barely walk. Legally they have to inform me as soon as I arrive, it's even noted in their policy. So both Dr. Hurt and the Chatham hospital staff failed to inform me of my right. They also prevented me and my family from communication.

They had some small and big lies in the record. A small lie was when I arrived in my dungeon room (which was another seclusion room), they wrote I was offered to go to a different room (the shared one) and that I said no I wanted to stay there. Of course I wouldn't want to stay in the creepy dungeon-torturous looking room. After saying I'd want to go home to my own room, I would've said "Yes please, help me up."

The nurse saying I could leave sometime after 7am the day I arrived was misrepresentation. I was held much much longer.

The hospital records conveniently left a lot out. Even simple things like there were three nurses that came in my shared room wanting to take my blood(nurse who elbowed me). So even when I tried to complain to the College of Nurses of Ontario (only after I found out about them in 2022) there was no documentation that he was in the same room with me. They only listed one female nurse.

How would I know the appearance, name, and dates, he worked that matched with their nursing schedule (which they also never gave me prior, I only got it after they sent it to the Health Board as their "proof".). It's not possible for me to know he worked the day he elbowed me and the day he brought me water (causing a panic attack). But the sad part is it seems companies (lookup the reviews yourself before they are changed), don't care about the victims. It gets swept under the rug as quick as possible and the victim doesn't get justice.

The Chatham hospital didn't even include the video surveillance evidence that was requested, and the College didn't push for it (just like they didn't with the nurse who abused me). If I didn't know my abuser's first name and lucked out finding him on social media, they would have ended it sooner and I wouldn't know the name of my attacker to put on legal forms. They withheld evidence.

The day the male nurse (I'll call him Nurse Bend) elbowed me in the chest, was the same day I arrived at the Chatham hospital, and the same day I was given a forced injection (right after). Legal terms: Nurse Bend caused assault and battery. Things I've heard on TV before so I know they are extremely serious. So why does simply telling the hospital, college, or a lawyer (not all), "He elbowed me in the left side of my chest so hard I fell to the ground and almost blacked out," not seem to be taken seriously at all? But say he assaulted me and caused battery, then suddenly more serious. They are the same, and it took me over half a year to recover from him hitting me combined with the hospital staff from the forced injection.

Ashes to Dust

It was so bad I couldn't even pull a empty cart, especially not with my left arm, or it'd cause such severe pain I'd have to let go because my arm and chest (left side) would hurt and I'd go weak. Sleeping was a nightmare. If I slept on my side (specifically my left) I would cough and it was so painful I could hardly breathe, it felt like I had a broken rib. Sometimes going up and down the stairs caused me to feel like I was having a heart attack, and breathing was too hard. Even standing could cause me breathing difficulties. It's hard to narrow down what side effects were a result of which abusive incident, as there was a lot the hospital did to me. From Nurse Bend causing me assault and battery, the forced injection side effects, and the staff and security who also caused assault and battery holding me down for the forced injection. That's all just the physical, not including the mental and psychological abuse that was done to me while there.

And no they weren't aware of things I've written about in this book like the events happening from the dehydration or even during my false imprisonment stay in their facilities. They obviously picked up on strange things I said like talking in "third person," but they didn't know anything else. And unfortunately they liked to make wrong assumptions like me not looking at a staff member (because I was terrified and remembering what they just did to me in that awful place), as seeing something that wasn't there. Not true. I wasn't aware at the time, that my mom was emotionally abusive, and neither was the hospital. They kept getting mixed up between my mom and her ex, and decided to write things that weren't true like, "mom hits them all," without specifying. And neither my mom nor her ex hit us all. The hospital also liked to write, "lesbian mom," which seemed uncalled for.

Even if somehow the hospital knew (again they didn't) all the stuff I was going through prior, and during the hospital false imprisonment, they still had no right to treat me the way they did; and it still would've been wrong all the same. Legally, and morally.

Ashes to Dust

My memoir cannot be used against me in a negative way without also having the abuse by the hospital acknowledged as proof and fact as well. Because it is. And my life has felt ruined by it ever since. There is no trying to justify what was done to me by using the "entertainment" parts of my book, because abuse is abuse. A hit is a hit. The pain it caused is fact, and real, and everlasting.

The forced injection could've killed me. They weren't aware of my heart condition, weight, prior gallbladder surgery, what medications I was taking that could interact, and my overall health at the time. I was already in their "care" for over five hours and not given anything to eat or drink, so I was still severely dehydrated. I was in that seclusion room without food, water, pads, or help, or any basic care warranted to me, for nearly eleven hours. I didn't realize it was so long until I saw the time they put me in and let me leave on the records they never sent me (they sent to the College). I could've easily gotten hypothermia since I was so severely dehydrated and the room was a ice box in the middle of winter with no blankets. I was freezing the entire time, and I never slept the entire time I was in there (though they falsely put I was sleeping multiple times).

The hospital staff twisted my body in ways it shouldn't go. After being injured by Nurse Bend, I was put in a double locked room (two doors locked) with no way out. I wasn't a danger to myself or others, yet staff and security came in, and twisted my body in ways it shouldn't go. They twisted my neck and back, and laughed at me when doing it, before finally using me as a stepping stool when they were finished.

The pain I felt I already wrote in the book. It may have seemed less serious in the context I wrote it in, because it was shrouded with the "entertainment" parts like the Universe, Loki, and Death. But it was serious, and no one helped me despite my pleas. I don't think I wrote that the first time someone called "Ash" through the door was Nurse Bend after he hurt me while I was in the bathroom crying

Ashes to Dust

uncontrollably. (No wonder my brain worked over time in it's dehydrated state to comfort me, which wasn't actually comforting. Ha.). Good thing I didn't have food or water in my system or I would've thrown it all up from the anti-psychotic they gave me. I found out it was olanzapine, and that they documented I was "sleeping" most of the time in the seclusion room. I never once fell asleep, that would require feeling safe and not being in excruciating pain with non stop crying. I even desperately waved in front of their camera, begging for help, but I guess that was also "sleeping."

Dr. Hurt had documented to keep a eye out for cardiovascular depression if giving me a anti-psychotic, yet no one bothered. I was alone, in pain. I say alone, but I'm sure you, the reader, remember it as the one-woman-show so not alone, but alone. And as it turns out, side effects for the drugs they gave me were personality changes, hallucinations, mood swings, and so much more.

It's no wonder it took me over 5 months to finally look in the mirror again (only after bleaching my hair) since I was trapped in the seclusion room all day with a shatter proof mirror showing my distorted and messy haired self. It was a unexplainable sad time for me. And I had no one at home for support, just my fabulous cat.

The hospital did take a X-ray after I was out of the seclusion room (according to their records). But they never documented it as Nurse Bend being the reason for my pain. None of the nurses reported Nurse Bend even though they witnessed it. They tried to say it was abuse at home (wasn't).

Turns out the involuntary head movements I suffered (still suffer) from were thankfully documented right after they released me from the seclusion room. Not that they'd admit anything but it's proof it started as a result of the trauma they caused me and the forced injection side effects.

Reading their notes it turns out they were drugging me without my knowledge or consent by crushing up anti-psychotics into my drinks

Ashes to Dust

(their favourite go-to was apple juice). So it's no wonder I was declining while there, on top of their abuse I endured by them. Antipsychotics have serious side effects especially for people who don't need it. Many. And since I was unknowingly being given these drugs since the Wallaceburg hospital, I never stood a chance at recovering from just dehydration unscathed. They added a shit ton more I didn't need affecting me more than the dehydration was. (As a kind CMHA worker had said, it's like a person stranded with no water in the desert, you start hallucinating from the dehydration.) No wonder it took almost two months or so to feel like I could think straight. They pumped me with too much mind-altering drugs that take a a long time to wear off.

The day my sister came to visit me was actually the day they legally had to let me leave because their invalid Form 1 was at a end. However they didn't let me leave with my sister when she asked, and she's not the firm-pushy type. They told her it was up to the doctor. Which is bullshit because even prisoners get released by the guards when it's their release day. Because they didn't release me on my or my family's wishes, this is forced imprisonment (yes I say that word a lot). Depriving me of my liberty, and right to freedom.

The next day I was still held against my will, but they made a false claim in their records that I was now voluntary for the last three days. Not only that but they made it seem I was "receptive" and happy to be there whenever my family complained after my release, or when I complained. In the documents, a big lie, they said I wanted to be there and it was good for me.

Oh yes, thank you so much for the life-long mental scarring, and physical side effects I still live with, and the many new issues I never had before like PTSD, anxiety, panic attacks, involuntary movements, and freeze responses (and possibly depression when released when I had a moment to process all they had done to me). So very fucking happy to have been abused mentally and physically by the hospitals.

Ashes to Dust

That-is-sarcasm. It was the worst hellhole of a experience in my life. I honestly think I would've noticed and felt worse if I wasn't so dehydrated, mixed with their drugs, and stuck in fight, flight, or freeze response where my brain just went to survival mode. Probably why I crashed so hard, lying in bed in pain and in quiet when I finally got home, because everything they did sunk in. That no one cared sunk in. That my family wasn't being kind on my return for sure caused that to deepen. That the hospital never reported Nurse Bend for hitting me, and he got away with it. They all did.

Me small, them big.

They didn't report a lot of things. Not when me and my roommate (Sad Girl) feared for our safety from the other two patients. Not me wanting to go home (thank fuck they wrote it just once, so it's proof, and it was on the day they claimed me "voluntary."). Not even simple things like Nurse Bend handing me water two days after he abused me and then walked me to my room where I had a severe panic attack (didn't know at the time, I had many in that hospital). His face and him walking so close to me triggered me.

The hospital even had the nerve to reply to a complaint by saying if I had have been hit I would've reported it and there would've been a record of it by staff or patient relations. Victim blaming at its finest. I did report it, but as most people who experience shock or abuse know, it can take you a while before it really sinks in and that only happens when you're safely away. I reported it and got X-rays, yet they never said the reason was their staff hit me. It shouldn't be the victim's responsibility, the nurses who witnessed it and the attacker, should've reported it right away. I will never get a apology from Nurse Bend. And even if I did out of the blue years later, I wouldn't accept it because it's meaningless now. Empty words don't heal wounds.

I told the Patient's Relation Specialist, I told my mom, I even told my doctor who sent me to a cardiologist to make sure Nurse Bend didn't damage my heart. I was so scared he injured it in a way that wasn't

Ashes to Dust

fixable. Thankfully no permanent damage to my heart was reported (that I'm aware of).

When I reported everything to the Patient Relations Specialist when I got home, they didn't document everything (like Nurse Bend), or staff violence for holding me down (she simply put I was "displeased" with some aspects of my care). She wrote only what she wanted so the hospital wouldn't look like they were ever in the wrong. Very unprofessional, going so far as to telling my mom over the phone that my mom abuses me.

1) You would never tell a suspected abuser that they are a abuser.

2) In this case it was not true, and they tried saying she was the reason I wasn't ok from everything, not the hospital. Apparently this is a typical angle hospitals go with to avoid being sued or held accountable.

All this did was make my mom suspicious of me. She got in my face and asked me if I was telling people she was abusive. At the time I wasn't on the phone so I didn't know where the fuck this came from, so I said no. But she didn't believe me and at that time I was going to counseling and not telling her, so she was constantly telling me I was a liar, being sneaky, throwing her under the bus, selfish, some more not nice words. It's why things got so much worse for me being home.

Still at the time I had no clue why she was doing this to me. I started thinking she just is like this to me now, maybe because I'm not cooking for her and everyone in he house anymore, or because I'm not telling her where I'm going. Which I didn't want to say was counseling for the hospital abuse, because I wanted one thing private. Especially how she had been behaving. But it was because of the P.R.S's false words she was acting out like this to me. Completely unfair to me by both of them. It caused me a lot of turmoil and me and my mom haven't been close since.

The P.R.S had no right to say that. Especially since I never said my mom was abusive to any hospital staff. Just the one drugged-without-

Ashes to Dust

my-consent day with a false memory which I took back well before the P.R.S talked to her.

I noticed the hospital records were disorganized and messy. They got confused and didn't establish if they were talking about my mom or her ex. Again like the random note that said lesbian mom hits them all. Doesn't say which person they are talking about. And my mom's ex is not my mom. So I think that's what happened which is really fucked up. Thanks for ruining my life further with your mistakes and violations again.

They ad-lib a lot in their documents, which doesn't make them factual. I never said to anyone, that my mom or ex, "hit us all." They didn't elaborate whom. I said my mom's ex punched her teen daughter in the face, but that's completely different. She's a very violent person for sure, but their document is still incorrect.

Unfortunately some of what they wrote escalated from there. Making shit up or maybe they were just confused on who they were talking about. Is it so hard to write "ex" and not be confused?

Doesn't matter if later on through counseling it turned out my mom was emotionally abusing me. What the hospital was writing wasn't true. They even incorrectly labeled me as having D.I.D (you know why) and I'm not sure how to fix that.

The P.R.S document was very quick to be closed. Our complaints were marked as mild, because we weren't involving lawyers or the news. So we weren't a "moderate" threat or the top. She didn't bother telling us we could go one step above her to complain, which she should have informed us about (it's even in their policy to do so). She didn't tell us about the Colleges either. But my mom did tell her she'd complain to the College of Doctors, which the P.R.S was quick to note and to inform the hospital and Dr. Hurt about. Very glad I focused on small claims instead of both since at the time I didn't know they had a heads up. I also didn't know that my mom told the P.R.S that she would sue them, and the P.R.S responded that the court systems were

Ashes to Dust

closed (2021)and backed up due to COVID so "good luck" getting a lawyer.

Since the Colleges and Health board do not work, and there's no proper system to protect me or others who have been abused by hospitals or their staff, I forged ahead with small claims. Two years to find a lawyer during COVID wasn't enough time especially since the first year everything was fresh. I have nothing to lose from trying to attempt justice for myself. It seems like I will only be listened to if money is on the line.

My cat is happy and great. I don't think I wrote about it, but what the hospital did to me also gave her trauma. She had never been separated from me before. So after they kept me involuntarily she was depressed, not eating, and my family scared me by saying if the hospital didn't release me they were worried she wouldn't make it because she was so thin. I thought calling her over the hospital phone (when they finally let me use it) to hear my voice would help, but it didn't, it made it worse because then she searched for a long time after trying to find me. When I finally got home, she was extremely light it scared me. I noticed her dishes weren't filled, and the upstairs one she always ate at was empty. It's probably because she is my cat, so I know her best, but she always likes the upstairs food dish. So I didn't know if she wasn't taken care of, or if my sister's cat ate her downstairs food, but I was upset. I got her back to a healthy weight again, but it took her almost half a year to become herself again. She was like super glue to me, and never wanted to play, just to stay wherever I was. It made me so sad to know she was traumatized and not her happy self, who barely did anything but stay by my side.

She's great now though thankfully. If I could've afforded it and had a bigger house I would've gotten her a new cat friend. But that may have been because when my mom wasn't being so nice to me, she kept mentioning how my cat would suffer if I moved because she'd be alone, and she's never been alone without other animals, etc. So she ear wormed it into my head that she might be lonely. I moved anyways. My cat was always in my room with me prior to moving, and I know what's best for my cat, especially when I saw how she was when I was away. It was just a way to try to make me not want to leave. But my cat is happy, and more free than she was there (since my mom started wanting me to lock her up in the bathroom at night). I also don't have to worry for her safety anymore like I did there with my mom's ex, or my cousin who would abuse the animals and swear at them if she was mad at someone or was in a bad mood. My cat was showing signs someone was abusing her because she would flinch. And I was the target when living there when my mom was mad at me when I got back from the hospital, which meant my cousin was mistreating my cat and no one stopped it.

   End of 2022 I had to get a endoscopy for my throat. Ended up having what I assumed was PTSD and a panic attack episode in the hospital even though it was in Windsor and not the Wallaceburg or Chatham ones where my abuse happened.

   The bed, the gown, wrist band, bed railings, all got too much once the nurse got close with a needle and I started bawling. I didn't want to make her uncomfortable so I tried to stop it and hold it in but that wasn't possible. She asked what was wrong and I said I have hospital PTSD. She was so nice, and unexpected (probably from my experience), and said, "I won't ask you about it." Which was the kindest thing I didn't know I needed to hear from her. She called another nurse and that nurse (also kind) tried to distract me while inserting the needle.

   What really surprised me was how well she (1st nurse) knew how to navigate my Aphantasia. She asked a question of if I have a pet. I said yes a cat. She said, "Do you love your cat?" I laughed because it was absurd and obvious so I said, "Of course I do." She said, "Good. Think about my silly question next time to make you laugh." That was her solution to not being able to visualize a happy place. I thought she was very clever.

When I was rolled in I was so nervous but I started laughing and smiling because the doctor and staff were chanting, "Rising Star, Rising Star." It was so nice to hear and a very positive thing to have as a memory when all other hospital memories were so horrible and full of pain. I'm thankful to those people at the Windsor hospital that worked that day. They went out of their way to comfort me in the most unexpected ways.

I'd like to say happy New Year 2023, I'm magically cured of everything they put me through! I'm not. It doesn't work like that. I'm able to do things I wasn't before (sounds silly but is a big deal) like gaming, and I even managed to sorta edit a manuscript a bit (yay me!).

I'm hoping music is next. Before the hospital incident I paid for a 30 day music production class, and even created a music business license. But the hospital took all that from me - all that hope and joy I had and excitement for my future. The class was at the same time I was in my false imprisonment so I missed too much and I wasn't in any shape to try to catch up after.

I was also learning a new editing program for my book literally before the hospital, which I never got to learn. If I hadn't been held against my will with my rights stripped, I would have at least one completed series (four books, I need to write the final two) and one partial to a new series that I was excited about. I would also have had music production knowledge and at least one full album completed. But I forgot a lot of basic things I learned because of the trauma, like music theory, even all the Japanese I learned before. It's like there was a block to the memory of who I was before, including some of the knowledge I learned before the hospital trauma, and it all just got replaced with trauma and misery. I haven't even been able to sing since the 2021 hospital incident. Partially because of the involuntary head movements that were happening a lot before 2022. So I haven't sang or really talked much since then. So if I want to try to finally become a singer, I'll have to hope I can start singing again, and not sound too bad recording while building my voice from square one.

Trauma is a bitch no doubt.

I'm stuck between trying to move forward but also trying to learn for more for small claims to get justice. It's tiring because I end up avoiding everything since it's trauma related, and it's not helpful. Not sure if I feel like I'm having a momentary hopeless moment when thinking about going against a professional lawyer and their team who are backing the hospital that abused me. All while I'm still struggling from what the hospital did to me, making me emotionally drained super fast.

I would love to have punitive damages where they have to better themselves, and Nurse Bend and Dr. Hurt actually get repercussions for their actions. Whether that be a few unpaid months to finish mandatory new schooling, or temporary suspension with no pay. And the actual hospitals themselves would need to undergo a lot to prevent this from happening again to someone else. I'd also want it stated on my record that my stay was not good and "receptive" but traumatizing, with a list of the intentional torts (assault, battery, false imprisonment, intentional infliction of mental and physical damage by staff) that happened to me there so they can't lie again saying it did me well. I want it on record, both my health record and their system, that Nurse Bend had hit me during my stay and is not allowed near me, and Dr. Hurt is not allowed to ever be the doctor in charge of my care even in emerge.

Ashes to Dust

I swear/affirm that the following is true:

Set out the facts in numbered paragraphs. If you learned a fact from someone else, you must give that person's name and state that you believe that fact to be true.

1. I am requesting video surveillance footage from the Chatham-Kent Health Alliance on [DATE REDACTED], 2021 from 7am - 11am, located in the hallway (right side, the side the kitchen is located).

2. The footage holds proof that [NAME REDACTED] was in fact interacting with me, despite the lack of paperwork. It will show video evidence of him elbowing me in the chest (assault and battery), and show the forced impact caused me to fall to the floor. It should also include the 2 female nurses (and anyone else unbeknownst to me) that witnessed the abuse and did not report it, and their collegue [NAME REDACTED]

Continued on next page

Ashes to Dust

> **FORM 15A**   **PAGE 4**   Claim No.
>
> AFFIDAVIT IN SUPPORT OF MOTION, continued
>
> 3. This footage was requested when I made a complaint to the College of Nurses. (Exhibit A) proves that the Chatham-Kent Health Alliance did not comply. Because they did not comply to the very serious abuse case, I decided to take things to small claims in hopes a judge will be able to make them submit the evidence and help me with closure. This being one of the serious torts.
>
> 4. I called before April 2022 by request of the College of Nurses, and the Chatham-Kent Health Alliance receptionist assured me the footage would not be deleted. So I know it is still available, and has been confirmed by the receptionist that they do not delete it. But I will need court help to obtain the proof that is illegally being withheld.

I filed for a motion (photos above, excluding the Exhibit A due to possible legal issues) to have the hospital give up their video surveillance footage of the hospital hallway to either me or the judge to be entered into evidence, as it was proof Nurse "Bend" elbowed me in the chest on the same day he worked. But the hospital tried to claim it's for "monitoring purposes" only, which doesn't make sense as they would need to record to show to police or to report a incident. Then they wanted me to revoke the motion request for the video footage for the morning of the day Nurse Bend hit me. I said no, and was suddenly hit with a new amended defense by their lawyer saying I didn't do the plaintiff's claim correctly and they wanted it dismissed with pay. With them working so hard to get my motion and case dismissed I spent weeks doing my best to redo the entire plaintiff's

Ashes to Dust

claim so it got done properly, despite the extreme hardship it caused me. Thankfully they cannot claim it was not done properly to get it dismissed anymore. I am the only one fighting for myself.

It turns out the Health Board doesn't even discipline the nurse. It's not even what I though it was. I was told they can only have the College of Ontario case be reviewed to see if they didn't do what they could with the case, and I would have to prove it sufficiently. So it seems more like the Health Board is there to critique the College's documentation of a case, and that's it. So it still isn't a way to get justice. We really are just discarded to fall through the cracks without a proper system to actually discipline the wrong-doers.

This book is all I have right now, and it's not like I can name names, or they would sue me. Even writing these personal last chapter entries the hospital may still go after me for shedding them in a negative (but true) light. But it's not out of malice. I'm just writing what really happened because I don't seem to be getting justice in any system. I'm only nervous about sharing the book while still tied up in Small Claims, because then they'd just use it in whatever ways they please, making me more miserable. I'm stuck where I don't know if I can speak out about stuff on social media or share this, or if I want to put myself out there. Because the one time I tried to reach out and say I needed legal help on social media, I was met with so much heartless negativity. And they didn't even know my situation, so I cringe now whenever I hear people say reach out for help (for anything) because I'm reminded of that. How can you reach out for help when people will take that outstretched arm and cut it up and send it back.

But I also want to move forward with my life. It really would've been easier if I could've afforded a lawyer so I didn't have to constantly re-traumatize myself and have mountains of stress. I hope things go great for me in the end. It's been misery because of what they've done and taken. I really want my life to start again. Not this loop.

Ashes to Dust

I'll end on a happier note. I am thankful to live with my cat with my freedom that was previously stolen. My whole life I'll be battling with what happened to me, whether it be a trigger by a show, food, smell, etc. But even if I have no one to share those happy moments with (my mom is not one, as I have written her reactions to my happy news … which wasn't good). I'm still glad for the small things. I no longer have to wake fearful that my mom's ex has come over and is trying to beat her, or hurting one of her kids, or threatening us (or worry for our animal's safety since her drug friends had decapitated a cat at her house before). I finally have my own space.

I hope to have happier moments to share one day too. Like published books and music. With COVID changing so much, I don't know if that means concerts will change further, but I'd love if I could figure out how to produce my music, and become one of the first VR concerts. Or live VR concerts so we can all enjoy from all over the world in the comfort of our homes. That technology may be years away though. I have positive thoughts about the future, it's just getting there that's difficult with this weight dragging me down.

Please don't claw up my vulnerable outstretched hand. Can you lift me up instead?

Thank you for reading.

www.ingramcontent.com/pod-product-compliance
Lightning Source LLC
Chambersburg PA
CBHW071114080526
44587CB00013B/1338